Medical Humanities, Sociology and the Suffering Self

Following criticisms of the traditionally polarised view of understanding suffering through either medicine or social justice, Lowe makes a compelling argument for how the medical humanities can help to go beyond the traditional biographical and epistemic breaks to see into the nature and properties of suffering and what is at stake.

Lowe demonstrates through analysis of major healthcare workforce issues and incidence of burnout how key policies and practices influence healthcare education and experiences of both patients and health professionals. By including first person narratives from health professionals as a tool and resource, she illustrates how dominant ideas about the self enter practice as a refusal of suffering. Demonstrating the relationship between personal experience, theory and research, Lowe argues for a pedagogy of suffering that shows how the moral anguish implicit in suffering is an ethical response of the emergent self.

This is an important read for all those interested in medical humanities, health professional education, person-centred care and the sociology of health and illness.

Wendy Lowe is a Senior Lecturer in Medical Sociology and Medical Education at Queen Mary University of London, UK.

Routledge Advances in the Medical Humanities

For more information about this series visit: www.routledge.com/Routledge-Advances-in-the-Medical-Humanities/book-series/RAMH

Medical Humanities, Sociology and the Suffering Self

Surviving Health

Wendy Lowe

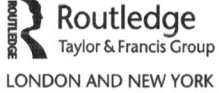
Routledge
Taylor & Francis Group

LONDON AND NEW YORK

First published 2021
by Routledge
2 Park Square, Milton Park, Abingdon, Oxon OX14 4RN

and by Routledge
52 Vanderbilt Avenue, New York, NY 10017

Routledge is an imprint of the Taylor & Francis Group, an informa business

British Library Cataloguing-in-Publication Data
A catalogue record for this book is available from the British Library

Library of Congress Cataloging-in-Publication Data
Names: Lowe, Wendy (Lecturer in medical sociology), author.
Title: Medical humanities, sociology and the suffering self: surviving health/Wendy Lowe.
Description: Abingdon, Oxon; New York, NY: Routledge, 2021. | Series: Routledge advances in medical humanities | Includes bibliographical references and index. | Contents: Stitching suffering together -- Patterns of suffering -- Suffering as foundational to health professional education -- Sorting the wood from the trees -- The suffering self and burning woman -- Pilgrimages - how can medical humanities think differently about suffering? -- Diving Down Deep. | Summary: "Following criticisms of the traditionally polarised view of understanding suffering through either medicine or social justice, Lowe argues that medical humanities can help to go beyond the traditional biographical and epistemic breaks to see into the nature and properties of suffering and what is at stake"-- Provided by publisher.
Identifiers: LCCN 2020032574 (print) | LCCN 2020032575 (ebook) | ISBN 9780367321413 (hardback) | ISBN 9780367672997 (paperback) | ISBN 9780429316937 (ebook)
Subjects: LCSH: Medicine and the humanities. | Suffering.
Classification: LCC R702.L69 2021 (print) | LCC R702 (ebook) | DDC 610--dc23 LC record available at https://lccn.loc.gov/2020032574 LC ebook record available at https://lccn.loc.gov/2020032575

ISBN 13: 978-0-367-32141-3 (hbk)
ISBN 13: 978-0-367-67299-7 (pbk)
ISBN 13: 978-0-429-31693-7 (ebk)

Typeset in Sabon
by MPS Limited, Dehradun

For Ellen and Lauren

Contents

Figures

Tables

Boxes

Preface

In the cool, darkened twilight of the Intensive Care Unit (ICU), I stand next to the bed, explaining to the patient why I'm there and what I'm to do. I run through everything we discussed pre-operatively, re-establishing our relationship in the strange confines of a steely, clattering, beeping, busy room. I place my hands gently on her chest, keeping my eyes on hers as I go through the physiotherapy techniques to help her clear her lungs post-operatively. She cannot speak as she has a tracheostomy to prevent lung complications. The amount that could go wrong is terrifying, which makes the work I do both extremely necessary, <u>and</u> dangerous, as well as painful for the patient.

She starts to look around, at other staff, her eyes beseeching them to get me to stop. She becomes agitated, wanting to escape me, indicating that she wants her small blackboard. She writes, "She's trying to kill me." I feel devastated and try lamely to reassure her while not being able to speak to what she is going through. While I know the clinical justification enables me to carry out this work, built on extensive preparation pre-operatively, continuing on feels like torture for both the patient and myself.

She makes a good recovery, we restore our therapeutic relationship post-ICU, when she returns to the surgical ward. At least she can speak by then, by placing her finger over her silver tracheostomy that remains in her neck. The torture, confusion, agitation, anguish and questioning seems a thing of the past for this patient, although I know I will be in many similar situations throughout my working life.

The wordlessness that characterises these extreme circumstances seems to be a part of the character of suffering (Cassell, 2004; Frank, 2004, 2013). I have heard clinicians asking what they could say in times of extreme suffering and death. In my research, a participant asked, "How do we even begin to ask the right questions?" These deep questions can be a source of suffering in themselves since rarely are they discussed within healthcare (Ferrell & Coyle, 2008). Suffering is an inherent part of healthcare; bearing witness to the suffering of patients and their families, as well as colleagues, means that clinicians will have more exposure to this in their lifetime, quite apart from any suffering experienced personally as a result of family and social circumstances.

Ferrell and Coyle (2008) hope to give voice to the suffering nurses witness. I too hope that "by making this suffering visible, we honor it and may learn from it" (Preface, not numbered). I am using a particular lens through which to view suffering, including a psychological (Cassell, 2004; Frank, 2004), sociological (Wilkinson, 2005) and philosophical perspectives (Nussbaum, 1986). By exploring suffering through these different perspectives, I hope to find the words to help <u>encounter</u> suffering whilst also knowing that a full description of suffering is not possible nor desirable (Frank, 2001).

Suffering is rarely mentioned in medical education, research or practice (Cassell, 2004). Perhaps this is due to the disconnection inherent in suffering (Frank, 2001): "Our suffering was why we could not talk. Our suffering was what we could not say" (p. 354). The unspeakable, experiencing yourself on the other side of life as it should be, the distress that threatens the intactness of the self by making that self absent, also contributes to the hole in what clinicians can say and do (Frank, 2001). Being able to encounter the hole, the gap, without turning patients or clinicians into objects of suffering, means being able to remain "silent in the face of what they could not speak" (Frank, 2001; p. 59).

Therefore this book has its genesis in the suffering in healthcare that I along with many others experienced at an early age, which has preoccupied me for many decades as I have yearned to find the lost words and absence of those experiences. The purpose of the book is to encounter suffering through the use of medical humanities and medical sociology. Medical humanities can be broadly understood as medicine reflecting on itself through the medium of the arts, whilst medical sociology is like someone holding up a mirror to medicine. If suffering is characterised by the unspeakable and incomprehensible (Frank, 2001), then we may need to listen to the "silence about those things we need to hear" (Rukeyser, 1996; p. 15). There is still so much we can explore on suffering whilst honouring the sense of muteness that descends in an encounter.

Suffering is an understorey (McFarlane, 2019) to medicine, the main event of healthcare, whose shock can render us mute:

> Everyone is shocked by how much suffering there is in the world, as if we really believe there could, or should, be much less. Indeed talking about justice or scientific progress are both ways of talking about potentially avoidable suffering. We need to believe that someone can intervene in our suffering and make a noticeable difference. (Phillips, 1999; p. 3)

Medicine is wracked by debates on scientific progress to find cures versus justice in reducing health inequities in those with the worst health outcomes. Both seemingly opposite, as they are often positioned, are in fact two sides of the same coin of suffering. How can we expect to understand unless we go through, encounter, endure experiences, to suffer as in the original meaning of the word? The word suffer comes from the Latin words "sub" – under, from below; and "ferre" – to bear; to form "suffere" – to undergo, bear or endure. The rhizomatic nature of suffering is at the root of medicine, forms the pathos – the suffering – at the heart of pathology.

Having been a health professional who went on to study sociology, one of the potential limitations of this book is in translating between different disciplines without having an exhaustive coverage of texts in the field. This is not specifically a medical humanities nor a sociology text but, rather, it is focussed on the conversation between them and the science of medicine. In particular, the focus is on the conversation between the individual and the world through the topic of suffering. In addition, this is also a philosophical matter, since to save lives, as healthcare does, is to ask questions about what it means to live and human excellence:

> The question of life-saving thus becomes a delicate and complicated one for any thinker of depth. It becomes, in effect, the question of the human good: how can it be reliably good and still be beautifully human? ... [T]hese questions are elicited and became part of the general question: who do we think we are, and where (under what sky) do we want to live? (Nussbaum, 1986; p. 3)

Given that the nature of suffering concerns the distress associated with events that threaten the intactness of a person, then who we think we are has relevance to the encounter of suffering in healthcare.

As clinicians, there are many times when we cause suffering as part of an intervention (Ferrell & Coyle, 2008). If we see ourselves as fixing or helping or saving, there is an implicit inequality, a moral judgment that increases the distance and disconnection between clinician and patient:

> In fixing there is an inequality of expertise that can easily become a moral distance. We cannot serve at a distance. We can serve only that to which we are profoundly connected, that which we are willing to touch ... we serve life not because it is broken but because it is holy. (Remen, 1996; p. 24 cited in Ferrell and Coyle, 2008; p. 109)

This change in the perspective of the sacredness of life with all its suffering reflects an ancient understanding of the body as a locus of personhood, something often disputed in sociology. That in an inclusive healthcare practice, we perhaps do not need to dismiss the person, their body, or experience of suffering as something outside life. Bynum states that "women understood the suffering that lay at the core of their lives to *be* both mystical ecstasy and active, innerwordly service of their fellow human beings" (1992;

p. 74, original emphasis). By taking suffering as laying at the core of life, this book explores the messy, rooted vulnerability of human lives as well as the aspiration to goodness and a liveable life (Butler, 2005; Nussbaum, 1986).

The scope of this book is to explore suffering through the conversations between humanities, sociology and science. This, through a persistent attention to and re-interpretation of concrete words, images and incidents:

> We reflect on an incident not by subsuming it under a general rule, not by assimilating its features to the terms of an elegant scientific procedure, but by burrowing down to the depths of the particular, finding images and connections that will permit us to see it more truly, describe it more richly; by combining this burrowing with a horizontal drawing of connections, so that every horizontal link contributes to the depth of our view of the particular, and every new depth creates new horizontal links. (Nussbaum, 1986; p. 69)

This entanglement (Fitzgerald & Callard, 2016), linking and hovering in thought and imagination is a restorative act, paying homage to "the enigmatic complexities of the seen particular" (Nussbaum, 1986; p. 69). A restorative act is in contrast to the "addictive idea of redemption – being saved from something or other" (Phillips, 1999; p. 145). A restorative act requires that we stay with, undergo, suffering in all its complexities and perhaps live to tell a deeper story.

Staying with suffering means being with the meeting place between clinician and patient, where some truth is shared (Foucault, 1973; Rukeyser, 1996). Whether that sharing is silent as in great suffering, or whether there are words to go with that experience may perhaps not matter so much:

> It is a great thing to say to our wordless, we will speak, in self-knowledge, in faith, at a beginning-place of many beginnings, in which none of these means is enough in itself, since each is an index to a beginning of the single spirit of the world; it is a great thing to come to the unbegun places of our living and to say: Now we will find the words. (Rukeyser, 1996; p. 132)

This book tries to come to the "unbegun places of living" in healthcare, where suffering is an understorey but rarely mentioned. This means encountering suffering, where there is a hole in saying and doing. Returning to the narrative at the start of the preface, starting a conversation with this "unbegun place of living" meant drawing a visual relationship between the patient, surroundings and myself, reminiscent of *The Scream* by Edvard Munch (1893) (Figure 0.1). *The Scream* is said to represent depersonalisation, which certainly resonates with Frank's (2001) experience of the absence of the person, or loss of intactness (Simeon & Abugel, 2006).

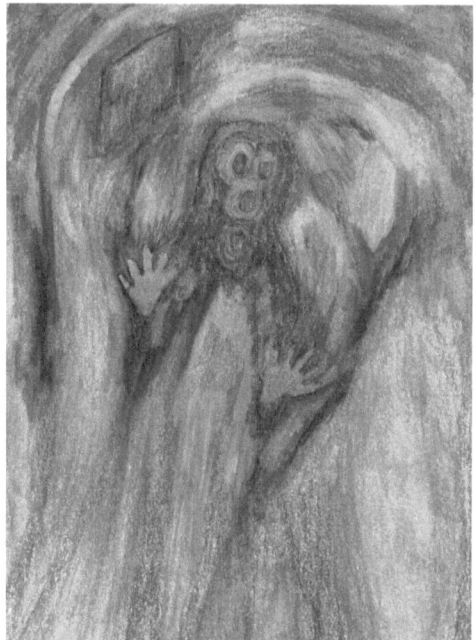

Figure 0.1 Lacunae of suffering

In Figure 0.1, what stood out for me were the holes, the lacunae, a term which cuts across both anatomy and sociology, as well as representing the holes in what can be said and done. Lacunae reside deep in bones where cell bodies of bone making cells sit; they are thus a nesting place for life and connections. Lacunae in sociology refer to the gaps and spaces in texts, and, unlike anatomy, there is no-thing in the centre of the empty spaces. These holes in speech, in carrying out healthcare tasks, where:

> I must constantly choose among competing and apparently incommensurable goods and that circumstances may force me to a position in which I cannot help being false to something or doing some wrong; that an event that simply happens to me may, without my consent, alter my life; ... all these I take to be not just the material of tragedy, but everyday facts of lived practical reason. (Nussbaum, 1986; p. 5)

By reflecting on the lacunae (Figure 0.1), I realise that these holes are a character of both suffering and healthcare. This is the material tragedy of healthcare as well as the everyday facts of lived practical reasoning. These everyday facts of lived practical reasoning are what contribute to a sense of depersonalisation both for patients and clinicians (Ferrell & Coyle, 2008;

Frank, 2001). Yet suffering is rarely mentioned, perhaps due to its inherent disconnect. Through exploring suffering, encountering and speaking suffering, we may make restorative acts through linking words, images and experiences, moving us beyond an addictive model of redemption from suffering.

Box 0.1 Reflection

In this encounter I struggle so much as a young professional with what I am required to do with another person. The humanity of the situation where I am required to perform a task and a role which produces in me an anguish since I see myself as inflicting harm on someone else's emotional and physical state. I am caught between two (at least) conflicting impulses of wanting to help according to established guidelines – I am required to do this – and of wanting to care, nurture, reassure the patient – my original motivation for applying for this role. I feel ashamed of my inadequacy; I hate myself for being in this harm inflicting role and of the authority that gives me the right to carry out this task on another person. I feel devastated that I cannot speak words which could ease the suffering of the person. I also regret the use of my hands which should be sources of comfort and care and instead are being used and perceived as instruments of inflicting harm. The institutional authority that gives me the right to do so seems cold comfort in the moment. I doubt my own knowledge, skills and capacity as well as the evidence base on which I carry out this intrusion on someone else's life. I question what circumstances led me to be in a situation where I as a human being can be inflicting pain and discomfort on someone else, another human being, and yet we cannot speak of this basic humanness of the situation; we are constrained by the words we have and the knowledge that is allowed. What is between us has a formative aspect in that, that experience changes me and, no doubt, the patient, too. There is something else going on between us at a very basic level of humanity; the transmission, or not, of trust, belief, truth and reality. There is also a sense of betrayal – no-one ever said practice was going to be like this or even mentioned the ethical conflict between one's role as a health professional and role as a human being, and what that does to your sense of self. Any ability to make sense of the experience is diminished and perhaps reduced to the notion of ICU delirium.
Questions for reflection

1. What are the somato-sensory, motor, symbolic, imaginal, verbal and intersubjective components of this example?
2. What are the relational hallmarks between professional and patient in this example?

3. As health professionals, by what right do we have the authority to convince patients of the "rightness" of our actions?
4. As health professionals, from where do we gain our sense of self, and what limits and benefits does that confer? What are some of the socially sanctioned major forms of identities of health professionals (archetypes)?
5. Who are we asked to be in the face of suffering?
6. How much of yourself should you include in your practice and what are some of the consequences of that?

Further Resources

    Alma D., Amiel K., Rosen M. (Eds). 2020. These Are The Hands: Poems from the Heart of the NHS Paperback.

References

Butler J. 2005. *Giving an Account of Oneself*. Fordham University Press: New York.

Bynum CW. 1991. *Fragmentation and Redemption. Essays on Gender and the Human Body in Medieval Religion*. MIT Press: New York.

Cassell EJ. 2004. *The Nature of Suffering and the Goals of medicine*. Oxford University Press: Oxford.

Ferrell BR., Coyle N. 2008. *The Nature of Suffering and the Goals of Nursing*. Oxford University Press: Oxford.

Fitzgerald D., Callard F. 2016. Entangling the medical humanities. In *The Edinburgh Companion to the Critical Medical Humanities*. Whitehead A, Woods A, Atkinson S, et al. (eds), Edinburgh (UK): Edinburgh University Press; 2016 Jun 30. Chapter 1. Available from: https://www.ncbi.nlm.nih.gov/books/NBK379264/

Foucault M. 1973. *The Birth of the Clinic – An Archeology of Medical Perception*. Vintage Books: New York.

Frank AW. 2001. Can we research suffering? *Qualitative Health Research*; 11(3):353-362.

Frank AW. 2004. *The Renewal of Generosity: Illness, Medicine and How to Live*. University of Chicago Press: Chicago, IL.

Frank AW. 2013. *The Wounded Storyteller: Body, Illness and Ethics*. Second Edition. The University of Chicago Press: Chicago.

McFarlane R. 2019. *Underland: A Deep Time Journey*. Penguin Random House: Milton Keynes.

Nussbaum MC. 1986. *The Fragility of Goodness: Luck and Ethics in Greek Tragedy and Philosophy*. Cambridge University Press: Cambridge.

Phillips A. 1999. *Darwin's worms. On life stories and death stories*.

Rukeyser M. 1996. *The Life of Poetry*. Paris Press: Connecticut.

Simeon D., Abugel J. 2006. *Feeling Unreal: Depersonalisation Disorder and the Loss of the Self*. Oxford University Press: Oxford.

Wilkinson I. 2005. *Suffering: A Sociological Introduction*. Polity Press: Cambridge.

1 Stitching suffering together

1.0 Introduction

The purpose of this book is to stitch together different lines of inquiry about suffering in order to have the means to more deeply understand the experience of suffering. Piecing together different texts on suffering from within different disciplines is necessary because, at present, knowledge about suffering tends to be collected in isolated texts and disciplinary journal enclaves with few integrated into medicine and healthcare generally. Suffering is rarely mentioned in medical education (Cassell, 2004), and the means to explore it less so (Frank, 2001). Yet some would say there is an epidemic of suffering in healthcare (Dempsey, 2018) – an epidemic which is currently becoming more visible, through the COVID-19 pandemic (Holmes et al., 2020).

There is a sense that some of the fear around the pandemic is from knowing a tidal wave is about to descend with little knowledge or understanding on how to navigate through the enormity of suffering that is personal, professional, economic and political. More than ever, health professionals are expressing their emotions and are checking whether their responses are normal, seeking validation that they should be responding in this way, on top of the already overwhelming affect they are feeling:

> Is it normal to keep bursting into tears? Driving home last night, I welled up. At work, several of us were crying. I am not as resilient as some of my tweets make me out, or as hard.[1]

On top of the feeling of suffering, there is also questioning and self-doubt about how one should feel in these circumstances, what is appropriate and what is normal. Now more than ever, there is an imperative to understand suffering and to know how to be with suffering in the best possible way, even to avoid unnecessary suffering if possible or to know whether to dive into the tsunami or run away.

There are specific models of compassionate care addressing suffering in healthcare, that of both patients and health professionals (Dempsey, 2018). These so-called "antidotes" to suffering provide an important avenue of pragmatic action whilst helping to raise the profile of suffering. I also believe there is a case for understanding or stitching together the fragmented disciplinary knowledge on suffering into our practice. I suggest that perhaps what has stymied the inclusion of learning about suffering in the medical field is the marginalisation of learning and knowledge from medical humanities, sociology and critical pedagogy. I feel incredulous that in a profound human experience such as that of suffering, there is not ready acknowledgment that we need all types of knowledge and understanding of suffering and that the last thing we need to do is to deny our capacity to, and the validity of, feeling suffering:

> ... a person 'who can still suffer over the suffering of others' cannot help feeling lonely, powerless, isolated in present-day society. He cannot help doubting himself and his own convictions, if not his sanity. He cannot help suffering, even though he can experience moments of joy and clarity that are absent in the life of his 'normal' contemporaries
>
> (Fromm, 1993; p.65)

Deepening our understanding of suffering means both a stitching together of these different lines of inquiry – a horizontal movement across disciplines – as well as a deepening understanding of the particular from the universal existential suffering that occurs. The in-depth exploration is less of a theoretical conceptual matter and more of an experiential affective orientation that seeks to recognise our common humanity. Both the horizontal and the vertical movements are necessary.

This chapter introduces basic definitions and properties of suffering and explores the need to have interdisciplinary perspectives from medical humanities, sociology and biomedicine. The point is that now more than ever we need to know explicitly how and what we are suffering. Perhaps this is the most important action we can take in the face of enormous suffering: to know and understand what form and shape this suffering takes. I explore how we stitch these interdisciplinary knowledges together and why the way we do this is important. I go on to explore who could benefit from this writing and when we need to think about on suffering in these terms – at what place in the trajectory of suffering is it of benefit to consider these issues? Similarly, where is the most benefit gained from understanding and knowing about suffering? Finally, I explore what assumptions underpin this work on suffering in order to bring critical thinking to the healthcare service understanding of suffering and signpost how this exploration will take place in the ensuing chapters.

1.1 Definitions and properties

As shown in the tweet above, health professionals often do not seem to know they are suffering and because of that can doubt their reactions to extremely difficult situations. Remembering that "[o]ur suffering was why we could not talk. Our suffering was what we could not say" (Frank, 2001; p. 354), it seems a service to health professionals and patients to try and describe suffering in more detail. The unspeakable, experiencing yourself on the other side of life as it should be, the distress that threatens the intactness of the self by making that self absent, also contributes to the hole in what clinicians can say and do (Frank, 2001). Feeling overwhelming distress may manifest as unpredictable weeping or a silent withdrawal from the world. Suffering is therefore an affective experience related to the language-based reflections we make about ourselves, others, our existential experience and experience of the world (Devisch et al, 2017). As such, suffering is a subjective experience, not self-evident and cannot be objectified. There are thought to be two orthogonal axes of suffering consisting of the relationship between self and other on the one hand and between languishing and acting on the other (Figure 1.1) (Devisch et al, 2017).

The orthogonal axes forms the basis for the following work where reflections, art, film, literature and theory are drawn upon in order to deepen understanding. These axes of self-other and languishing-acting are the starting point for stitching together, and form the core of, the work in successive chapters. Frank's (2001) desire not to be treated as an object and the points of Devisch et al (2017) about the sufferer's withdrawal from the world and lack of ability to trust are the points where health professionals and patients intersect. The closer to the intersection of these axes, where these different aspects collide, is where most real-world problems exist and where understanding is most necessary (Wilson, 1998).

Suffering is thought of as occurring inherently as a result of bearing witness to and living through existential circumstances and events that overwhelm and that can lead to despair. The relational aspect to this occurs in the relationship a person has between their suffering and the world. That is, suffering occurs as a result of being in the world. Yet one of the

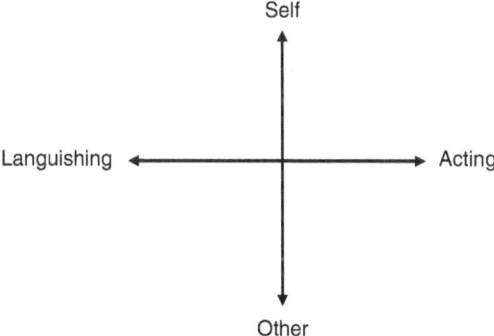

Figure 1.1 Mental suffering based on observations from Ricoeur (Devisch et al, 2017).

paradoxes of suffering is that people can withdraw and suffer in isolation as a result of the speechlessness inherent in suffering:

> Suffering consists of withdrawing from the bond with the other. Persons who suffer frequently feel isolated and undergo the misery they feel overwhelmed by [alone]. Suffering throws people back on their own; locked up with experiences they can hardly tolerate, life turns into hell.
>
> (Devisch et al, 2017; p. 261)

Part of the reason why suffering people withdraw is because they feel they cannot trust other people to understand what they are going through. This in turn makes attending to any suffering more challenging. Signs of suffering include ceaseless weeping, continuous restlessness, agonised crying or self-wounding as a way to manage overwhelming affects that are experienced as intolerable (Devisch et al, 2017). Clearly there are implications here for a medical model based on diagnosis and treatment of a range of conditions for which the guidance from the Diagnostic and Statistical Manual of Mental Disorders Version 5 is not always clear (Vanheule & Devisch, 2014). Ideas around normality arise and this is where the social milieu in which an individual is embedded is crucial and where health professionals are implicated. Ideas around the self-other in suffering begin with an individual and move towards health professional response in how an individual manages suffering.

In addition to the self-other axis, there is also the continuum of languishing-acting. This dimension refers to the "impossibility of performing an act that transforms one's self-experience" (Devisch et al, 2017; p. 261). There are thought to be four levels to this dimension:

1   Suffering is characterised by impossibility at the level of speech – paradoxically while people may want to talk about what they live through, they may not be able to find the words.
2   The passivity characterising suffering is borne out of the belief that nothing can be done, that suffering must just be endured, which reinforces the circle that acting is impossible.
3   Suffering is experienced as a break in the narrative thread; therefore, people are not able to tell stories about nor bring organisation or integration to their suffering.
4   Suffering brings about an impossibility in valuing one's self which again makes acting an impossibility. Performance of an act to transform one's suffering is possible only if people think of themselves as agents that are capable of making accurate judgments: "uncertain as they are, suffering individuals no longer trust their own opinions" (Devisch et al, 2017; p. 261).

Therefore the languishing-acting continuum is inherently connected to a person's self-experience. The focus of an ethical debriefing, for example, is on the existential components of suffering to enable people to move from unbearable to bearable suffering in their experience of self (Devisch et al, 2017). A crucial area of intervention is to provide information about suffering – that these are normal reactions to abnormal situations – and normalisation of the experience of suffering.

The ideas around normality are particularly crucial because people who suffer experience themselves on the wrong side of the fault line of life (Frank, 2001). Thus a major property of suffering is that it calls into question what is normal and what is right. Any response by healthcare professionals to patients and each other must therefore be aware of this property since there is potential to inflict further suffering by not attending to this. In a recent workshop, a group of doctors identified that suffering was a part of life characterised by isolation, loneliness and helplessness on the part of both patient and doctor; physical, mental and emotional pain; fear and guilt on the part of the doctor when treatment did not work or there was an unexpected death; overwhelm in medical students when left on their own to deal with circumstances that were well beyond their capacity; and that sometimes there was just too much protracted pain and suffering, which could end in suicide. Part of the "too much" pain and suffering was seen as coming from the impoverishment and numbing in doctors that accompanied prolonged exposure to multiple causes of suffering. Acting as an advocate for patients in order to provide/facilitate social justice was one way in which doctors thought they could attend to suffering. Being on the front line of service provision and experiencing the high level of suffering without having recourse to do much about it was perceived as being excruciating. The participants clearly identified that while no-one was immune to suffering, there were constraints in attending to this suffering.

However, not speaking about suffering can contribute to a feeling of alienation that is at the root of suffering. Suffering involves a loss of the intactness of the self, an absence, that we are required to encounter (Frank, 2001). By not speaking about suffering, we are carrying on while the elephant in the room only looms larger. Yet it is difficult to talk about suffering for, on the one hand, fear of being detached and abstract through categorisation of experiences best left in their particularity (Frank, 2001) or, on the other hand, fear of becoming mired in an engulfing helplessness from which health professionals fear they could not recover or be able to function (Orange, 2011). Categories of bodily, mental, social and existential suffering (Hofmann, 2015) may provide a piecemeal approach to individual suffering when the context is not considered. That is, the individual is seen to suffer separately from and as not shaped by their environment, including healthcare. That being said, there are ways to explore suffering that take on board the context of definitions and categorisation whilst always keeping an eye on who is best served by these definitions and categories. There is a balance required between providing structured guiding rails to hold onto before letting go and fully immersing oneself in the experience of suffering.

Given that the experience of suffering is widespread within healthcare services and healthcare professionals are generally unprepared for this work and phenomena, I suggest that we need to do more to understand the speechlessness between self-other and the continuum between languishing and acting. My basic theses are that (1) whilst individual health professionals look to go beyond basic medical science in their understanding and practice of healthcare, there is little to guide them in how to integrate new understandings – how do health professionals stitch together new/any medical humanities or sociological understandings in relation to suffering? (2) The absence of integration of sociological and medical humanities thought into practice may increase suffering experienced by patients and health professionals unwittingly by increasing the hole in what we can say and do. This was evidenced during my data collection for my PhD when health professionals asked, "How do we even begin to ask them the right questions?" or "What do you say when …?" in a situation of extreme suffering. (3) This absence as a hole in practice is of value to explore; yet holes, absences, lacks, as causes of anything are generally viewed askance philosophically even though an absence, as in suffering, may be an essential feature of the causal situation (Mumford, 2012). To explore the subject of nothing is to engage in a tangle, philosophically speaking (Mumford, 2012). And finally, (4) unacknowledged suffering may surface in other forms such as Post Traumatic Stress Disorder (PTSD), Dissociative Identity Disorder (DID), Depersonalisation Disorder (DPD), Moral Injury (MI) or as stress or burnout for both patients and health professionals. De Certeau (1984) believes that the eliminated will come back in disguise.

In order to stitch together these different lines of inquiry, a different approach to the range of perspectives is required. Since exploring the dimensions of suffering includes a horizontal movement across disciplines as well as across languishing-acting, and in addition, a vertical understanding of the nature of responses to suffering, the approach I take in this book is as an interpretive *bricoleur* in order to try to bring a psychological, emotional and theoretical unity – a pattern – to an interpretive experience of suffering (Denzin & Lincoln, 2005). This approach is how I will answer the question of how do we understand suffering? And how does our understanding inform how we practice as health professionals *and* have a livable life (Butler, 2005)? Perhaps by understanding suffering more, healthcare professionals will be able to understand their own guilt, self-blame, shame, sense of self-responsibility and fear around suffering.

1.2 Stitching interdisciplinary knowledges together in the service of suffering

In this section, I will explore what I mean by medical humanities and sociology and how I intend to relate them to each other. It is important to make this explicit since how suffering is written will impact how it is understood and therefore how the different disciplines are related to each other. It seems to me that in the face of overwhelming suffering, the one thing we can do is deepen our perspective on suffering. Deepening our perspective means taking into account literature from medical humanities and sociology including critical race studies since this tends not to be integrated into mainstream medicine and is crucial for a fuller understanding of suffering. The sociology of health and illness tends to look at patterns of ill-health in society (Armstrong, 2002; Scambler, 2008) by stepping back and using the sociological imagination to gain a wider perspective (Mills, 2000).

However, moving from the universal to the particular is not usually a feature in medical sociology. For that, medical humanities and philosophy have a more articulate way of describing the lived experience of people who suffer and offer critical thinking on crossing the gap between the social and the individual (Kristeva et al, 2018). For all that, neither sociology nor medical humanities on their own are able to stitch together the diverse approaches and studies to provide a way of acknowledging the different dimensions and properties of suffering. Nor do they tend to acknowledge the epistemic injustice inherent in predominantly white ways of knowing (Fricker, 2007). I will describe more about the importance of the way this stitching is carried out in the next section. For now, I will describe features of the stitching together of different disciplines.

In order to outline features of stitching together knowledge and understandings from different disciplines, as mentioned above, I draw on the concept of a bricoleur. The concept of a bricoleur has echoes in both qualitative research and philosophy. A bricoleur stitches together the individual and social aspects of life in order to reclaim this life from institutional structures (de Certeau, 1984). An interpretive and theoretical bricoleur produces a bricolage, a quilt, of "a pieced together set of representations that is fitted to the specifics of a complex situation" (Denzin & Lincoln, 2005; p. 4). This pragmatic, strategic and self-reflexive approach aims to pull together the threads of medical humanities, sociology and medical education through the unifying experience of suffering. The combination of these different perspectives is intended as a strategy to add height, breadth, complexity, richness and depth by stressing "the dialectical and hermeneutic nature of interdisciplinary inquiry, knowing that the boundaries that previously separated traditional disciplines no longer hold" (Denzin & Lincoln, 2005; p. 6). By relating these different disciplines to each other, there is the hope that knowledge and experience of suffering can be extended to understand the fabric of that experience.

By pulling together the threads of medical humanities, sociology and medical education in order to reach beyond the boundaries of each, there is an explicit acceptance of each of their contributions in order to develop new conversations and awareness about suffering. At the moment, there is little said about suffering, and this could be because of constraints enacted by disciplinary silos. These boundaries, silos, are normative; that is, they impart rules and regulations, often implicit, about what can be discussed about suffering. Rules and regulations are institutional habits or structures that produce features such as an aspirational culture that denies the presence of grief and suffering; reversals in knowledge accumulation and loss; forgetting; paradoxical situations of lauding the heroic National Health Service (NHS) workers whilst at the same time failing to provide adequate protection from the spread of a contagion (McCartney, 2020). Yet mostly these habits of culture and institution are rarely discussed even though they are formative in how we respond to suffering. The culture of healthcare tends to be stoic under the remit of professionalism, yet there is room for some fluidity here, certainly in exploration of the matter.

Whilst respecting stoicism there is a precision required for each thread and stitch as it is placed in the matrix of the quilt. By precisely placing threads and stitches in this bricolage, I hope to reach the heart of the matter of suffering and therefore how we think about suffering. For example, a quilt is amenable to reversals, to showing its other side. Acknowledging reversals as a part of healthcare, looking at the underside, is crucial to understanding what is happening and including the full range of experiences within our theory and practice. De Certeau (1984) believes that unless we do this, the eliminated will come back in disguise. The denial of the hole in suffering allows that suffering to become an understorey of medicine even while the main explicit purpose of medicine is to relieve suffering (Gordon, 2005). This is a difficult notion to understand and requires further explanation.

To show how health professionals can be in the business of both providing care and withdrawing it at the same time, to leave an absence, the unnameable, I will draw on de Certeau (1984) as well as practical current examples. Michel de Certeau was a French philosopher who wrote about everyday life and how to reclaim that from institutional strategies and structures of power. Reclaiming the everyday life meant to engage with the poetics of making do; using art as a "way of making" circumscribed institutional rules or norms, "an art of combination which cannot be dissociated from an art of using" (de Certeau 1984; p. xv). Citizens engage in the art of activity, which at the same time "organizes a network of relations, poetic ways of 'making do' (bricolage), and a re-use of marketing structures" (de Certeau, 1984; p. xv). Through drawing on an art of practice circumscribed by the institution of healthcare, health professionals are organising networks of relations, using institutional regulations and losing some information at the same time. These activities usually go unremarked and health professionals tend to remain unaware of the absence in their practice. Making do means that health professionals provide care in a socially standardized way which can often mean that people who do not fit the social norm are left with an absence in their care related to culture or language or bureaucratic homogenisation.

For example, currently some doctors are quietly rejoicing in the fact that the onset of the COVID-19 pandemic has meant a sweeping away of some bureaucratic obstacles which in turn means that they are able to do what they have always wanted to do and be with patients in an unencumbered way (Brindley, 2020; McCartney, 2020):

> The NHS is threadbare of resources and cut to the quick of beds. The scars left after all the NHS contract negotiations are still visible, if healed at all. Yet the professional contract is not, at heart, with government, but with patients. This explains much professional discontent, when clinicians feel that the work stipulated serves a political agenda, not a clinical one. It also means that in times of crisis, liberated from the shackles of other peoples' priorities, we can get back to the core meaning of being a health-care professional.
>
> (McCartney, 2020; p. 2)

> Things that would have taken years in healthcare can now get greenlighted in a few days. Humour and common sense are returning to institutions that were previously, in my opinion at least, held back by excessive political-correctness and bureaucracy. Administration is now listening to clinicians, and just as shocking, clinicians are listening back.
>
> (Brindley, 2020; p. 1)

> We healthcare workers are scared but, in some ways, we are also lucky. We have the best chance to relearn that human contact is lovely, that caring for others matters, and that finding humour in the everyday is glorious.
>
> (Brindley, 2020; p. 1)

This reversal of the bureaucratic status quo means that health professionals seem to be more at ease with their making do of their work. In this sense, after years of austerity in the NHS, health professionals are finding their own path and reclaiming what they once knew.

Losing information whilst in the business of providing care means that health professionals are left to their own devices on how to manage suffering *in extremis* beyond scientific medical intervention. Health professionals could be seen as "silent discoverers of their own paths in the jungle of functional rationalists ... something that might be considered similar to the 'wandering lines'" (de Certeau, 1984; p. xviii), indicating their awareness of traversing these rules and regulation, but who are yet to come into speech. What is left out of their training and work are the forms and phrasing of practices:

> Statistical investigation grasps the material of these practices, but not their form; it determines the elements used, but not the "phrasing"

produced by the *bricolage* (the artisan-like inventiveness) and the discursiveness that combines these elements, which are all in general circulation and rather drab. Statistical inquiry, in breaking down these "efficacious meanderings" into units that it defines itself, in reorganizing the results of its analyses according to its own codes, "finds" only the homogenous. The power of its calculation lies in its ability to divide, but it is precisely through this ana-lytic fragmentation that it loses sight of what it claims to seek and to represent.

(de Certeau, 1984; p. xviii; emphasis original)

Thus it is that health professionals can ostensibly be engaged in providing the best scientific evidence based care for patients; yet at the same time losing touch with the form, phrasing or tone of their practices, particularly in relation to suffering.

De Certeau (1984) argues that the "scientific" discourse has driven out of its "own" field and constituted as "other" different knowledges, for example, medical humanities. This driving out of knowledges was justified by the life and death nature of medicine. He saw the break between life and death, where death is seen as a defeat by medicine, as organising knowledge in relation to poverty and suffering. This is a stitch between the practice of medicine and the types of knowledges admitted to the field through existential matters of life and death. The organising was around the in-between space between life and death; the silence of the subjects themselves always in relation to the *other* that precedes the subject and is constantly occurring; the other being death, the index of alterity or otherness (de Certeau, 1984; p. 194). Illness is transformed into a scientific and linguistic object, which is perceived as foreign to everyday life, producing a darkness, a falling outside the *thinkable*, which is identified as what one can *do*.

The dying man is the lapse of this discourse. He is, and can only be, ob-scene. And hence censured, deprived of language, wrapped up in a shroud of silence: the unnameable.

(de Certeau, 1984; p. 191)

Driving the speaking about death and suffering outside the thinkable has a function in that it protects a place. The place and health professionals are protected by what they are not. In this way, the denial of suffering, at the same time, creates a nothing, a space, a lacunae, in the loss of speech and provides an uncrossable space that articulates two different presences, both of which are related to each other by the fragility of knowledge.

This uncrossable space, a nothing, is a loss from which writing can be formed, although this is difficult. The uncrossable space, a silence, asks of writing to come from speechlessness – "Why write if not in the name of impossible speech?" (de Certeau, 1984; p. 194). This impossible speech is a feature of suffering (Cassell, 2004; Devisch et al, 2017). Therefore medical humanities have a crucial role in navigating this space which scientific medicine cannot. How we think about suffering is influenced by the speech we have available to us and the writing we are able to do. Writing from this perspective makes the uncrossable space explicit, an inherent part of the work to do, and a key feature of the bricolage of medical humanities, sociology and medical education.

The writer moves towards a presence it cannot reach, is indefinitely linked to an untethered absolute response, that of the other. Yet at the same time, the difficulty of writing asserts itself as participating in an illusion that suffering and death are elsewhere – "The reversal begins in the very work of writing, whose representations are only its result and/or waste product" (de Certeau, 1984; p. 194). Therefore another stitch to add to our bricolage is that of reversal. To know that as we try to cross that space, we will be performing an absence if writing from a place that asserts suffering is elsewhere than us.

> Writing repeats this lack in each of its graphs, the relics of a walk through language. It spells out an absence that is its precondition and its goal. It proceeds by successive abandonments of occupied places, and it articulates itself on an exteriority that eludes it, on its addressee come from abroad, a visitor who is expected but never heard on the scriptural paths that the travels of a desire have traced on the page.
>
> (de Certeau, 1984; p. 195)

This absence, nothing, is one that affords protection to place and health professionals, usually through a reversal, as suffering is perceived as something elsewhere. That is, both a provision of care and a withdrawing of care at the same time, loss of information, a poetics of making do, losing touch with the form, phrasing or tone of their practices; the break between life and death, where death is seen as a defeat by medicine, as organising knowledge in relation to poverty and suffering are all features of healthcare practice that tend towards suffering being an understorey in medicine. This uncrossable space that articulates two different presences, both of which are related to each other by the fragility of knowledge, is the form or tone of this writing, where we begin to write about suffering even though this is philosophically challenging.

I hope I have demonstrated sufficiently the necessity of exploring the absences of suffering through the use of knowledges outside the typical teaching, learning and practice of medicine. In part, these absences are created by health professional practice, in part by the exclusion of knowledge that doesn't fit within the biomedical realm, in part as a need for protection of place and denial of the existence of these absences as well as by the speechlessness that accompanies suffering alongside the circumstances themselves. So far, these features of bricolage have been fairly general and spoken mainly from a white epistemology. The necessity for exploring suffering from a diverse epistemological perspective cannot be emphasised enough, as without doing so there is the danger of epistemic injustice (Fricker, 2007).

1.3 Epistemic injustice

Epistemic injustice or disadvantage are terms used to describe the injustice or disadvantage experienced by persons in their capacity as knowers, which causes them further suffering (Dowrick, 2018; Fricker, 2007). Conveying knowledge about and making sense of one's experience are primary life tasks and capacities, ones that can go first when someone is suffering (Devisch, 2017). In addition to the personal loss of capacity, there is also the social rendering of muteness due to prejudice and stereotyping of what constitutes legitimate knowledge (Fricker, 2007). Particular marginalised groups, according to age, gender, race, ethnicity, socioeconomic status and disability, are more likely to encounter this disbelief of their experience and therefore suffer the additional wounding of injustice. In these situations, their knowledge forms what is abject or outside mainstream society.

Therefore exploring absences in suffering also requires that we acknowledge or perceive what is abject from a moral and ethical imperative; for all that is abject in our society, there is an associated collapse (Kristeva, 1982). This collapse into itself stems from the violence of absence, the forgotten space of blackness; as an example,

> [L]anguage of analysis begins from the violence of her absence, and it is clear the film operates within a logic that cannot apprehend her suffering. How she is written into the film and the film's inability to comprehend her suffering are part of the orthography of the wake. The forgotten space is blackness, and as Jackson is conjured to fill it she appears as a spectre.
>
> (Sharpe, 2016; p. 29)

The language of analysis, logic and writing creates Jackson as "the ejection, the abjection, by, on, through, which the system reimagines and constitutes itself" (p. 29). This gratuitous violence at the level of structure creates a nothingness, which constitutes the black as the constitutive outside (Sharpe, 2016). Any text that does not engage with critical race theory is reinforcing structural violence, antiblackness and thus epistemic injustice, thereby strengthening the status quo.

The moral and ethical imperatives to explore antiblackness and suffering through the violence of abjection requires that we take on this difficult, profound work. We can no longer ignore critical race theorists when educating health professionals; there is so much to say here, which will be explored throughout this book as a persistent, necessary theme. When stitching in critical race theory to the work on suffering, ruptures are a possibility:

> What happens when instead of becoming enraged and shocked every time a Black person is killed in the United States, we recognize Black death as a predictable constitutive aspect of this democracy? What will happen then if instead of demanding justice we recognize (or at least consider) that the very notion of justice ... produces and requires Black exclusion and death as normative.
>
> (James & Costa Vargas, 2012; p. 193 cited in Sharpe, 2016; p. 7)

Sharpe asks that we proceed from this point, as if we know this antiblackness to be the ground on which we stand before we begin to speak as a knowing caring subject.

Writing as if we are aware of antiblackness, with the suffering and death that brings, requires us to think twice (Butt, 2002). Writing with an ethical and moral imperative means we must examine a morality which has itself been shaped and conditioned by the social roots of democracy that enforce this abjection, this reversal. Butt asks, "What are the real roots of justice if the notions of 'health equity' and 'access' are rooted in the neoliberal economic policies?" (p. 13):

> We are far more implicated in the lives of others than can be realized by reading stories of suffering strangers. Just because suffering appears to be universal does not free those who experience it from being exposed to the abuse and manipulation that can follow from any claim to universality.
>
> (Butt, 2002; p. 16)

There are nuances to be aware of in the examination of suffering by health professionals. Butt (2002) warns against tokenism, distancing and using stories of suffering strangers as a rhetorical device that only further entwines the scholar with the perceived needy in a circle of spiralling dependencies, where the "haves" improve the lot of the "have nots." Instead, she recommends that "fully embracing the humanity of others and letting their suffering fracture our own existence is the most difficult and most important thing we have to do" (p. 4).

By not attending to suffering, or attending to it in rhetorical form, we become abstracted from our own lives and those around us. We live on the edge of our experience. Yet writing about suffering, stitching together lines of inquiry about suffering in order to more fully explore the experience of suffering, is difficult because of the challenges of writing about holes and absences. These difficulties come with caveats of rupture and fracture, of avoiding tokenism and making sure we always think twice to include critical race studies in our analytic, for our nothings may just about be someone else's something. This something from people who have been traditionally confined to the nothing may be what is needed to make new progress on understanding suffering. This book is unique in that it attempts to stitch together critical race studies with health professional education through medical humanities and sociology in the belief that including those who are traditionally excluded may lessen the reinscribing of further avoidable suffering.

1.3.1 Summary of section

Key features of stitching these knowledges together is the epistemic break between life and death, where death is seen as a defeat by medicine, which in turn organises knowledge in relation to poverty and suffering; death as an index of alterity/otherness which produced a rejection of anything "unscientific" or not "objective" – a jettison which in turn created a space for suffering; partly this abjection was to protect time, people and place; reversals in the status quo with concomitant forgetting of information; reversals when speaking and writing as if from a place where suffering was not; and a lack of inclusion of critical race studies as providing a counterpoint to the quilting of mainstream epistemology.

1.4 Why is the way knowledge about suffering stitched together important?

Bleakley (2017) argues that the worry is not how we knit together the medical humanities with medicine "but whether or not we can find compelling topics that act as encompassing vehicles for collaboration between differing approaches of thinking and making" (p. 46). However, I argue that the art of combination, the stitching together, is the key point. How we think about these matters in combination and how we put them together are crucial to connect the dots and a feature of critical thinking. The lack of connectivity seems to be what has stymied the integration of medical humanities into/with medicine. In this section, I will explore what is lacking in terms of depth and imagination to provide cohesion of a fragmented field.

A compelling topic such as suffering shows how the way scholars think about suffering lacks imagination from a critical medical humanities perspective. Sociology and critical race studies show how the hole in suffering can be a consequence of the dominant normative mindset. Stitching these together and deepening our understanding seem all that is possible when there is little else to do, as a manifestation of suffering itself. That is the point where suffering can be most stark, and that is where the boundary needs pushing in order to stitch together lines of enquiry about suffering.

Given our enormous resources, it is surprising that we have not progressed more in our thinking about suffering.

For example, if one of the primary features of suffering is the hole in what can be said or done, and feeling as if you are on the wrong side of a fault line (Frank, 2001), then we need to integrate these very perceptions into our practice from the perspective of marginalised people. If attending to suffering is the core business of medicine, then why aren't we devoting more time and effort attending to the way we think about suffering? Part of the reason for this could be the view that everybody knows implicitly that suffering is there: "I guess it's because everybody's facing the same thing. So therefore you don't talk about it," stated one participant in my research on health professional education when talking about and showing the distress inherent in her work.

Biomedicine tends to be seen as limiting and fragmenting discussion about suffering; therefore one of the ways in which this fragmentation can be addressed is by paying attention to how we stitch our thinking together. By deepening our attention to stitching, thinking about our thinking on suffering, a new feminist epistemology, complementary to the masculinist emphasis on knowing for doing, can be developed. I have found that by making deepening an explicit part of my scholarly practice, I can find a sanctuary in the middle of suffering.

Wilson (1998) advocates for consilience – the unity of knowledge – to link together the sciences and humanity. He sees the fragmentation of knowledge and the resulting chaos as artefacts of scholarship that has failed to find common groundwork of explanation. Linking the four domains of ethics, biology, social science and environmental policy through a quadrant, he highlights the place of intersection of axes as being an increasingly unstable and disorienting region and the place where most real-life problems exist. But no maps exist for this place, and fewer concepts and words. It is only in the imagination that we can travel around these domains in order to link them together. Both science and the humanities transmit information; science by breaking phenomena into entities that can be measured and arranged, concepts formed, detection of patterns and use of predictive models, not necessarily in a linear fashion but always creative (Wilson, 1998). The humanities' strength is in explaining and transmitting information about the particular, the lived experience, through pattern recognition of affects as well as cognition. The common property of art and science is the transmission of information.

In linking together the four domains of scholarly practice surveyed in this book, the quadrant shows biology (biomedicine); social sciences (public health, social determinants of health, syndemic suffering); environmental policy (Black Anthropocene, consumerism); and ethics (humanities). The threads running through this patchwork quilt are sources of self, the hole in what could be said for the surviving self, the

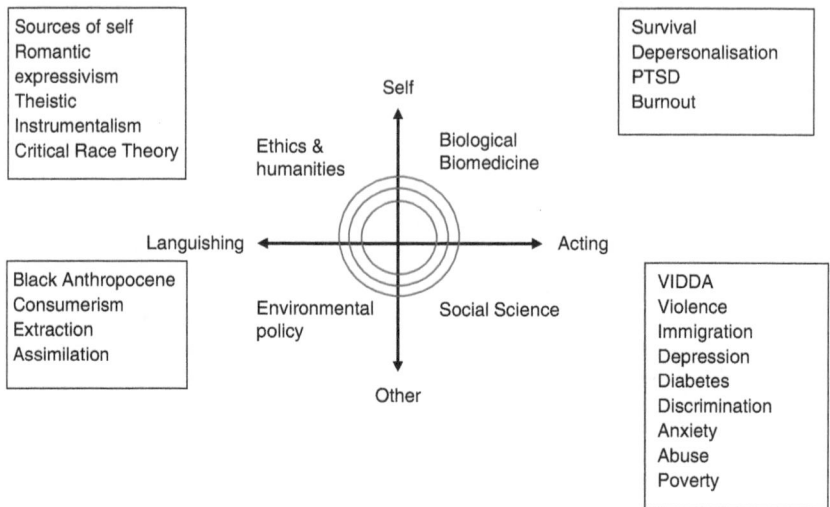

Figure 1.2 Consilience of suffering.
(Source: Adapted from Wilson, 1998).

syndemics of suffering using the "Violence Immigration Depression Diabetes Abuse" (VIDDA) model, critical race theory and the Black Anthropocene, and the moral-ethical anguish of fusion of self and role. The dilemma for health professionals and patients when working close to the intersection of axes are ideas around choice, control and responsibility, especially in relation to health professional advice and public health ideals of health promotion. The circles at the centre represent the ways of travelling around the map, where we are perhaps pushed onto the edges of our experience and knowing when we don't acknowledge suffering.

1.5 My motivation

Continuing on from the last section, my main motivation for writing this book was about wanting to stitch together critical medical humanities, sociology and biomedicine through the lens of suffering in order to improve health professional education along with patient experience and health outcomes. Each discipline plays a crucial role in these processes. Yet knowing how and when to draw on each in a complementary fashion is still a real challenge (Bleakley, 2017). Instead of complementarity, disciplines tend to retreat to their silos and argue competitively from the margins about the value of their particular contribution. In this section, I will discuss the issues involved in integrating these different disciplines from a personal professional perspective. This perspective regards the interaction between the external environment and the internal representation of that environment as key to understanding how to stitch together these different disciplines and as such necessarily involves the discussion of some theory that has informed me.

Integrating social sciences and biomedicine arouses anxiety – the fear of getting lost in the psychological and sociological underbrush (Herman, 2001) – particularly around the overlap between subject and object (Devereaux, 1967) and polarisation of subjectivity and objectivity (Kristeva et al, 2018).

> In short, behavioural science data arouse anxieties, which are warded off by a countertransference inspired pseudo methodology; this man-oeuvre is responsible for nearly all the defects of behavioural science.
>
> (Devereaux, 1967; p. xvii)

An effective behavioural science methodology treats disturbances, produced between observer and subject, as the most significant and characteristic data (Devereaux, 1967). These disturbances, including suffering, which im-plicate both patient and health professional (Orange, 2011; Butt, 2002), must be raised as the primary method for integrating different disciplines. These disturbances have been a key feature of my practice as a health professional, educator and researcher.

As a health professional, I knew there was something amiss with the scientific approach we were trained in, that of "the invisible man desperately trying not to be seen seeing other men, while academic psychology and sociology are even farther down the primrose path of Newtonian epistemology" (Weston Le Barre in Devereaux, 1967; p. viii). The alleged invisibility of us observational scien-tists in pursuit of the best available evidenced-based healthcare was part of the problem of poor healthcare paradoxically, it seemed to me. That is, by not acknowledging suffering and our shared humanity in that suffering, as a pri-mary force in healthcare, we are missing the point.

In a radical turn, Devereux suggests that the partition between humans, ignored usually in the hope that this "will just go away" (p. xviii), is the point of intervention:

> Not the study of the subject, but that of the observer gives us access to the *essence* of the observational *situation*.

The data of behavioural science are, thus, threefold:

1   The behaviour of the subject.
2   The "disturbances" produced by the existence and observational activities of the observer.
3   The behaviour of the observer: his anxieties, his "decisions" (= his attribution of a meaning to his observations) (Devereaux, 1967; p. xviii; emphasis original).

While writing my motivation for this book, therefore, I have been acutely aware of my own disturbances – the need to classify and categorise different knowledges in order to make sense of a multitude of data. The process of classification is worth considering in depth and I spend time doing so in this section. In addition, the subjects of healthcare – both patients and health professionals – are disturbed by and through suffering. There are inherent relations between all of these factors that I have seen played out many times, although not usually acknowledged explicitly, as well as experiencing them myself.

I have wanted to go down deeply into this matter because of the belief that analysis in depth of a single phenomenon may produce just as many insights as analysis of a range of phenomena (Devereaux, 1967). Of course, suffering is not just one phenomenon – there is a range within this. Having seen a range of suffering within healthcare, as well as in the community, I have been amazed at how little this is explored in the literature. Perhaps this is because suffering is not seen as enticing as scientific studies. Partly I think this is the result of how we have been educated: to not dwell on particularities or be deep in our thinking or ask difficult questions. Culturally, we are advised to aim for aspirational goals and to rise above any suffering in a transcendent model of being. There seems to be a prohibition generally on speaking about matters in depth.

After graduating, both under- and post-graduate study, I started trying to piece together all the different information I'd "received" in order to try and make sense of it all. Specifically, I was focused on the links between learning and health because, it seemed to me in hindsight, this was the point of intervention where the partition between the observer and the subject, health professional and patient, was most strong. Health professionals operated on the assumption that the link between learning and health was most straightforward; all that we needed to do was provide information to patients, and they would then be able to carry out the correct activities to improve their health. Yet obviously with all the literature on adherence, compliance, behaviour change, social determinants of health, etc., this is clearly not a straightforward transaction. Nor does suffering enter into this equation of transaction.

In that frame of mind, I approached what I had been taught and learned, to try and piece together the fragments of knowledge, in order to be clear about my toolbox and what I could draw on to help specific patients and situations. I set out a number of times different linear frameworks, influenced no doubt by different mapping techniques, including task analysis, to try and have an index of approaches. I think I was also influenced by biology with its taxonomy of genus and species, which showed where everything belonged in a family of organisms and also, implicitly, in relation to the environment – that is, the recognition that the structure of organisms and systems determines and is determined by their interactions with specific configurations of the environment, which in turn can trigger structural changes in those organisms and systems, a reciprocal bi-directional movement. However, the coding of these sorts of classifications relies inherently on binary logic, which limits the stitching together to a linear in and out pattern more reminiscent of a causal chain than a quilt.

Semantic representations of knowledge fall into two models, that of the dictionary and that of the encyclopedia (Eco, 2014). From Aristotle, the rules governing classification of knowledge followed a dictionary model based on logic:

> In defining a term (and its corresponding concept), the *dictionary* model is expected to take into account only those properties *necessary and sufficient* to distinguish that particular concept from others; in other words, it ought to contain only those properties defined by Kant as *analytical* (analytical being that a priori judgment in which the concept functioning as a predicate can be deduced from the definition of the subject).
>
> (Eco, 2014; p. 3)

Properties which fell outside the distinguishing capacity of the model were believed to be knowledge of the world more generally and therefore a matter for the *encyclopedia*. The definitional model was seen as the tree of knowledge and conceived of as a representation of logical relationships. Differences may be divisive or constitutive, or they could conceivably be both at the same time, depending on the context. I believe it is important for health professionals to understand that the very way knowledge is structured and written about produces the type of knowledge relied upon – that seeing the way knowledge is represented in our systems determines our interactions with patients and vice versa. And in order to provide any unity, we need to be able to stand outside these systems of classification to see the impact they have on our practice.

Classification through difference, or differential diagnosis, is how medicine is operationalised (Seth, 2018). Yet this process is not finite nor pure and risks exploding into a dust cloud of differences (Eco, 2014) and fragmentation (Bohm, 2002). The tree model of definition assumes a logic of representation that is decontextualised; every branch on the classification is potentially a pointer to another realm of knowledge. However, representation itself assumes an objectivity and neutrality on the part of the observer, which is often not the case in healthcare. The objectivity means that there is a perception that our nervous system works by generating representations of an outside world, in which there is a direct translation of the outside world into knowledge into maps in our minds. However, there is no evidence to suggest that this is case.

The alternative view, a cognitive solipsism, portends that all we know is generated internally by our nervous system and that all is relative. A third way sees both as being partially true and that unity is provided by an "outside" observer who correlates both the partial and perspectival and the objective reality. Feminist researchers would argue that no-one is outside the social milieu in which they work and live. But that does not mean that researchers and workers will not position themselves as being outside in order to obtain a presumed objectivity. These assumptions and points of view are crucial to understanding what happens between healthcare professionals and patients, when patients feel objectivised in their suffering (Frank, 2001). There has been a great deal more written about the impact of the penetrability of the medical gaze on patients by Foucault (1973), but for now I will focus on difference and the classification of knowledge.

The notions of difference stems from and provides the analytical basis for this way of classifying knowledge, yet it is not without its controversies (Seth, 2018). Thomas Aquinas noted that "what defines substantial form is difference as an accident" (Eco, 2014; p. 16). To explain further,

> There exist essential differences; but which and what they are we do not know; what we know as specific differences are not the essential differences themselves, but are, so to speak, signs of them, symptoms, clues, superficial manifestations of the being of something else we cannot know. We infer the presence of essential differences through a semiotic process, with knowable accidents as our point of departure.
>
> (Eco, 2014; p. 16–17)

Thomas Aquinas' assumption was that the effect was the sign of the cause. These assumptions and explanations show the difficulty of adopting a tree model of representation of knowledge in an endeavour as inherently complex as healthcare. Yet mostly this is what modern-day heuristics are based on.

I struggled with this difficulty and frustration because always at the heart of that struggle was the person who was suffering and who was potentially undermined by healthcare's system of knowledge. Not only were they suffering due to a condition and social circumstances or events that made dealing with this condition worse, they were often met by health professionals who demonstrated that their suffering did not fit in with their models of learning. Or with ones who simply could not identify with or relate to suffering as an absence.

When I started my PhD, again an attempt to pull together the pieces of knowledge I had accumulated along the way, I drew on the metaphor of a labyrinth to bring together an adaptation of Habermas' lines of inquiry – predictive, understanding, emancipatory – and I added a fourth of deconstruction (Lather, 1991). I've since found out that this way of stitching knowledge together belongs to the encyclopedia model of representation (Eco, 2014). Whilst an encyclopedia depends on a tree of knowledge classification for its organisation, it is also larger than that and able to move beyond the binary subdivision of the tree:

> It was some time, however, before the "plan" of an encyclopedia began to constitute an object of reflection or meta-encyclopedic comment. For the reader, the encyclopedia appeared as a "map" of different territories whose edges were jagged and often imprecise, so that one had the impression of moving through it as if it were a labyrinth that allowed one to choose paths that were constantly new, without feeling obliged to stick to a route leading from the general to the particular.
>
> (Eco, 2014; p. 26)

The point of the encyclopedia is not to register what exists in an evidence-based manner; but to register what people traditionally believe exists. In this way, the encyclopedia moves beyond a mere biological index to include the critical medical humanities and sociology, for example.

The move from the Renaissance and Baroque eras to developing encyclopedic containers of content has also drawn on the forest and related this to the labyrinth: "A forest is not ordered according to clear binary disjunctions; instead it is a labyrinth" (Eco, 2014; p. 36). The meaning of using a labyrinth is to discover something new or to see a relationship between two or more things that were previously hidden from awareness. Crucially, traversing a labyrinth relied on the embodied experience of walking or moving through the paths; a journey which could often end in a dead end by relying on just one faculty or discipline of knowledge. Francis Bacon transformed the idea of an inventory of knowledge to discovering something new, to construct "a bricolage, discovering new syntheses, connections and dovetailings among other things that at first sight did not appear to have any reciprocal relationship" (Eco, 2014; p. 38). Wilson (1998) also suggests a labyrinth for providing a unity of knowledge. However, both the dictionary and encyclopedia with its labyrinth were still predominantly masculinist forms of classifying knowledge.

Drawing on the metaphor of a labyrinth during my PhD research, I hoped to stitch together different understandings and learning. This was not an abstract endeavour for me. This was a practical, pragmatic, conscious strategy to help me through implicit suffering in healthcare. To me, these schemata felt containing and were something I could hitch experiences to. The "encyclopedia" helped me to see relations between concepts and events and was a bridge between task focused doing and decontextualised embodied suffering – or, that is, between cognitive representations and internal lived experience. These connections in a field like healthcare are vital to help prevent further suffering such as that where cultural and racial groups are treated differently according to stereotypes perpetuated by medicine in a form of sanctioned institutional racism (Seth, 2018).

Further motivation for writing this book, in addition to understanding how different lines of inquiry are stitched together in order to provide the means for understanding the experience of suffering more, is simply but most importantly to survive. That is, health professionals spend their working lives with patients who are suffering; if there is not a strong understanding of suffering, then it is difficult to see how health professionals can maintain their work in a connected way. Inherent in this understanding is an awareness of the self and other (Devisch et al, 2017). Not understanding others in their suffering as well as one's own suffering means by default that existential issues and their responses such as transcendence, salvation, redemption and petition are disavowed or denied, whereas restorative attendance to suffering can mean linking of images, words, music and experiences in a way that addresses the hole or the absence and helps the person through to a bearable state of suffering – to be able to survive the onslaught that healthcare can be at times (Dempsey, 2018). Since there is so little written on suffering, it is my hope that this collection of material will provide a resource for further reflection and understanding.

Finally, in my quest for understanding suffering, I have drawn on the arts, literature and film as a form of solace and resonance in the world, where perhaps I have received a nuanced acknowledgement of suffering. The art to me is how this reflection is put together; the critical thinking about how to stitch together different lines of inquiry. I have been struck by a number of films where women voluntarily surrender to the deep water and survive, such as *Whale Rider, The Piano, Moonacre, The Shape of Water,* and *Iris.* My motivation has therefore been fuelled by my desire to dive deeply to go beyond current scripts. This is what I have found, that to find a way out of the labyrinth required me to go down through the portal of suffering, to the underland: the only way out is down, into the abyss.

Therefore, in summary, my motivation for writing stems largely from a need to stitch together bodies of knowledge to provide a container for both objective facts and subjective experiences, to understand how both critical medical humanities and biomedicine can both be true at the same time and be different in their fundamental assumptions and operational practices. Stitching together allows me then to explore understanding and experience of suffering, with both the health professional and patient inherently in that together. This is a challenging task: to reiterate – "fully embracing the humanity of others and letting their suffering fracture our own existence is the most difficult and most important thing we have to do" (Butt, 2002; p. 4). Absences must be explored (Paton et al, 2020). It is no longer enough to medicate away suffering or objectify it behind a health professional uniform.

1.6 Theoretical struggles of writing

As can be seen from above, the theoretical struggles of this writing stem from the way knowledge is classified and categorised, from the tree to the encyclopedia. That is, a binary classification of scientific classes and families of knowledge serves to exclude some knowledge, including some at the expense of others. This initial struggle affects what knowledge is counted as legitimate; what disciplinary boundaries are enforced and how; and therefore what theories, concept, frameworks and assumptions are included. A further theoretical challenge is therefore that the goalposts are constantly shifting according to changing contexts, competencies and circumstances (Eco, 2014). Knowing that this is the case has the potential to bring awareness to the process of stitching together what has not yet been demonstrated in relation to suffering. An encyclopedia representation of knowledge is potentially transformative:

> Every result of this action on the world must, however, be interpreted in its turn, and in this way the circle of semiosis is on the one hand constantly opening up to what lies outside and on the other constantly reproducing itself within.
>
> (Eco, 2014; p. 51)

This constant opening up to what lies outside and reproducing itself within is a hallmark of the dynamic nature of knowledge production and legitimation. The most obvious recent example of this is the knowledge production around COVID-19 with an increasing recognition that all knowledge, not just biomedical, is necessary to contain and manage the pandemic (Holmes et al, 2020; Michie et al, 2020; Wang et al, 2020).

For example, while the focus has been on providing trends in death and infection rates, as well as developing vaccines and treatments, there has been more information available about public health, epidemiological concepts such as "flattening the curve" to reduce the likelihood of overwhelming the NHS, national government policy mandating social distancing and washing of hands, stigma when people are from a particular race or when they don't comply with lockdown recommendations, the disproportionate deaths in Black Asian and Minority Ethnic (BAME) groups globally, stress and grief in health professional workers, the higher rate of death in health workers particularly those with a BAME background, the logistics necessary to set up field hospitals in two weeks, availability and access to ventilators and personal protective equipment (PPE), ethical issues around prioritising patient access to ventilators in the event of a shortage of machines and staff, ethical issues around patients and families being able to communicate for the last time before the patient is sedated for intensive care procedures, from which they may not recover, and so on (Arie, 2020; Shanafelt et al, 2020). Clearly, each of these different knowledges has its place in the armamentarium against a pandemic. But what does it mean to engage with methodological plurality? The following subsections each focus on a specific theoretical challenge – how to integrate methodological plurality, relational theory, the role of the body and the use of metaphors.

1.6.1 Integrating methodological plurality – the causal problematic

In understanding suffering, the challenge is to link different knowledges together to see how they could work to enhance understanding. I have mentioned before that disciplinary knowledge tends to operate in silos. To put this more explicitly, these knowledge silos are abstracted from people and relationships as if they are standalone entities. There is therefore a lack of plurality and relationality, where causality is seen as the sole arbiter in deciding the legitimacy of knowledge. There has been a lack of understanding at this fundamental level, which could help to explain why the medical humanities has not progressed and been more integrated into medicine. These sorts of issues – of understanding the basic assumptions underpinning practice – are curricular issues specific to medical education where the integration of the humanity into practice requires careful thinking through.

An example of careful thinking through is provided by Rocca and Anjum (2020) in their analysis of causal evidence and dispositions in medicine and public health. Causal dispositionalism takes contextual factors that influence outcomes as causes themselves. These causal mechanisms are believed to have intrinsic properties, otherwise known as dispositions or causal powers or capacities, and they fund the knowledge on the hows and whys of phenomena. Properties or potentialities are stable capacities that cause the phenomenon in its context and that require mutual manifestation partners for the phenomenon to appear. Figure 1.3 shows the process of a dispositionalist approach to methodological pluralism (Rocco & Anjum, 2020) using a diagram relating suffering to this approach. Both the biomedical and a deeper understanding are required and are complementary to each other. The diagram of suffering shows that medical humanities and sociology are both necessary steps in this process and that we should not shy away from this methodological pluralism.

An example of methodological pluralism that enhances understanding of suffering is the work by Mendenhall (2019). Her work is a landmark for thinking about causal dispositionalism and linking lived experience with clinical research. *Rethinking Diabetes* is an astonishing achievement for both its breadth in mapping lived experiences for both men and women around diabetes over four locations, whilst teasing out the differences between those locations, and for its depths in understanding how diabetes is both a contributor to and effect of trauma, poverty, immigration, isolation and other health conditions. Mendenhall (2019) provides real-life examples of dilemmas experienced by participants in taking care of oneself in the context of chronic illnesses, poverty, violence, discrimination and displacement or immigration. She draws centrally on the concept of syndemic suffering to explain what is subjectively defined, contextually rooted and communicated through the mind and body:

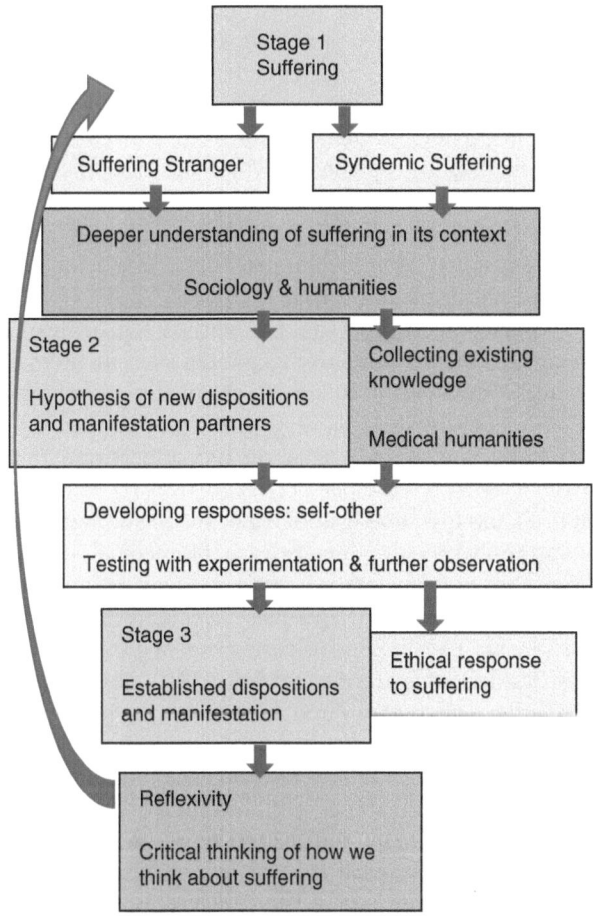

Figure 1.3 A dispositionalist approach to methodological pluralism for causal
evidencing in medicine and public health (Rocco & Anjum, 2020) and
relating suffering to this approach.
(Source: Adapted from Rocco & Anjum, 2020).

A syndemic embodies the *synergies* of epi*demics*, whereby two or more
conditions cluster together within a community, interact at the
biological, psychological, or social level, and are driven by social or
political factors.

(p. 24) (original emphasis)

The clustering together of conditions is the point about the research, that
suffering is far worse and more difficult to grasp when these clusters occur
and for the most part health professionals have little understanding of this
combinatory effect, which can make matters worse for patients. Her key

arguments are that (1) diabetes must be understood as a disease of poverty without obscuring this fact and concomitant health inequities through a misjudged focus on modernity; (2) diabetes is always syndemic; (3) a diagnosis transforms how people perceive and experience their physical condition; (4) the social life of diabetes is significant across contexts; (5) interventions should employ syndemic thinking for both upstream and downstream locations; and, finally, (6) the clinical world has oversold the individual behavioural interventions of diet and exercise, often to ill effect, without considering the conditions of peoples' lives such as poverty and isolation. In thinking about causality, Mendenhall provides a blueprint for understanding suffering in all its forms and tones.

Mendenhall (2019) draws on powerful personal narratives that identify the contingencies of structural violence underlying poor health including inequities, discrimination and stigma practiced at both the macro and micro level. These fault lines of inequality and poverty are compounded by healthcare systems both locally and globally that do not understand the meaning of structuring from a social science perspective. By this I mean that she connects the inherent grief and loss, and lack of legal, social and familial protection, to what constitutes women's illnesses in a biomedical sense. Including the lived experience of participants is a powerful way to link the larger social forces with the circumstances of peoples' lives and their way of coping with a chronic illness. The linking of categories of illness with biomedical measurements, models of suffering, patterns of ill-health and social-cultural meaning have the potential to pave the way for the inclusion of sociology and medical humanities in medicine.

However, whilst the VIDDA model links poverty, violence, immigration and isolation, depression, diabetes and abuse with healthcare practice – showing how the dispositions of each compound the worse health outcomes and thereby form stable properties or capacities – there are some gaps in understanding how social structures contribute to these dispositions. That is, in linking the macro with the micro, there is a gap in understanding the concrete processes and epistemological effects. Sewell (1992) explores the term structure in great detail, understanding that its use is problematic within the social sciences. "The metaphor of structure implies stability" (p. 2), and "moving from questions of stability to questions of change tends to involve awkward epistemological shifts" (p. 3). Sewell understands human agency – the ability to take effective action and respond to circumstances – as inherently implicated in social patterning of ill-health. Therefore, structures must be seen as dynamic processes and not a static phenomenon. He debates whether social structures are not just simply the practices and rules of social systems; they are also the principles of these practices (Sewell, 1992):

> [S]tructure is to practice as *langue* (the abstract rules that make possible the production of grammatical sentences) is to *parole* (speech, or the production of actual sentences; 1976, pp. 118–22). Hence

structure, like *langue*, is a complex set of rules with a "virtual" existence while practice, like speech, is an enactment of these rules in space and time.

(Sewell, 1992; p. 6)

The relationship of the abstract to the concrete is of primary importance. Here is precisely where medical humanities is inserted into sociology and medicine. Social systems are observable, intertwining and relatively bounded social practices that link persons across time and space (Sewell, 1992). Note that the word relationship does not figure in this description. Actors are knowledgeable of these rules and therefore capable of action – the culture of a social system can be explored deeply in order to move beyond the recurrent patterns of binary opposition – and this knowledgeability includes the use of informal and unconscious schemas, metaphors or assumptions presupposed by formal statements (Sewell, 1992). The generalizability or transposability of schemas is the reason why they must be understood as principles or virtual. Therefore, structure is dynamic and the continually evolving outcome of resources and processes in a matrix of processes of social interaction; in other words, of relationships.

1.6.2 *Relational theory*

Understanding structures, matrices and the relationship between these and medical humanities, sociology and medicine is the key theoretical challenge of this work. This is the key challenge that gets played out between health professionals and patients and where there is such little guidance from either sociology or medical humanities. Knowledge is presented from all disciplines as if in a silo or in isolation from the key actors in the healthcare setting. This is the hole in the understanding of health professionals and where/how they feel unable to respond to suffering because they do not recognise, or at least refuse to recognise, the importance of relationship and response in implementing knowledge. This recognition goes far beyond empathy and compassion. The recognition is in knowing that relationships inform and are formed by knowledge and context; they are not an afterthought or an optional extra. There is little demonstration of a granular understanding of the importance of relationship in medicine, medical education or sociology; between Foucault's (1973) disembodied gaze or Freire's (2000) binary in the pedagogy of the oppressed, there is little in between.

In order to understand the importance of relational models, we need to turn to Fiske (1993) and Haslam (2012). These two authors lay out four relational models that include decision procedures, social values and domains of how people relate to each other that has been found to be applicable across cultures. I have included these because they are inherent to an understanding of suffering and responses to that. Medical humanities and sociology both play a key part in these models; medical humanities in its use and acknowledgement of metaphors (Bleakley, 2017) and sociology in its understanding of social structures – here is the link between the individual and the social. The four models are summarised in Table 1.1 but basically form a continuum between a communal consensual approach, authoritarian, democracy or egalitarian and capitalistic market-driven approach. There is also the null approach which is antisocial, anarchic and not perceived to be relational (Fiske, 1993; Haslam, 2012). With each model, there are different types of social relationships and these are expressed through metaphor, amongst other mediators, as Sewell (1992) indicated. Each model has a different response to suffering according to the perspective of different persons, whether they see themselves as having transgressed an unwritten rule or a punitive authoritarian figure or perhaps just suffering the consequences of their own choices and actions. These properties are the dispositions that must be taken into account when advocating methodological pluralism through medical humanities and sociology.

To return to Figure 1.3 showing methodological pluralism, a focus on purely experimental and observational science without acknowledging the relational embeddedness of that science, is to create a void. The void is perpetuated by a distinction between the objectivity of science and the subjectivity of culture whereby health is seen as a definitive state outside the laboratory as well as the biography and life context of individual patients (Kristeva et al, 2018). In this perspective, critical medical humanities

> should rather be seen as *a cross-disciplinary and cross-cultural space for a bidirectional critical interrogation of both biomedicine (simplistic reductions of life to biology) and the humanities (simplistic reductions of suffering and health injustice to cultural relativism).*
> (Kristeva et al, 2018; p. 2; emphasis original)

However, I would go further and state that critical medical humanities requires an understanding of relational theory in which all activities are embedded and which is particularly relevant to understanding suffering. The void in what can be said could be positioned as of the social – a reflection that health professionals have been trained to be scientific, objective and detached and so cannot relate at this level to what patients have to say about their suffering. This creation of a void by health professional training by not making suffering a foundational aspect of that training could be a sixth category of relational absence that is just characterised by a vacuum (see last column in Table 1.1).

Zooming in from macro arrangements of knowledge to the relationship between them requires an understanding of the mediators of that cross-disciplinary and cross-cultural space. It is not enough to state that there are

Table 1.1 Basic modes and properties of relationships (Fiske, 1993; Haslam, 2012) in relation to suffering – final column (various authors)

Domain	Communal Sharing	Authority Ranking	Equality Matching	Market Pricing	Null	Suffering
Decision making	Community consensus, e.g., Quakers	Leader Authority Wise	Referendum Ballots	Demand-supply	No joint socially organised decision at all Anarchic	Self-Other Languishing-Acting dimensions No longer trust their own opinions
Reflection & discussion	Moral & political – pull together; values	Biblical or paramount being	Take in turns Flipping a coin Reciprocity	Benefits, costs, risks & temporal discounts	Terror, coercion Sexual inducements Threatening Asocial Arbitrary violence	Withdrawal from relationship Isolation Unbearable experiences Other people just don't get it
Ideological	Based on need Kindness Collective sharing	Loyalty, Awe, Moral reasoning Obeying Defer	Equality Fairness Moral axioms	Freedom of choice Moral value of each person making their own choice & living with the consequences	No social organisation of social responsibilities	Finding oneself on the wrong side of the fault line Despair Vicious circle Existential layer challenged
Benefits	Belonging to the relevant group or being the right type of person	Specific benefactor Respect Deference Loyalty Obedience	Equality Reciprocal arrangements	Due proportionality Get what you are willing to pay for	?	Dialogic inherent in loss of self Social crisis, ritual, & process of subject formation

(Continued)

Table 1.1 (Continued)

Domain	Communal Sharing	Authority Ranking	Equality Matching	Market Pricing	Null	Suffering
	entitles one to free access to resources					Linking concrete actions to experience can help, listening, understanding Void
Making sociomoral sense of their experience of suffering	Don't know Breach of collectivity Jinxed Polluted Don't know what to say – a violation of unity, solidarity & wholeness of community Jonahs, pariahs	Why would God do this to them? Forsaken Punishment Angered protector Shame Anger Guilt	It isn't fair, why is this happening to me? Search for something they've done wrong	Consequences of a calculated choice, or related to responsibilities inherent in a contract; risk based on value-free choice among alternatives, rational comparison of expected costs & benefits		Impossibility of performing an act – speechlessness, despair, rupture in narrative thread, impossibility of valuing one's self, unable to trust one's self, overwhelmed & devastated by excess of information (Devisch 2017; Macnaughton Whitehead

Mediators	Consubstantial assimilation indexical, metonymic	Social physics Iconic, metaphoric	Concrete operations procedural	Arbitrary signs Symbolic	2016, Mendenhall 2019; Frank, 2001; Cassell, 2004) Cultural melancholy – holy trinity of avowed affect, hidden affect & disavowed loss of self, unconscious displacement of loss onto ego (Singleton, 2015) Chiasma – (Merleau-Ponty, 1968; Levin, 1991) Suffering
Examples	Burnout	Moral Injury	PTSD	Stress	PTSD

these gaps and spaces. The mediators are what connects the figures and the different people within the disciplines. I will provide an example of this relation between health professionals and people with the worst health outcomes as described by Mendenhall (2019) in order to show the matrix (Gerada, 2019) between and within and how these all relate to the suffering self. Further, the epistemological injustices inherent in these matrices require elucidation and stitching in – this in itself provides a theoretical challenge since writers in both the white and black epistemologies tend not to cross-fertilise each other's ideas. Trying to stitch them together can come across as disjointed if attention is not paid to the unifying experiences linking both these locations and others. Unifying experiences, such as the absence or the hole in what can be said, depersonalisation and finding oneself on the wrong side of the fault line, for example, link both health professional and patient.

Fiske (1993) builds on work from Piaget to link cognitive development to relational contextual understanding. Cognitive development and expression are therefore mediated by sensorimotor, concrete operations and procedural information, as well as through the use of metaphors, metonyms and symbols in language. Making sense of an experience of suffering is related to each of the types of relations, thereby providing an overview for processing and responding to suffering. Medical humanities has a role here to provide understanding at the metaphorical and interpretive level whilst also still critically analysing the cross-disciplinary and cross-cultural space. The fabric of the bricolage requires that we understand social patterns and absences in which these relationships take place. These key theoretical challenges of causality, methodological plurality and relationships in understanding suffering form the fabric of the quilt. However, in order to provide a more concrete example, I am going to draw on a metaphor of bone and will provide an example of this in relation to healthcare practice and suffering. I will also provide more granulation to this metaphor as I proceed.

The theoretical framework here lends itself to the metaphor of lacunae, with the connecting canaliculi, paths between the lacunae, in bone. I have chosen this metaphor to show the social matrix and connections between medical humanities, sociology and suffering in order to demonstrate the polydimensional nature of these. The lacunae or spaces I see as more reflective of the social void in understanding; the lack of response to injustice and perpetuation, indeed widening, of inequalities. I have chosen to write the text with its emphasis on lacunae, the unbegun places of living, where suffering is an understorey and we ask "who do we think we are, and where (under what sky) do we want to live?" (Nussbaum, 1986; p. 3). To me, the lacunae (Figure 1.4) with radiating lines (the canaliculi) emanating from each show alignment with writers who offer up suffering as a racialised phenomenon and a source of epistemic injustice along fault lines (Section 1.3). That is, the blackness, the othering, of the hole in speech of what we can say about suffering is fundamental to understanding this experience. For example,

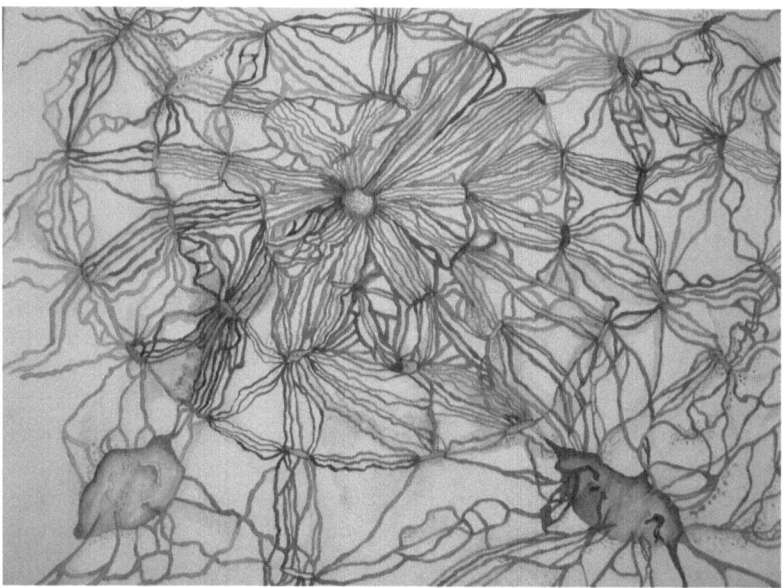

Figure 1.4 Lacunae representation of theoretical framework on suffering.

Singleton (2015) weaves together critical race studies, psychoanalysis, queer theory, and performance studies to acknowledge hidden dialogues, making explicit the interplay between psychic and social, personal and political, individual and collective in order to emphasise the work necessary for racial grieving, critical race consciousness and collective agency.

Therefore, any writing on suffering would not be complete without acknowledging and trying to understand how race and culture already always inform our experiences of suffering through a process of colonisation, even though this may not be explicit (Desai & Sanya, 2016). For example, Mukandi (2015) states:

> The architectonics of their work are derived from and must remain intelligible to the colonial *centre* if they are to go by the title "philosophy." Philosophy – not thought itself, not necessarily, if only because thought and philosophy are not reducible to one another – the academic discipline is part of a global system of relations that are ultimately colonial.
>
> (Mukandi, 2015; p. 527) (my emphasis)

The global systems of relations that are ultimately colonial predate relational theory. He goes on to describe the "tragic situation of the thinker belonging to a colonised group: we are submerged under colonialism and everything that we produce is inevitably complicit with the colonial project" (p. 528). I write about who I think I am and under what sky I want to live to acknowledge my complicity with colonialism and know that any writing will necessarily unfortunately be a part of that academic system. Therefore in contrast to other books on medical humanities, I state this upfront since I know that these are not value free endeavours.

Furthermore, I draw on black women writers who know what it is like to have to try and speak from within the academy whilst at the same time as being perceived as outside the mainstream (Anzaldua, 1999; Behar, 1997; hooks, 1994; Sharpe, 2016). "Only by remaining flexible is she able to stretch the psyche horizontally and vertically" (Anzaldúa, 1999; p. 100–101). Attending to these voices has meant that more of the gaps in theorising have been crossed than would have been possible otherwise. There is constant movement in this attempt, and for this the bone matrix must be seen as a flexible, alive process of continued growth and development, as it is in the live body. The temporal and spatial dimensions are important factors to consider in subjectivity – "the co-articulation of the space of experience and the horizon of expectation is interlaced with the biographical dimension" (Venn, 2002; p. 58). These knots in a network or, perhaps the cell body within the lacunae, occur at temporal, spatial and biographical points in relationship with others (Bingham, 2004; Venn, 2002):

> In this way, every self is sutured in history. But this suturing, or folding requires the participation of others: as *interlocutors*, imagined or not, as models or ideal egos, as those in the gaze of whom recognition is bestowed or refused, as elements of the lifeworld that validate particular selves.
>
> (Venn, 2002; p. 58) (my emphasis)

This intersubjective network of interactions means that we must always counter the sovereign ideal of the autonomous independent individual with an understanding of the other who always helps to form our experiential horizon.

The work requires the constant stretches between vertical and horizontal fault lines as shown between the lacunae in a three-dimensional manner. The vertical lines of suffering are marked by religious notions of redemption, salvation, transgression or transcendence as a response to suffering. The horizontal lines are the fault lines set through intersections of race, ethnicity, gender, poverty, violence and immigration (Mendenhall, 2019). The relationship between self-other (Devisch et al, 2017) is also a vertical-horizontal dimension in both the type of (vertical) relation (Fiske, 1993) and horizontal across repetitions of metonym, metaphor, concrete and symbolic manifestations of agency of the self, in the context of these fault lines and matrix of society. For example, authority or authorising "happens on the fault line between the psychic and the intersubjective, [and] we must consider it to be a relational activity that begins in the psyche but ends up in the real world where humans have agency" (Bingham, 2004; p. 31). I would also say that the reverse process across fault lines between the social and the individual is also true although the debate from internalisation of social/psychic phenomena is far from over (O'Grady, 2005; Sawicki, 1991; Venn, 2002). However, the co-creation of and articulation between the social and the individual along these fault lines is crucial to understanding suffering in both the health professional and patient. This co-creative work requires that we examine our ways or articulations of knowing and look actively for examples of epistemic violence (Sharpe, 2016). This is as true in medical humanities as it is in sociology.

1.6.3 *The theoretical challenge of the body*

The plurality of knowledge and disciplines required to understand suffering is not complete without understanding the body. Therefore, the knowledge, theory and understanding necessary to explore how the body is stitched into the fabric of suffering presents another theoretical challenge of this writing. Addressing this theoretical challenge is vital because at present there is no unity in the field in relation to suffering; there is the biomedical biological body, the structured body in relation to inequalities, bodies across the lifecourse, the mortal body (Williams, 2003), the absent body (Leder, 1990), the postmodern body (Fox, 1999), the disciplined body (Foucault, 1973), the cultural body (Lupton, 2012), the body multiple (Mol, 2002), the diseased body (Sontag, 1991), the body in pain (Bourke, 2014; Scarry, 1985), the distressed body (Leder, 2016), the breathless body (Macnaughton & Carel, 2016), the metaphorical body (Bleakley, 2017) and the embodied body (Sawicki, 1991). Medical sociology and the medical humanities have contributed to understanding the ways in which the body is experienced, understood and represented in medicine. The methodologies of these disciplines range from anthropology, hermeneutics, narratives, phenomenology, psychoanalysis, critical race studies and queer and feminist studies to philosophy. I have chosen to draw on phenomenology because of Merleau Ponty's description of the relationship between self and other in terms of the chiasma (Levin, 1991).

Levin (1991) argues that Merleau Ponty's vision of the use of phenomenology is vital to understand our relationality and, conversely, our ability to self-isolate, both of which are relevant for suffering. Particularly, though, it is through our social embodiment that we know social justice and this is the key reason for using this theory. Furthermore, we have already noted with de Certeau (1984) the reversal that occurs – whereby the absence around suffering is one that affords protection to place and health professionals, usually through a reversal, as suffering is perceived as something elsewhere – and this has an echo in phenomenology where both the individualisation and the socialisation that occurs is through a reversibility of sight, hearing, touch and other communicative activities – a relation of flesh to flesh (Levin, 1991); "my eyes which see, my hands which touch, can also be seen and touched" (p. 66). Levin argues that the flesh is the formative medium or matrix of the object and subject, the dimensionality of our being. With this inseparability between the self and other, with mirroring and echoing of our basic primary relationality, we have capacities to feel pain and perceive suffering in others, which claim us morally and which we cannot disregard. The reciprocity and reversibility forms the basis of Merleau Ponty's chiasma, which means that we require, in the flesh, the means to be able to respond to suffering and issues of social justice and that this embodied sense provides the impetus and grounds to respond to suffering in others (Levin, 1991).

There are, however, nuances to this approach to understanding the relation to/with self and other which I will explore in later chapters. Suffice to say at the moment, in relation to suffering and how it is encountered in healthcare, the matrix of the socialisation of healthcare professionals does not always lend itself to social justice issues within the professionals (Gerada, 2019). The reversibility and reciprocity has not always been available for staff in the past and this may account for some of the absences I encountered when carrying out my research with health professionals. Bleakley (2017) argues that the body is a machinic assemblage with the capacity for both colluding and resisting socialised health, and debate about health, within an industrial war complex relying on burnt out heroes in under-resourced and dysfunctional organisational systems. In such a description as this, it is difficult to imagine social justice, reciprocity or reversibility. For now though, an explanation of the use of metaphors is necessary.

1.6.4 The use of metaphors

I am including a section on the use of a metaphor for three reasons: (1) To provide the epistemological validity of the use of metaphors through relations, (2) providing a vehicle for contemplation and exploring subject matter of suffering more deeply and more inwardly and (3) as a tool for survival during circumstances beyond our control as a way through suffering. I include a short review of selected literature in order to relate how metaphors work and what their effects are. Since metaphors are a feature of cognition, learning and teaching, relations and the imagination, they are one of the tethering or anchor points between layers of understanding in both the horizontal and vertical sense.

The use of lacunae arose initially from my first picture as shown in the preface and was a way of providing continuity to the writing. It captured the meaning of spaces and of lakes, bodies of water that allowed for a deep dive into the matter in hand. The word lacunae comes from the Latin *lacunae* for gap, vacancy, space or hole, a diminutive form of Latin *lacus* meaning *pool* or *lake*. Rauch (2003) suggests that lacunae, especially when not explored or known, can act as determinate in that knowledge will always reconstitute itself in terms of meaning, visibility, significance and consequences in their absence. Cultural studies concentrate on the contexts that surround lacunae, calling attention to ideologies that perpetuate the existence of these spaces unnoticed or unchallenged:

[P]ostcolonial studies have made an effort not only to have readers understand the role and the position of 'the other', but to have us consider this category as defining rather than defined.

(Rauch, 2003; p. 210)

These ideologies work not because lacunae are not important, but because they are. That is, societal patterns of behaviour or health may exist because of the absence of noticing or responding appropriately. He suggests that "the absence of a curriculum that addresses – at least from a conceptual perspective – how lacunae might impinge on their apprehension and re-presentation of the world, is perhaps the most notable lacuna to be addressed here" (Rauch, 2003; p. 214). His emphasis on the determinative factor of absent and invisible lacunae and the way we skirt around them and don't see them has relevance for understanding suffering. Resisting social responsibility by excluding social knowledge from encyclopedia creates boundaries in particular ways and locations.

Metaphors abound in the use of encyclopedia due to the transformative creative work necessary to develop new texts (Eco, 2014). Metaphors perform a cognitive function or recognition or construction of similarity with an added dimension of learning in a new way whilst arousing wonder and pleasure. Learning in a new way requires us to reorganise our categories and our opinions or definitions, especially in relation to cause and effects. Associative chains or interconnections are created which orient viewers and synthesises knowledge and thinking about a subject.

Eco (2014) argues that culturally we are inclined to forget knowledge when working from a labyrinth model of knowledge and that one of the functions of a metaphor is to enable us to remember what we do not know yet. Culturally, there is a switch, based on a need for survival, that acts as an imperative to forget and impose silence. This has particular relevance to suffering where already the experience is hallmarked by speechlessness. Perhaps this forgetting and speechlessness are why the field of study about suffering has not progressed as much as it could have given the prevalence of suffering in the world. There may be a latency of knowledge about suffering that could be identified once we start to make links between different properties and dimensions of suffering.

I see this as a critical role for medical humanities and one that cannot be emphasised enough. That medical humanities can assist in the remembering and bringing into speech the words around lacunae of suffering. By going through the portal of suffering, stepping into deeper spaces or bodies of water, there is a chance we will remember something that will help us to survive these difficult times. This is about finding the tools for contemplation of our mind in the midst of suffering:

> 'At the end of my suffering
> there was a door'.
> "The Wild Iris"

Louise Glück (2011; p. 406)

Remembering, stepping through portals into different worlds and surviving complements the use of metaphors as cognitive devices to cross gaps in logic. However, inherent in all these strategies is the use of metaphors as both process and product (Bleakley, 2017): "A metaphor is, then, a link between two previously unconnected things, usually acting as a catalyst for a deeper understanding. A metaphor is not only the link itself (a linguistic product of cognition) but also the means by which we appreciate, value and understand this link (embodied and social cognition" (p. 8). Bleakley (2017) states four functions of metaphors as knowledge representations – naming, remembering, analogical reasoning and learning – as workhorses of cognition. His comprehensive account of the use of metaphors in medicine includes the acknowledgment of sensorimotor grounding as intrinsic to metaphor enhanced cognition almost as if they acted as a turbo booster to the thinking process.

Perhaps this is an appeal to the cognitive, logical rational nature of medicine. However, he also suggests that metaphors can be transformative and emergent or fluid in promoting understanding, in order to reverse the thinking that metaphors are peripheral to conceptual thinking and metaphysics, and that in fact they are the core from which cognition arises. Metaphors can be structural (one concept is structured in terms of another), orientational (structured spatially – happy is up) and ontological (shapes experiences in terms of forms such as containers – I feel hemmed in) (Bleakley, 2017). Having very briefly reviewed some work on metaphors, the inherent purpose of which is to bridge two worlds, the value in providing structure and process in understanding suffering through the metaphor of lacunae and bone structure can be seen. The two worlds that need bridging are that between health professional and patient in the context of suffering. I will now provide an example of how these two worlds collide and what this means in terms of understanding suffering.

1.6.5 Example of the theoretical challenges in understanding suffering

Movements towards understanding and exploring suffering, of stitching together different knowledges about suffering, have been stymied for a number of reasons, some of which have already been explained. There is another reason for this theoretical challenge and that lies in the different matrices that both health professional and patient occupy. The different matrices provide differing selves and identities as well as different theories. Health professionals rely on objective detachment for their knowledge base, whereas patients tend to rely on their subjective lived experience for their understanding of their conditions. These do not always match and are not legitimated by the different groups of people. In the context of medical education and suffering, Gerada (2019) explains how their training has made doctors detached as a way of controlling their feelings, refraining from excessive involvement and not over-identifying with their patients.

The medical self is developed during training to accommodate the high level of responsibilities that permeate doctors' lives. The medical matrix is the collective identity formed by rules and regulations, culture, socialisation, physical manifestations and the lifelong burden of working so closely to distress that doctors develop collective defences which include depersonalisation, sublimation and denial of vulnerability:

> It is this medical self, located within the medical matrix, which acts during work to mask the doctor's suffering, and protect them from subjective feelings of guilt, fear and hopelessness.
>
> (Gerada, 2019; p. 355)

The way of thinking and being – being able to bear witness to a large amount of suffering – means that doctors carry suffering for others, whereby society uses "chosen subgroups" to delegate unpalatable tasks such as dealing with death and dying (Gerada, 2019). This unpalatable material then is hidden from sight, becomes the social unconscious whereby both patient and doctor, as well as society at large, collude to prevent the unpalatable from being visible. Gerada (2019) warns against psychological singletons who suffer from disconnection from their groups and believes that the medical matrix and medical self both contribute to the increasing rates of medical mental ill-health as well as the camaraderie that can protect doctors from this suffering.

If we return to the last section on the theoretical challenges of the body, we are reminded of the necessity for reciprocity and reversibility for the social process between self and other. If we also link this understanding with that provided by Mendenhall (2019) for syndemic suffering, we can see that the major themes of syndemic suffering were isolation, immigration, violence, depression, anxiety, poverty, diabetes and abuse. Expecting doctors and all health professionals to meet suffering when they have been trained to be detached and objective, whilst engaging with defences such as depersonalisation, sublimation and denial of vulnerability, is it any wonder then that health professionals rely on a clinical model as that is all that has been taught while what remains hidden is the collusion on denying the unpalatable and uncertainty of illness and death?

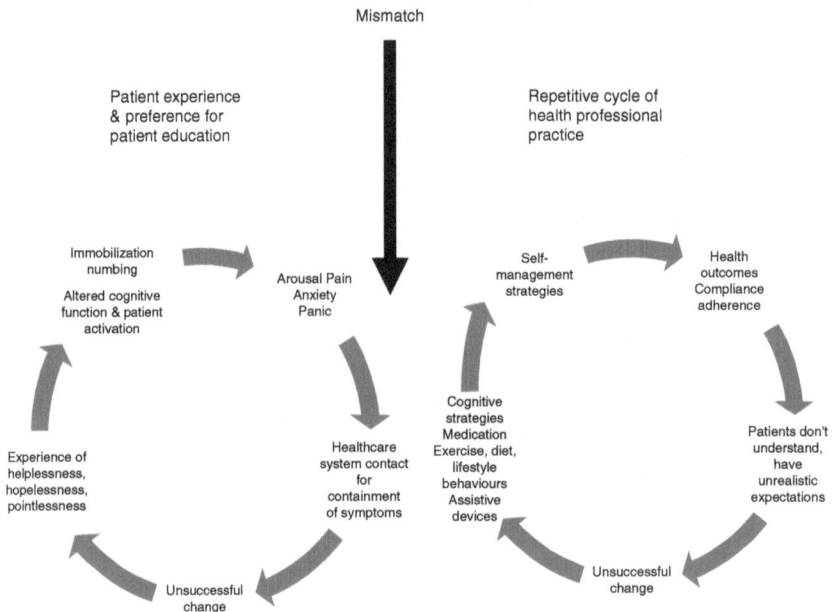

Figure 1.5 Mismatch in experiences of patients and health professionals related to musculoskeletal suffering (Lowe et al, 2014).

Whilst conducting research on musculoskeletal pain and suffering, the difference in perception between patients and health professionals was stark (Lowe et al, 2014). The health professional reliance on cognitive strategies for containment of patients' unrelenting symptoms, compared with patients who wanted better outcomes, if not a cure, but who were perceived by health professionals as therefore not understanding the cognitive content of their illness resulted in a mismatch between expectations on both sides (see Figure 1.5). The research showed limited reciprocity and understanding of patient narratives about pain. This research supported Mendenhall's thesis that health professionals relied too much on their clinical interventions without understanding the impact of the conditions of patients' lives. However, given the account by Gerada (2019) of the medical matrix and self with associated problems, there seems to be a great gap in understanding suffering on both the public's as well as health professionals' part. The distress associated with being a clinician has been characterised by depersonalisation, moral dilemmas, distress, injury and burnout due to the challenges inherent in navigating a system in an effort to provide good care, whereby clinicians reach a state of learned helplessness and give up (Dean et al, 2020). Understanding suffering on both sides of the clinical divide is necessary if we are to progress beyond repetitive cycles that frustrate both patients and health professionals alike. It is hard to see how doctors can attend to suffering when they have not been educated on suffering – both their own and patients'.

Writing these words on suffering, stitching them together one by one, has meant facing the understanding that in suffering, we are as much a product and function of society as we are of our own selves and our own doing. And in those selves, embedded in society, we are full of holes, absences and reversals, as well as breaks, in the space between life and death; the ultimate other. Suffering is therefore a relational linking concept as well as a verb which requires that we employ diverse knowledges and methods to truly undergo or endure it. Linking the self and other in that relational space through concepts, metaphors, symbolism, affect, narratives and a meta-analysis of our approaches to suffering requires much more than medicine in the traditional sense. How we organise knowledge in relation to poverty, suffering and death has perhaps become more crucial to how we operate than ever before.

1.7 Why a book on suffering, medical humanities and sociology now?

On the surface of it, there has never been a more salient time to talk about suffering right now as the global stage is dominated by the COVID-19 pandemic. This pandemic has exacerbated the inequities in healthcare and health outcomes as well as highlighting deficiencies in social care and government policy. In this section, I describe the components that make up the matrix of the health environment and how that relates to suffering. Considering the effects and prevalence of suffering, the role of healthcare workers and how medical humanities and sociology can help in understanding both the micro lived experience and the macro social patterns of suffering, as well as the relationship between them, means getting to grips with the interaction between health professionals and patients. Sociology is crucial to understand social patterns, discourse analysis and health inequities whilst medical humanities is crucial to processing and visualising information in different ways – a full range of which is needed in order to facilitate equitable access to information and healthcare. I will start with a sociological perspective then move, through a crossover, to looking at how health professionals are affected by working in these conditions with people who are suffering, before finally moving on to the most current circumstances due to the COVID-19 pandemic.

The two main reasons for writing this now, which will be unpacked further throughout the book but particularly in Chapter Two, are that conditions of living are worsening for the most vulnerable in our society and health professionals are on the front line of working with this increased level of suffering. For those in the most deprived areas, poverty is worsening and the chances of "lifting themselves out of poverty" are ever diminishing (Akala, 2018). Global political struggles are racialised and becoming more pronounced which could create a resurgence of extreme racism and discrimination as well as opportunities to address this racialisation which is no longer hidden from view.

The second main reason is that for the most part health professionals tend not to understand the lived experience of people who suffer from poverty, which makes engagement from both sides very difficult (McGarvey, 2017). Honest conversations seem impossible:

> I always just thought that the aim was to dismantle the poverty. However, once you see the mechanics of the poverty industry up close, you realise it's in a state of permanent growth and that without individuals, families and communities in crisis there would no longer be a role for these massive institutions.
>
> (p. 106)

> Not even the stark reality of child abuse, the inexorable rise of crime, the ubiquity of violence, the horror of domestic abuse, the scourge of homelessness as the tragic inevitability of alcoholism or addiction that underscores so much of it is enough to humble us into showing some contrition in the face of this issue.
>
> (McGarvey, 2017; p. 108)

The core issue seems to be understanding the role of structural oppressions of Western society, the symbolic violence inherent in capitalism and the link between these and the emotional stress, illness, lifestyle behaviours and the demoralising compulsion of these which people really struggle with (McGarvey, 2017). Then there is the fact that "every problem is discussed like it's beyond the expertise of the average person"; the externalisation of the responsibility of poverty and the whitewash of the subtleties of poverty at the ground level. "Those who shape the discussion about poverty often lack the necessary insight to accurately represent the issue. This creates a gulf between the people who want to sort it and the people who experience it" (McGarvey, 2017; p. 122). The gulf creates a feeling of exclusion along the lines of class, race, income, gender and location. The reasons for writing this now do not seem as if they will be going away anytime soon and in fact seem to be worsening due to the current pandemic.

1.8 Who is this book for?

Any health professional who is looking for an in-depth exploration of suffering and wants to be able to relate this understanding to their practice, to the wider perspective of sociology and the deeper perspective of medical humanities may find this book useful. It is for people who want to take on suffering and scratch beneath the surface, who want to acknowledge the place of suffering in our lives, to legitimate its presence as a worthy subject and object of inquiry, to go beyond surface rhetoric, platitudes and over-rehearsed scripts. If we consider the task of giving an account of oneself (Butler, 2005); there is no self-formation outside the matrix of norms and codes of conduct. Yet if we are to give an account of ourselves as a possible causal agent in suffering both to or of ourselves and others, then how are we to do this given that one of the cultural norms of medicine is to remain largely silent on suffering? If suffering is made to form an understorey in medicine, then how does that impact on our self-making activities, including giving an account of ourselves – knowing where we end and the world begins – and thereby live a livable life? Surely, by making suffering a silent trespass, we are doomed to not live a livable life because we cannot account for suffering?

This book is also for academics who are interested in exploring how medical humanities and sociology intersect with biomedicine and how each contributes to the current status quo. The thesis that there can be a unity of knowledge across medical humanities, sociology and medicine is shown by the complex stitching across the subject through consistent threads of epistemology in each chapter. Suffering itself provides a unifying force across the disciplines as significant terms appear for both patients and suffering to provide more words to the experience.

1.9 How is the remainder of the book structured?

This book is in two parts. The first part outlines the major issues and theories concerned with the suffering self, medical humanities and sociology, and encompasses Chapters One to Five. The second part (Chapters Six and Seven) then goes on to develop some new ideas in terms of pilgrimages and mermaids in order to find a way through the dilemmas outlined in previous chapters. Each chapter has a theme around the relational theory and epistemology as outlined in this chapter. Each chapter also has an image and a reflective piece at the end to deepen reflection on the issues discussed. Having outlined the major concerns of any exploration of the suffering self, medical humanities and sociology, Chapter Two will go on to describe the current situation of health inequities, poverty and the NHS. The proposal is made that patients and health professionals are inherently bound up in the inequities since people who are sick more often and more severely will come to the hospital and general practice surgeries more often. The chapter then goes on to describe how health professionals manage in terms of burnout, PTSD and depersonalisation. Therefore there is a benefit to health professionals in understanding suffering more since not only will that understanding assist their patients, it may also help them.

Chapter Three goes on to explore the work on suffering in greater detail. Different perspectives will be explored as well as the difficulty that sociology has with developing a theory of suffering. Included in this chapter is the work by Singleton (2015) on cultural melancholy as this has been the most in-depth exploration I have found that brings together ideas on both mainstream and marginalised groups of people. Following this, theory is reviewed that can manage the relational aspects of encountering suffering strangers (Orange, 2011) and finally what this means from a phenomenological perspective (Levin, 1991). A framework for exploring suffering is suggested that encourages a new way of thinking about suffering and how critical medical humanities can contribute to that. Key to understanding is the idea of reversal and how by making suffering a foundational aspect of our experience, we could perhaps make a difference rather than trying to override our consciousness about this.

Chapter Four then explores the art and science of medicine and how this relates to epistemological crises as well as the current state of both medical humanities and sociology by laying out the current challenges within each field and how they can be used to complement each other's search for legitimacy within medicine. The art and the science of medicine will be discussed, drawing on a range of literature in order to reach a perspective that enables further exploration without foreclosing on a premature identity for each. Breaking out of the circular thinking surrounding medical humanities and science seems an imperative in order to provide unity in knowledge formations.

Chapter Five goes on to explore in greater detail the idea of the self and in particular the suffering self. Suffering is historically bound up in ideas of redemption and salvation (Bourke, 2014). These historical ideas are explored through medieval women's religiosity and the embodied self as a way of obtaining a theistic source of self. Health professionals' ideas on suffering are then explored in relation to an instrumentalist source of self and how the fusion of self and role may contribute to the hole encountered in suffering. In particular, the organisation of healthcare seems to encourage a kind of disembodiment which then makes responding to suffering difficult. Working at the limits of the constructed self, on the edges of experience, is considered as a way of highlighting medical humanities contribution.

This leads on to the second part of the book. Chapter Six is where the predominant forms of suffering in health professionals are explored in greater depth in order to bring out the threads linking them all – burnout, depersonalisation and PTSD are explored from a medical humanities and sociology perspective. The theme of songlines and wandering lines is used here as a way of walking and connecting with suffering – pilgrimages – across the horizontal fault lines. The theme here is of a source of self through romantic expressivism, which is where medical humanities traditionally finds its home. Affects are integrated into epistemology by considering different experiences of the void. The moral anguish of fusion of self and role is considered through an example not unlike that covered in the preface. Knowing on the inside is explored and a pedagogy of suffering is suggested with principles and aims to assist in developing a curriculum that rests on acknowledging suffering.

Chapter Seven brings together all the different threads and themes to reflect on the bricolage created by this work by using the metaphor of mermaids in order to look at vertical ways of traversing the depth that now seems so overlain with suffering. Whilst suffering is both an individual experience and a social construction and therefore draws on different theories often positioned at odds with each other, suffering also provides a sense of unity that can provide coherence to these different theories and approaches. Diving deep into suffering may be the only choice we have when a wave crashes over us.

Box 1.1   Reflection

In the face of a pandemic, nobody knows how we *should* react emotionally. Furthermore, questions abound from people in all walks of life whether the emotional and somatic responses they do have are normal. There was a level of overwhelm as well as initial burst of adrenalin to combat this disease. Behavioural guidelines were instigated with penalties for not complying. Social institutions responded by closing or furloughing staff as people were mandated to work from home wherever possible. The streets became empty. There was concern about the health service capacity to deal with a wave of incoming patients with COVID. There was an emphasis in the NHS on compassionate care in the face of quarantine measures which prevented people from being with their loved ones as they died and who faced their last hours alone, save for the staff, in ICU, not knowing whether they would come out of the sedation they were put under in order to be able to tolerate the invasive experience of being on a ventilator.

Large NHS Nightingale hospitals were set up within a few weeks to enhance the NHS's capacity to ventilate patients. Yet the strict inclusion criteria for transfer of patients to these sites, due to their limited resources including staff, meant that they were not made use of as much as had perhaps been anticipated, given that the potential for capacity was 4000 beds in London, for example. Instead, patients were kept closer to home in the usual NHS which had also scrambled to increase its ICU capacity. Perhaps NHS staff were reluctant to transfer patients into the unknown spaces of the Nightingale hospitals and this social relational lore became a bigger determinant of how the extra facilities were to be used.

There were many workforce issues concerned with PPE supply and demand, the disparity between different racial groups in infection and death from COVID-19 particularly amongst NHS workers; blame and stigmatisation were also a feature of the pandemic, and there were many examples of community spirit and care.

I found myself caught up in a strange world of adrenalin fuelled wanting to go out and make a difference through the only avenue I had available that seemed socially validated – as a health professional – and

being at home in a somewhat virtual environment through online meetings which I never imagined myself being in at the height of what seemed like an apocalypse.
Questions for reflection

1   What reversals and ruptures were there in the above reflection?
2   What uncrossable space formed for patients and their families and how did health professionals navigate that with families?
3   Where can the difference between a binary dictionary model of knowledge formation and encyclopedic model be seen as playing out in the formation and use of Nightingale hospitals? How could this have impacted patients?
4   What examples of causal dispositional knowledge were evident in the above reflection? How do these impact suffering?
5   How did clusters of symptoms and patients form in a syndemic perspective of suffering communities?
6   What sort of relational mode of decision making occurs across nations and how did this impact making sociomoral sense of suffering?
7   What image or metaphor do you have for this time of dealing with the pandemic? How has that helped you or not make sense of this time?
8   How has the time of enforced isolation changed your sense of self?

Further Resources
   Astley N. 2011. *Staying Alive: Real Poems for Unreal Times.* BloodAxe Books: New York.
   Fromm E. 1993. *The Art of Being.* Robinson: London.

Note

1   https://twitter.com/EmergMedDr/status/1244542238404816896?s=20; 30th March, 2020.

References

Akala 2018. *Natives: Race and Class in the Ruins of Empire.* Hodder & Staughton: London.
Anzaldúa G. 1999. *Borderlands La Frontera; The New Mestiza.* Aunt Lute Books: San Francisco.
Armstrong D. 2002. *A New History of Identity: A Sociology of Medical Knowledge.* Palgrave: Basingstoke.
Arie S. 2020. Covid-19: Can France's ethical support units help doctors make challenging decisions? *BMJ*; 369:M129. doi: //doi.org/10.1136/bmj.m1291.

Behar R. 1997. The Vulnerable Observer. *Anthropology that Breaks Your Heart*. Penguin Random House: New York.

Bingham C. 2004. Let's treat authority relationally. Chapter 4 in *No Education Without Relation*. Bingham C., Sidorkin M (eds). Peter Lang Publishing Inc: New York.

Bleakley A. 2017. Thinking with Metaphors in Medicine: *The State of the Art (Routledge Advances in the Medical Humanities)*. Routledge: London.

Bohm D. 2002. *Wholeness and the Implicate Order*. Routledge Classics: London.

Bourke J. 2014. *The Story of Pain: From Prayer to Painkillers*. Oxford University Press: Oxford.

Brindley P. Opinion: Covid-19—Healthcare workers are scared but, in some ways, also lucky. *BMJ*. 31 March 2020. //blogs.bmj.com/bmj/2020/03/31/peter-brindley-covid-19-healthcare-workers-are-scared-but-in-some-ways-also-lucky/.

Butler J. 2005. *Giving an Account of Oneself*. Fordham University Press: USA.

Butt L. 2002. The suffering stranger: Medical anthropology and international morality. *Medical Anthropology*; 21(1):1–24; discussion 25–33. doi: 10.1080/01459740210619.

Cassell E.J. 2004. *The Nature of Suffering and the Goals of Medicine*. Oxford University Press: Oxford.

Daly K. 2018. *Natives: Race and Class in the Ruins of Empire*. Hodder & Stoughton Ltd: London.

de Certeau M. 1984. *The Practice of Everyday Life*. University of California Press: California.

Dean W., Talbot S.G., Caplan A. 2020. Clarifying the language of clinician distress. *JAMA*; 323(10):923–924.

Dempsey C. 2018. *The Antidote to Suffering: How Compassionate Connected Care Can Improve Safety, Quality and Experience*. McGraw-Hill: New York.

Denzin N.K., Lincoln Y.S. 2005. *Handbook of Qualitative Research*. Sage Publications: London.

Desai K., Sanya B.N. 2016. Towards decolonial praxis: Reconfiguring the human and the curriculum, *Gender and Education*; 28(6):710–724.

Devereaux G. 1967. *From Anxiety to Method in the Behavioural Sciences*. Mouton & Co: Paris.

Devisch I., Vanheule S., Deveugele M. Nola I., Civaner M., Pype P. 2017. Victims of disaster: Can ethical debriefings be of help to care for their suffering? *Medical Health Care and Philosophy*; 20:257–267.

Eco U. 2014. *From the Tree to the Labyrinth: Historical Studies on the Sign and Interpretation*. Harvard University Press: New York.

Fiske A.P. 1993. *Structures of Social Life: The Four Elementary Forms of Human Relations*. The Free Press: New York.

Foucault M. 1973. *Birth of the Clinic: An Archeology of Medical Knowledge*. Vintage Books: New York.

Fox N.J. 1999. *Beyond Health: Postmodernism and Embodiment*. Free Association Books.: London.

Frank A.W. 2001. Can we research suffering? *Qualitative Health Research*; 11(3): 353–362.

Freire P. (2000). *Pedagogy of the Oppressed. 30th Anniversary Edition*. The Continuum International Publishing Group Ltd: New York.

Fricker M. 2007. *Epistemic Injustice: Power and the Ethics of Knowing*. Oxford University Press: Oxford.

Gerada C. 2019. The making of a doctor: The matrix and self. *Group Analysis*; 52(3):350–361. doi: 10.1177/0533316418823117.

Glück L. 2011. The wild Iris. In Astley N (ed). *Staying Alive: Real Poems for Unreal Times*. BloodAxe Books: New York.

Gordon J. 2005. Medical humanities: To cure sometimes, to relieve often, to comfort always. *Medical Journal of Australia*; 182(1):5–8.

Haslam N. (Ed) 2012. *Relational Models Theory: A Contemporary Overview*. Routledge: London.

Herman J. 2001. Medicine: The science and the art. *BMJ Medical Humanities*; 27:42–46.

Hofmann B. 2015. Suffering: Harm to bodies, minds, and persons. In Edwards S., Schramme T. (eds). *Handbook of Concepts in the Philosophy of Medicine*. Springer: Berlin.

Holmes E.A., O'Connor R.C., Perry V.H. et al. 2020. *Multidisciplinary research priorities for the COVID-19 pandemic: A call for action for mental health science. The Lancet Psychiatry*. doi: 10.1016/S2215-0366(20)30168-1.

hooks B. 1994. *Teaching to Transgress: Education as the Practice of Freedom*. Routledge: New York.

Kristeva J. 1982. *Powers of Horror – An Essay on Abjection*. Columbia University Press: New York.

Kristeva J., Moro M.R., Ødemark J., Engebretsen E. 2018. Cultural crossings of care: an appeal to the medical humanities. *BMJ Medical Humanities*; 44:55–58.

Lather P. 1991. *Getting Smart: Feminist Epistemologies*. Routledge, Chapman and Hall: New York.

Leder D. 2016. *The Distressed Body: Rethinking Illness, Imprisonment, and Healing*. The University of Chicago Press: London.

Leder D. 1990. *The Absent Body*. The University of Chicago Press: London.

Levin D.M. 1991. Visions of Narcissism: Intersubjectivity and the reversals of reflection. Chapter 3 in *Merleau Ponty Vivant*. Dillon M.C (ed). State University of New York Press: Albany.

Lowe W.A., Adams J., Ballinger C., Armstrong R., Lueddeke J., Protheroe J., McAffery K., Nutbeam D., Russell C. 2014. *Patients' and health professionals' views, preferences and experiences of lower levels of literacy and musculoskeletal patient education: A qualitative analysis. Arthritis Research UK Report*.

Lupton D. 2012. *Medicine as Culture: Illness, Disease and the Body*. Third Edition. Sage Publishing: Sydney.

McCartney M. 2020. The art of medicine. Perspectives. Medicine: Before COVID-19, and after. *The Lancet. March 31, 2020*. doi: 10.1016/S0140-6736(20)30756-X.

McGarvey D. 2017. *Poverty Safari: Understanding the Anger of Britain's Underclass*. Picador: Edinburgh.

Macnaughton J., Carel H. 2016. Breathing and breathlessness in clinic and culture: using critical medical humanities to bridge an epistemic gap. Chapter 16 in Whitehead A., Woods A., Atkinson S., et al. (eds). *The Edinburgh Companion to the Critical Medical Humanities*. Edinburgh University Press; Edinburgh.

Mendenhall E. 2019. *Rethinking Diabetes: Entanglement with Trauma, Poverty and HIV*. Cornell University Press: London.

Merleau-Ponty JMM. 1968. *The Visible and the Invisible*. Northwestern University Press: Evanston, IL.

Michie S., West R., Amlot R. 2020. Behavioural strategies for reducing covid-19 transmission in the general population. *BMJ*. https://blogs.bmj.com/bmj/2020/03/03/behavioural-strategies-for-reducing-covid-19-transmission-in-the-general-population/.

Mol A. 2002. *The Body Multiple: Ontology in Medical Practice*. Duke University Press: Durham.

Mumford S. 2012. *Metaphysics: A Very Short Introduction*. Oxford University Press: Oxford.

Mukandi B. 2015. Chester Himes, Jacques Derrida and inescapable colonialism: Reflections on African philosophy from the diaspora. *South African Journal of Philosophy*; 34(4):526–537.

Nussbaum M.C. 1986 *The Fragility of Goodness: Luck and Ethics in Greek Tragedy and Philosophy*. Cambridge University Press: Cambridge.

O'Grady H. 2005. Woman's Relationship with Herself – Gender, *Foucault and Therapy*. Routledge: London.

Orange D.M. 2011. *The Suffering Stranger: Hermeneutics for Everyday Clinical Practice*. Routledge: New York.

Paton M., Kuper A., Paradis E., Feilchenfeld Z., Whitehead C.R. 2020. *Tackling the void: The importance of absences in the field of health professions education research. Advances in Health Sciences Education*.

Rauch A. 2003. The lacunae of science: Observing the unobserved in the practices of knowledge. *Interdisciplinary Science Reviews*; 28(3):209–216.

Rocca E., Anjum R.I.. 2020. Causal evidence and dispositions in medicine and public health. *International Journal of Environmental Research and Public Health*; 17:1813.

Sawicki J. 1991. *Disciplining Foucault – Feminism, Power, and the Body*. Routledge: New York.

Scambler G. (Ed). 2008. *Sociology as Applied to Medicine*. Sixth Edition. Saunders Elsevier: London.

Scarry E. 1985. *The Body in Pain: The Making and Unmaking of the World*. Oxford University Press: Oxford.

Seth S. 2018. Difference and Disease: Medicine, Race, and the Eighteenth-Century British Empire. *Global Health Histories*. Cambridge University Press.

Sewell W.H. 1992. A theory of structure: Duality, agency and transformation. *American Journal of Sociology*; 98(1):1–29.

Shanafelt T., Ripp J., Trockel M. 2020. *Understanding and Addressing Sources of Anxiety Among Health Care Professionals During the COVID-19 Pandemic. JAMA*. Published online April 7, 2020. doi:10.1001/jama.2020.5893.

Sharpe C. 2016. In the Wake: *On Blackness and Being*. Duke University Press: Durham.

Singleton J. 2015. *Cultural Melancholy: Readings of Race, Impossible Mourning, and African American Ritual*. University of Illinois Press.

Sontag S. 1991. *Illness as Metaphor*. Penguin Classics: London.

Vanheule S., Devisch I. 2014. Mental suffering and the DSM-5: A critical review. *Journal of Evaluation in Clinical Practice*, 20, 975–980. 10.1111/jep.12163.

Venn C. 2002. Refiguring Subjectivity after Modernity. Chapter Four in Challenging Subjects: *Critical Psychology for a New Millenium*. Walkerdine V (ed). Palgrave: Hampshire.

Wang W., He Q., Liu M., Wang M., Sun X. Covid-19: lack of knowledge is driving public panic. *BMJ*. https://blogs.bmj.com/bmj/2020/02/28/communicating-research-evidence-about-covid-19-to-reduce-public-panic/.

Williams S.J. 2003. *Medicine and the Body*. Sage Publications: London.

Wilson E.O. 1998. *Consilience: The Unity of Knowledge*. Abacus: London.

Wright Mills C. 2000. The Sociological Imagination. *Fortieth Anniversary Edition*. Oxford University Press: Oxford.

2   Patterns of suffering

2.0 Introduction

Suffering happens in a context – it is both an individual experience and socially constructed. There is thus a dialogic relationship between the individual and context which is co-determining. "A dialogic understanding, in a hermeneutics of trust, forms the hospitable response to the suffering stranger demanded by the ethics of infinite responsibility" (Orange, 2011, p. 15). This means shifting the focus from pathology to understanding the human that suffers. This chapter reviews the statistics and patterns of suffering but is mindful that there are humans behind these figures and statistics. Concepts associated with suffering are also reviewed, but there is again a need to remember the humans behind them. Finding the balance between knowing patterns of inequity and not wanting to make them worse, whilst also wanting to promote health through the judicious use of healthy lifestyle promotion, is a challenge that can impact on health professionals' practice and hence well-being. This chapter explores the challenge of an ethical response that necessarily involves both objective rationality and subjectivity.

Inherent in the review of patterns and concepts are notions of objective rationality – the rationality of conventional morality – and subjectivity – the experiential ethics necessary to engage with a dialogic understanding of the other. Whilst we may know that people represent particular groups at risk of particular conditions and invoke healthy lifestyle advice (Petersen & Lupton, 2000), there are lives behind these conditions and advice. The question is how much empathy with current experiences in peoples' lives is mustered versus advice about healthy lifestyles and running the risk of coming across as cold-hearted.

Medical humanities has typically been invoked to teach empathy to medical students; empathy itself is an ethical issue in the face of unremitting increasing inequalities (Guttman, 2017). That is, empathy can seem somewhat shallow, objectifying and patronising when no effort is made to reduce the conditions that are causing suffering in the first place. Disempowered individuals may turn to those in authority for help who may then empathise more from a perspective of colonialist superiority. There is still a sense of salvation and redemption about empathy when conditions are only worsening for a significant segment of the population. That is, the appeal to be saved occurs through the mechanics of internalisation – perfection of performance, competence and compliance along with internalised negative characteristics of marginalised devalued groups of people applies to patients as well as health professionals. Since identity is constructed from the outside as well as internally, health education is an experience of being governed from the outside and a request for self-discipline (Gastaldo, 1997).

Lifestyle advice and terms interfere with the choices individuals may make in relation to their healthcare and are thus a form of biopower (Gastaldo, 1997). Biopower (power over life) in health education promotes behaviours that should and "ought" to be adopted by the entire population, is educational in nature and interferes with individual choice. Providing information to foster "healthy" lifestyles is a form of normalisation; biopower is a code of normalisation since it promotes norms of behaviours. Health education represents a singular contribution to the exercise of biopower – the biological and political existence start to interface with each other in a web of micropowers that are subtle, continuous and ubiquitous (Gastaldo, 1997). When patients or health professionals are unable to meet these norms or "oughts" because of what "is" in their lives, they may suffer from stigmatisation. This implies an internalisation of failure in meeting norms as well as an internalisation of surveillance medicine and is a form of Othering (where persons are made different and distant by mainstream categorising), where blaming and judgment can occur. This is where moral and ethical responses originate – from the dynamic relation between co-operation and defection (Wilson, 1998).

In order to make change, objective rationally based concepts and measurements are necessary to present a case for justice as well as understanding the lived experience rather than just relying on a transcended notion of what it means to be a human being. Strategic essentialism takes on the idea of essences of human being even though from a post-structuralist perspective, essences are difficult to sustain both ontologically and epistemologically (Buchanan, 2018). That is, in considering identity, theorists argue that there is no such thing as a true self (Hutton, 1988) and that identity markers such as gender and race are social performances (Butler, 1993). Yet the more that concepts such as race and gender are deconstructed, the more one sees that there is nothing behind them which makes establishing common ground necessary to pursue social justice difficult. Strategic essentialism proposes to use concepts of race, gender, ethnicity and class in order to highlight injustices and therefore take political action – it is strategic in the sense that strategies are devised to address social injustice and are essential in that these categories, whilst recognised as not being inherent to humans, are necessary for the cause. However, while these may seem like dry concepts and abstractions, what is behind them is the lived experience of discrimination and marginalisation as well as the affect of the dialogic encounter with suffering. Medical humanities is the vehicle for understanding and transmitting affects (Deleuze & Guattari, 2009).

Figure 2.1 is presented for reflection on the role of transcendental approaches to healthcare. This approach in itself may be one of the structures – in a dynamic understanding of that – perpetuating inequities. Through the chrysalis can be seen a portal. As we immerse ourselves in suffering there may be a way through, a portal, provided by this immersion. Medical humanities can provide a way of thinking differently about the concepts, thoughts, emotions and context (Eichbaum, 2014) about suffering given that this is embedded in a colonialist transcended redemptive background.

2.1 Patterns of inequity and the NHS

Patterns of inequity have been well known for decades since at least the start of the NHS in 1948, confirmed again by the Black Report in 1979 (Townsend & Davidson, 1982) and have been exacerbated again over the last 10 years (CSDH, 2008; Joyce & Xu, 2019; Marmot et al, 2020). There

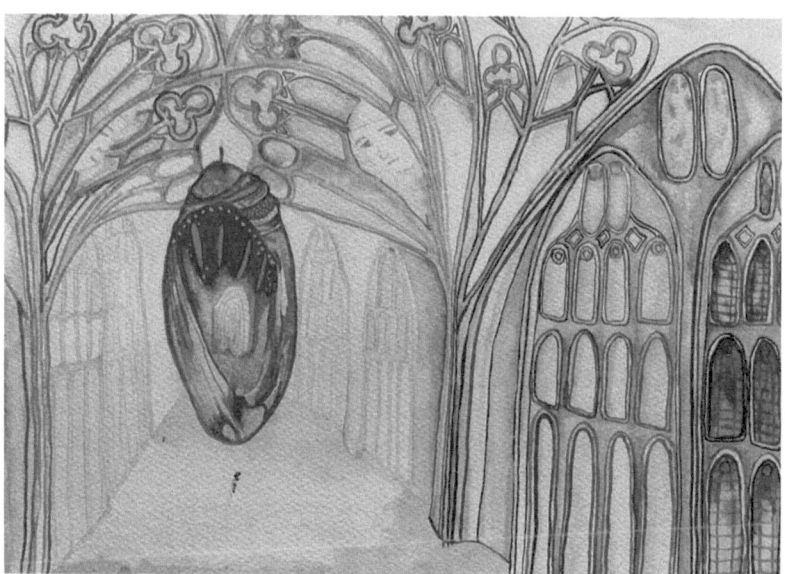

Figure 2.1 Cloisters of redemption and portals through suffering.

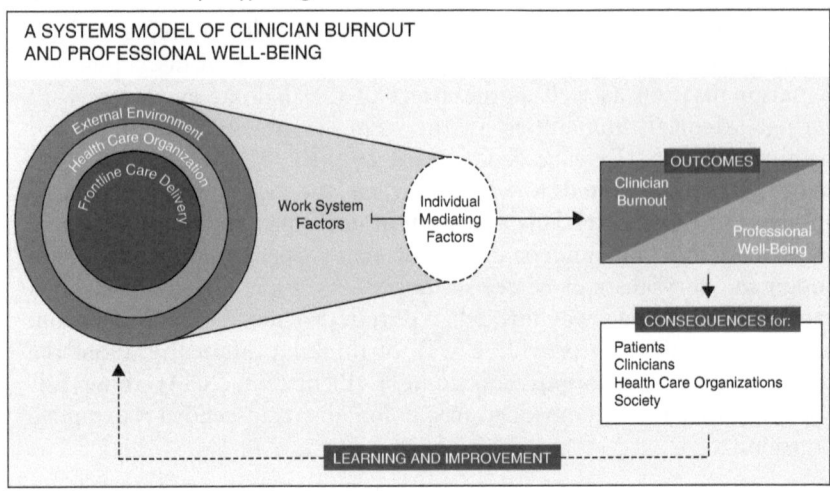

Figure 2.2 A systems model of clinician burnout and professional well-being (NAM, 2020).

are plenty of data to demonstrate that those with the worst health have been experiencing the worst health outcomes, prolonged periods of ill-health and a levelling off of life expectancies with some groups – women in deprived neighbourhoods – actually going in to reverse (Marmot et al, 2020). Health workers can be implicated in suffering and healthcare can be compromised through the work they do; excess deaths, distress related to poverty and the associated narratives, individualisation of responsibility for health, medicalisation of poverty distress, extremes of poverty such as homelessness, and the stigma associated with a medically termed "epidemic" of obesity form the social matrix in which health professionals' work. The context includes factors such as the bed crisis in the NHS, the clustering of conditions in multimorbidities with poverty, lower expenditure on the NHS, lower staff to patient ratios and betrayals by the political system, bullying and harassment within the NHS and focusing on clinical trial outcomes rather than equity of access means that the delivery of healthcare becomes about higher levels of individual responsibility and risk. The social matrix and the individualising context as well as the constant change are all ways in which health workers are caught up in suffering.. These sociological patterns of suffering are not new; the following detail provides evidence of the type of language in use about this state of affairs.

Geographically, areas showing excess deaths continue to do so – Glasgow and Tower Hamlets in the UK for example (Annual Public Health Report of the Director of Public Health, 2018; Walsh et al, 2016) – while there have been pockets of increased deaths by suicide – so-called deaths of despair – for white middle-aged men in the UK (Thomas et al, 2019) and the US (Case & Deaton, 2020). Poverty, deprivation, deindustrialisation, displacement and destabilisation are thought to increase peoples' vulnerability to violence, trauma, despair and the use of alcohol and drugs (Walsh et al, 2016). There is an epidemic of opioid use (Mars, 2012), and the use of antidepressants in order to treat rising levels of depression and anxiety in a medicalisation of distress (Thomas et al, 2019). Each of these distressing situations related to poverty and deprivation comes with associated stigma and moral judgment; adding to the lack of opportunity in secure employment, poor housing, social isolation, welfare reforms and an upsurge in social sanctioning (Thomas et al, 2019).

People who suffer from these circumstances demonstrated three interlinked types of narratives – a neoliberal narrative whereby people who have distress related to their circumstances are seen as having social or behavioural problems they need to attend to in order to seen as responsible citizens, thereby adding to guilt, shame and helplessness; a shame narrative whereby people who are seen as not contributing to society are seen as engaging in reckless and irresponsible behaviour, thereby leading to a fear of being judged and therefore avoidance of seeking help; and a medicalisation narrative in which mental distress from these circumstances was seen as a medical issue requiring medical intervention (Thomas et al, 2019). Therefore these narratives show how destructive circumstances are on people's sense of self, willingness and trust to seek support and how health professionals are implicated in the perpetuation of health inequities through the medicalisation of distress:

> At the heart of these issues are questions about where responsibility for health and wellbeing should lie. Governments can facilitate responsibility in citizens when they provide the material and structural resources required for this to become feasible. Yet, within the current neo-liberally oriented era, government and popular rhetoric around individual responsibility feed directly into strategies aimed at reducing welfare support, blaming and shaming individuals and communities, and deflecting attention from the responsibilities of those with the power and remit to effect positive change. Such a situation is clearly inequitable and in fact damaging to people's mental health and wellbeing.
>
> (Thomas et al, 2019, p. 20)

Thus health professionals become implicated in government policy by the very nature of medicalisation of symptoms of poverty. The increasingly punitive nature of the welfare reforms means that health professionals directly encounter the increased vulnerability to mental distress though the reduction of benefit entitlement, whilst at the same time questioning and delegitimising people's medical or disability status, a dehumanising experience and repercussion of dealing with the system itself (Thomas et al, 2019).

Health professionals are often seen as part of the system with the lack of trust and judgment that involves.

If we drill down further into the segments of the community that perhaps suffer the most from all of the above, there has been an increase in homelessness over the last decade (Hassanally & Asaeia, 2018; Watton & Gallivan, 2013), with hospitals ill-prepared to treat the complexity of problems that arise, due to cuts in social care funding (Aldridge, 2019). The political determinants of homelessness, including child poverty, poor education and employment opportunities, criminalisation, invisibility and stigma come home to roost in the accident and emergency department of hospitals (Bowen et al, 2019). Mortality rates and health inequities are high for this group of people (Wadhera et al, 2019). The rising levels of homelessness are seen as a barometer for social justice and require a serious governmental response beyond the Homelessness Reduction Act 2017, public health and NHS response (Fransham & Dorling, 2018; Public Health England [PHE], 2018; Reynolds, 2018; Watton & Gallivan, 2013). The suffering inherent in being homeless has perhaps been best described by the notion of those who are abject from society (Kristeva, 1982).

Further examples or manifestations of suffering that are on the rise include the so-called obesity epidemic, often most prevalent in those communities with the great deprivation and poverty (WHO, 2020). This has meant that local authorities have channelled their efforts into promoting weight loss, exercise and diabetes management (see, for example, Tower Hamlets Health & Well-being Board, 2017). However, these sorts of measures have only served to increase the judgment and consequent bias towards different people who are already in distress and suffering: disgust, anger, blame and dislike, awkwardness, unattractiveness, ugliness and non-compliance felt by and directed towards patients (Alimoradi et al, 2019). Conceptual challenges around obesity impact the way we think about obesity and they have an impact on policies and patients. Attributing weight issues to behavioural influences alone produces bias and stigma (Phelan et al, 2015). Weight related stigma causes psychological distress which only exacerbates the problem of obesity. Ethical response to patients requires that we understand fully the implications of our theoretical frameworks and biases. Clinical interventions have oversold the benefits of diet and exercise in lieu of understanding the context, confounders and mechanisms of obesity. There is no doubt that this interaction between health professionals and patients where clinical interventions predominate has the potential to cause more suffering if not handled adequately. These examples demonstrate that with each of these life-limiting circumstances and conditions, there are associated stigma and discrimination, not the least of which has been the concomitant decrease in social care funding which could have kept people out of hospital and in the community (McCartney, 2016).

Every winter for the past decade or so, the NHS has been in a crisis over the lack of beds and increased waiting time to be seen in Accident and

Emergency, placing patients, their families and healthcare providers under great stress (The King's Fund, 2019a). The prolonged funding squeeze over the last decade has meant that staff have had to cope with financial constraints as well as severe workforce shortages alongside a rising demand for care (The King's Fund, 2019b). Population growth, an ageing population with complex long term co-morbidities and technological advances mean that with the rising demand comes an increased pressure for efficiency and effectiveness of healthcare services. General practitioners have been overwhelmed and the accessibility for appointments has decreased, which has only placed more pressure on hospital services (McCartney, 2016). Threaded throughout all these crises are inequities in access and health outcomes by race, ethnicity, income level or poverty, age, gender and geographic location (Marmot et al, 2020). Mental health in particular shows an increase in diagnosis, higher use of care services or rates of compulsory assessment and treatment in some ethnic minority groups (Bhui et al, 2018).

Often patients have multiple complex conditions so that when they are seen, there is a multitude of issues to contend with. Multi-morbidity and complexity are the main characteristics of modern day healthcare. Poverty impacts the efficacy of treatment (Thomas et al, 2019) with concerns over the low levels of adherence to medication (World Health Organisation, 2003) driving the desire to find better ways to manage and treat those with multiple long term conditions (The King's Fund, 2015). Medicine's success in treating the leading causes of death such as cardiovascular disease, lung disease, cancer and diabetes has meant that chronically ill people are living with a longer period of ill-health called pre-death (Warraich, 2017). Therefore, these complexities and longevity of conditions come at an increased cost to the NHS, resulting in budget deficits of up to £2.3 billion in 2016 (The King's Fund, 2019b).

The expenditure on the NHS is low compared with other European countries like France, Portugal or Greece. UK healthcare spending per person (£2989) was the second lowest, with the highest spenders being France (£3737), Germany (£4432) and the United States (£7736) (Office for National Statistics [ONS], 2019). Whilst other European countries were spending more on their health, UK healthcare spending fell from 9.8% GDP in 2013 to 9.6% GDP in 2017 (Office for National Statistics ONS, 2019). However, the amount spent is important because it shows that expenditure on healthcare services (up to the amount of £2500 per person) is directly related to improving health outcomes. According to The King's Fund (2020a) the total number of NHS hospital beds in England, including general and acute, mental illness, learning disability, maternity and day-only beds, has more than halved over the past 30 years, from around 299,000 in 1987–1988 to 141,000 in 2018–2019, while the number of patients treated has increased significantly. Bed occupancy averages around 90.2% and exceeds 95% in winter. Most of the reduction in beds has come from the outsourcing of care to the community and private sector for services for the ageing, learning disability and mental illness (The King's Fund, 2020). The one area to go against this trend is the area of critical care which has seen the total number of critical care beds in England increase from around 5400 critical care beds in 2011–2012, to 5900 by 2019–2020 (The King's Fund, 2020a).

Despite these trends in spending and reduction of beds, the UK has actually slightly increased the number of doctors to 2.8 per every 1000 people (Moberly, 2017). This is lower than most other countries in the Organisation for Economic Co-operation and Development (OECD), where the UK ranks 22nd in terms of doctors per head of population (Moberly, 2017). This equates to areas of good performance in health service outcomes but overall, spending, patient safety and population health are all below average. In order to address these deficits, more may need to be spent on increasing the supply of labour and long term care as well as reducing the decline in social spending (Papanicolas et al, 2019). Over the last 10 years of austerity, the NHS has been asked to cut expenditure by £22 billion in efficiency savings, announced in 2014 and to be met by 2020 (NHS England, 2016). These efficiency savings were not expected to compromise patient care. However, across the NHS, there have been staff retention issues as many have left and were not replaced. Morale was further worsened by the junior doctor strike in 2016, where many felt they were being betrayed by working in an underfunded system and the trauma that involved (anonymous doctor, 2016). At the same time, junior doctors were also being scapegoated by the "7 Day NHS" ideology (McCartney, 2016).

Health professionals feel a betrayal by not being listened to when they have the expertise and evidence to contribute to the development and management of healthcare services, yet policy makers insist on policies that are not based on evidence and are more likely to be based on a political agenda of privatisation. The constant change over the last 10 years, with the introduction of the Health and Social Care Act 2012, as well as the Sustainability and Transformation Partnerships, have destabilised the NHS and reduced workers to technicians passively carrying out government policy (McCartney, 2016). Many (almost a fifth) are thinking of voting with their feet, particularly with the influence of Brexit, and leaving (British Medical Association [BMA], 2018a).

In the atmosphere of the NHS are pervasive amounts of bullying and harassment (British Medical Association [BMA], 2018b), fear of consequences of missed targets, stress from staff shortages, fatigue, propping up a failing system by working beyond contracted hours, humiliation from the Care Quality Commission Scores (McCartney, 2016) and low morale from public failings such as that highlighted by the Staffordshire Inquiry (Francis, 2013). Cynicism over continual politically motivated change leads to poor teamwork and a desire to withdraw from the workplace (Firth-Cozens, 2020; McCartney, 2016). On top of all that, staff see work outsourced to private companies who then turn around and sue the NHS for not being awarded a contract (Matthews-King, 2017). It is difficult to know where to begin to think about these issues, compounded by the fact that thinking about them is often ignored given the current climate.

For example, in spite of advocacy on behalf of marginalised groups, researchers have had to turn to the medical humanities to take on the struggles in health policy, particularly in relation to uncertainty and how that is used to exacerbate inequalities in access to treatment and prevention of HIV by pre-exposure prophylaxis (PrEP) (Nagington & Sandset, 2020). Introducing notions of uncertainty by focusing on clinical trial outcomes rather than equity of access means that the delivery of healthcare becomes about individual responsibility and level of risk. This is paradoxical because it is the state intervention that creates the rhetoric around uncertainty of eligibility and then withholds treatment on what has been argued as dubious ethical and ideological grounds (Nagington & Sandset, 2020). Uncertainty can lead to innovation, as Scotland has demonstrated in its rollout of PrEP, to improve access to treatment for trans people, black-British communities, certain migrant communities and sex workers (Nagington & Sandset, 2020). This example shows the value of thinking differently about current issues within the NHS that medical humanities is able to facilitate, in order to lessen avoidable suffering.

Health professionals often find themselves caught up in delivery of healthcare that can perpetuate inequities in health outcomes and struggle to understand how to change this (Lowe, 2014). By having the tools to think differently about such issues, they may be able to mitigate the individualisation of responsibility and choice through the rhetoric of risk by understanding in the first instance that they are not at fault:

> Oh yeah, I can remember a few years ago I really umm, you know I nearly worked myself into a major depression. And then one day I woke up and I thought "hey this isn't about me, it's not my fault that I can't see all these people" so I stopped short of actually hitting rock bottom, which was an amazing thing. You can only do what you can do. Oh yeah, I was doing the 4 o'clock, you know, wake up being really tired and going to bed and then wake up feeling bad but then I thought this is ridiculous, it's actually not my fault.
>
> (Gill) (Lowe, 2010)

The higher level of responsibility that health professionals are trained to take on means that they can struggle with being able to think differently about their work and the challenges they come across. As Gill showed, it was an amazing thing for her to realise that this situation wasn't her fault. Given that the healthcare workload is only increasing in complexity and in level of health burden for patients, it seems as if health professionals need to be able to think differently, specifically about not individualising challenging situations in healthcare.

However, this is often easier said than done as the following excerpt shows, when a health professional tried to speak up and make changes:

And you're a cog in the wheel .... And I tried to fight it then and I just got burnt so badly ... ummm, and I thought, I'll never do that again because you can't change that huge wheel.

(Donna) (Lowe, 2010)

On the one hand, health professionals talk about compliance with standards, evidence based practice, professional values and organisational policies which demonstrate their enculturation into the social matrix and perhaps slippage of personal self in service of a professional self. And on the other hand, health professionals draw from an expertise and talk about empowerment, choice, control and autonomy in relation to their patients but fail to see that they themselves are caught up in the social matrix as much as patients are. It is theoretically challenging to know how to manage sociological patterns of health, organisational politics, low morale, increasing demands on time and capacity without lapsing into despair or becoming an unwitting victim. However, it seems necessary now more than ever that this must be done whilst thinking of new ways forward in order to be able to change the status quo.

Perhaps one way forward is to theorise differently by working in an interdisciplinary manner and including the body in that theorising. I have already stated in Section 1.6.3 that one of the theoretical challenges is including the body in a model of suffering, with its inherent relation to the Other, and the perceptions of suffering that claim us morally, which we cannot disregard. Through this reciprocity and reversibility – the chiasma – we lean on ideas about social justice and equity (Levin, 1991) yet often don't know how to embody them, as shown by the health professional quotes above. There is an awareness of social and individual suffering, yet often health professionals feel unable to do anything about this. Worse, they may also feel that because they have not been able to change conditions of suffering, they are somehow complicit in perpetuating suffering (Zembylas, 2019).

This is a really important epistemological point about suffering and healthcare because it connects the health professional with patients directly whilst providing the basis for taking embodiment and relationality as primary means of understanding suffering. The connection here between health professionals and patients is the crossover point where much can be learned and thinking about how we think about suffering can be different. Johnston (2013) argues that since health professionals have a higher risk of encountering suffering due to their work, they are at a higher risk of burnout. She also believes that because of the heightened suffering encountered, health professionals are more likely to engage in acts that are at expense to themselves and that therefore we need new sophisticated educational strategies that engage directly with the suffering to develop practical wisdom borne out of situated experience. This is where the medical humanities come in by providing different avenues of exploration and forms of knowledge making to complement the biomedical approach.

Sophisticated educational strategies need to be able to take into account the embodied and relational forms of knowledge. What this means, in the context of suffering, is to directly acknowledge feelings of shame about one's perceived complicity in Others' suffering: the shame at being human and shame of the world at not being able to reduce suffering (Zembylas, 2019). Living with this impossibility is believed to be crucial because out of this impossibility something new may emerge to disrupt the dominant logic. That this is necessary now more than ever because this dominant logic is part and parcel of the production of health inequities, social injustice and suffering (Zembylas, 2019). Invoking transcendental moral questions is thought to be inadequate since by becoming decontextualised and disembodied, the questions become abstracted from the particularities of peoples' lives. New educational strategies such as a pedagogy of shame on suffering means neither avoiding shame nor fetishising it but rather aiming towards a reparative understanding of and response to shame and suffering (Zembylas, 2019). This inclusion of shame as a relational solidarity with the Other in suffering is an attempt to bridge the epistemic gap between health professionals and patients in order to be able to understand both.

2.2 Health professionals' health and suffering

Crossing over into the state of health professionals' health and why a book on suffering is necessary now, the research shows that not only are doctors in distress (Gerada, 2019), they also have higher rates of mental illness than other groups and the general population, higher suicide rates (especially women) (Andrew & Brenner, 2018; Dutheil et al, 2019; Milner et al, 2016) and higher levels of alcohol consumption (Medisauskaite & Kamau, 2019). The trauma produced by the level of responsibility carried by health professionals whilst at the same time being placed in conditions that make the meeting of that responsibility a severe challenge tends not to be addressed with the result that many health professionals suffer from stress related illnesses (McManus, 2007), their ability to look after their own health is not effective (IPSOS MORI Social research Institute 2009) and their adherence to health promotion messages is minimal (Needle et al, 2011). The assumption that health professionals are invincible and are not vulnerable to the stresses and strains of everyday life (Hawton et al, 2001; Miller et al, 2000; Schwenk et al, 2010) may have something to do in part with the notion of maintaining a professional approach. Maintaining a professional approach in this context is a heroic task of monumental proportions for which training has not prepared them.

Sinclair's (1997) seminal work "Making Doctors" boldly states that "mental illness is not simply an occupational hazard, but a professional probability caused by training" (p. 301). The training individualises health; that is, the major focus of the training is on the individual as the locus of responsibility, choice and control. The language acquired in training emphasises scientific objectivity in knowledge, emotional detachment in experience and mature judgment in the ownership and action of responsibility (Sinclair, 1997). These three mechanisms of training influence the ability to be aware of social or structural factors. They work through the avoidance of internal conflict, the distinction between care and competence with an emphasis on the latter and the discomfort with seemingly abstract notions such as feelings and experiences (Sinclair, 1997). The individualisation of health may contribute to the emergence of psychological distress (Squiers et al, 2017), yet this notion has been neglected for decades. Moreover, certainly in the past, the culture and process of training in a variety of health professions has seemed to require that students suffer (Gillepsie et al, 2017; Monrouxe & Rees, 2012; Olasoji, 2018; Rahman, 2016; Rios, 2016).

These factors, beginning in training, mean that health professionals are more than likely to suffer and have less resources to manage suffering. Therefore, it seems an imperative to further explore suffering in depth. However, in doing so, we enter on the horns of a dilemma from both a medical humanities and sociology perspective. Generally, research on how health professionals suffer tends to attribute symptoms of distress to individual biological representations as this is relatable and understandable (Kamel & Hashish, 2015; Walsh et al, 2010); this is the Scylla of the dilemma (Levin, 1991). That is, it is the individual's mind and body that suffer from burnout, moral injury, depersonalisation or PTSD. Some of this suffering may well be related to workplace conditions in a human factors approach to well-being. This is the Charybdis of historism (Levin, 1991); workplaces and educational institutions have traditionally historically been sources of stress for workers and students as the effects of power on the body discipline and regulate the individual (Foucault, 1973). What is missing from these accounts is a way of riding the knife edge between a psychological biological monster of representationalism focused on the individual and a historical regulatory whirlpool of ever decreasing cycles of thinking about workplace conditions of distress, with particular relevance for suffering in healthcare. Medical humanities and sociology get caught up in these two dilemmas, and this could account for why little progress has been made in integrating either of them into medicine or in changing conditions in workplaces. Finding a way through these two horns of the dilemma means grappling with ideas about how we know what we know (epistemology), the nature of reality (ontology and metaphysics) and what it means to be human.

Ultimately the dilemma comes down to the causal problematic (Kristeva et al, 2018). For example, Gerada (2019) posits the collapse of the traditional medical social matrix, the loss of support, alongside worsening workplace conditions as a cause of the rise in doctors' distress. This may well be so, and there is no argument against this here. However, what I argue for is a fundamental re-think of the way the psychological isolate (Gerada, 2019) has relied on the external social support as a sole mechanism for survival within healthcare when it has often fallen short. There are many issues to unpick here around basic assumptions of the self, the role of the workplace in supporting an already separated worker, the role of the NHS as a part of the so-called Nanny State (Coggon, 2018) and issues of power and authority that mean we have to think very differently in order to make any progress.

The resistance to writing about this from a psychological point of view, where the "problem" is located within the mind of the individual, comes from understanding that both psychology and sociology have gained their credibility from aligning with the biomedical model (Ogden, 2001). This type of thinking sets up a particular type of relationship of authority with the self at the same time as trying to obtain therapeutic results, a situation which is not always conducive to productive outcomes. With this caveat in place, I will now review the literature on health professionals' psychological distress, the nearest that suffering comes in being mentioned.

Clarifying the language of clinician distress is important because without knowing the precise language it is difficult to know what acts as an artefact of the psychological biomedical approach and what is suffering as an existential concern in healthcare. Furthermore, language can reflect people's experience and the more generally this language resonates with experience, the more alignment between concepts may occur. It may be that some of the psychological language used to describe clinician distress works to obscure the suffering that takes place within clinicians on behalf of or in relation to patients and their families.

Clinician distress has been described in terms of moral dilemmas, moral distress, moral injury and burnout (Dean et al, 2020). Moral dilemmas are predictable, anticipated (in the course of working as a health professional) and challenging decisions made about the choice of treatment (or not) for particular patients. Moral distress occurs when health professionals believe they know the right thing to do but institutional or political constraints make it difficult to do what is right (Dean et al, 2020). Moral distress occurs at the intersection between individuals' own intact moral frameworks and the healthcare system values. Moral residue is the unresolved emotional and psychological conflicts left over from moral distress. These can accumulate to produce moral injury. Moral injury implies damage to or erosion of an individual's moral framework as a result of single or multiple transgressions of that framework (Dean et al, 2020). Transgressing can mean perpetuating, failing to prevent or bearing witness to acts that offend deeply held moral beliefs and expectations. In healthcare, the deepest belief is the oath physicians take to provide the best possible care for patients and to make patients' needs their priority, for example (Dean et al, 2020). If these types of injuries occur frequently, then a health professional may progress to burnout.

Clinician burnout is when a person is physically and emotionally exhausted from navigating and struggling within a challenging system whilst trying to provide the best possible care, to the state where they reach learned helplessness and give up (Bendix, 2019; Dean et al, 2020). The clinicians may feel their actions are futile, feel emotionally distanced, or depersonalised or detached, "to tolerate inescapable exposure to his or her patients' suffering" (Dean et al, 2020, p. 924). Thus it can be seen that the progress from moral dilemmas to injury, and finally to burnout, is framed as "a coping strategy to withstand an intolerable, inescapable situation" (Dean et al, 2020, p. 924). The treatment is to eliminate unnecessary barriers that interfere with delivering good healthcare with the patients, in what can be seen as a relational experiential context.

It is important to be precise in terminology for another reason. The reason for the need for precision is in order to relate what approaches to patient healthcare relate specifically to healthcare workers' suffering. The whole approach to healthcare is provided by a compass of enhanced patient experience, improving population health, reducing cost and improving the work life of healthcare providers since the latter impacts on the former three aims (Bodenheimer & Sinsky, 2014). With rising expectations of healthcare providers, there is a recognition that these providers need to be resourced to provide excellent healthcare, yet the gap between societal expectations and professional reality is believed to set the stage for at least half of physicians to experience burnout, thereby reducing physician adherence to treatment plans and lower levels of empathy and patient safety (Bodenheimer & Sinsky, 2014). Healthcare providers' and patients' well-being, and therefore suffering, can be seen as intimately related.

Moral distress has been delineated from suffering in that sadness and grief are seen as normal emotions in response to suffering and loss, whereas moral distress is characterised by powerlessness, an inability to fix a wrong, frustration and anger (Epstein & Hamric, 2009). There are believed to be three patterns of response to moral residue crescendo – a numbing of moral sensitivity, withdrawal from ethically challenging patient situations; conscientious objection; and burnout followed by leaving a position or profession (Epstein & Hamric, 2009). However, the crisis of burnout in healthcare professions has been resistant to solutions, with clinicians citing a subtle, elusive disconnect between what they have experienced and what they perceive as encapsulated by definitions of burnout (Dean et al, 2019). Part of this disconnect may be due to having to serve many masters at the same time – management, disciplinary hierarchies, patients and families and policy.

The term burnout, used to denote a syndrome consisting of emotional exhaustion, depersonalisation (disengagement) and a low sense of personal accomplishment from work driven factors within the work environment, has been around for about 50 years (National Academies of Sciences Engineering, and Medicine, 2019). Rates of burnout among nurses range between 35% and 45%, whereas that for physicians in the US range between 40% and 54%, over the past decade. Those percentages are just under double for those of the general population in the US

(Shanafelt et al, 2015). Specialities in medicine with the highest risk of burnout are those at the front line of the health care delivery system such as emergency medicine, family medicine, general intern medicine and neurology. Younger workers, women and those with significant life events show higher levels of risk of burnout (National Academies of Sciences Engineering, and Medicine, 2019). In Australia, five areas of stress were identified as demands on time, professional development and training, delivery demands, interpersonal demands and administration/organisational issues, with about half of trainees (49.5%) scoring highly in emotional exhaustion or depersonalisation and 23.4% scoring highly in both (Leung & Rioseco, 2017). It is difficult to establish causality since there are no long term studies (Amoafa et al, 2015).

In the UK, junior doctors and women in particular were likely to suffer from burnout, perceived to be due to a work-life imbalance, lack of social support outside work due to long hours and constantly moving workplaces (Rich et al, 2016). Low morale and harm to well-being in terms of feeling exploited by employers and the government, led to a sense of dehumanisation and overt gender, family, and part-time work discrimination. The emphasis on remediating these conditions was on change of structural work factors rather than focusing on individual pathology (Rich et al, 2016). The belief was that the workplace did not fit the workers and this is what needed to change.

Also in the UK, behavioural and health problems associated with occupational stress included high rates of insomnia, binge eating, drinking alcohol, substance use and ill-health (Medisauskaite & Kamau, 2019). Forty-four percent of doctors binge drank (consuming six or more drinks on one occasion) with 5% meeting the criteria for alcohol dependence. A range of 20%–61% of doctors had some type of sleeping problem. Not surprisingly, doctors who reacted to stress by blaming themselves were more likely to use substances to get themselves through periods of high stress.

In a systematic review that included burnout, but was not solely limited to it, nine research studies were found (with 10,702 unique participants) on surgeons that demonstrated the difficulties experienced by them after complications from surgery in patients, a concept of the consequences of adverse events or second victim phenomenon (Srinivasa et al, 2019). Surgeons were affected emotionally (anxiety, guilt, sadness and shame) as well as experiencing interference with professional and leisure activities; they used coping mechanisms such as limited discussions with colleagues, exercise, artistic or creative outlets, alcohol or substance abuse; had some institutional support, as well as perceiving that emotional distress could be seen as a personal weakness; and there were believed to be impacts on future clinical practice. Acute traumatic stress was of a concern when self-distraction was used as a coping strategy. One of the most pertinent findings was the lack of evidence on this topic, which after all encapsulates moral distress, injury and burnout.

There are many suggestions to deal with occupational burnout aimed at institutional and political levels, as well as patient interactions, although evidence is lacking (Montgomery et al, 2019; National Academies of Sciences Engineering, and Medicine, 2019). Practicing grim storytelling in the making of life or death decisions (Alison & Shortland, 2019); addressing the disconnect in medicine that promotes depersonalisation through training – seen as being our problem with human suffering, through compassionate care (Martinek, 2017); resilience training in medical education (Chan & Dennis, 2019); organising to fight burnout (Eisenstein, 2018) and using Trauma Informed Care (Kuehn, 2020) are all suggestions to lessen the burden of burnout.

Burnout has also been associated with an increased risk of suicidal ideation in healthcare workers with an increased risk of up to 200% in physicians (National Academies of Sciences Engineering, and Medicine, 2019). This increased risk is believed to start in training so there is a constant theme of burnout, depression and anxiety that must be addressed. In a recent international systematic review, the prevalence rates for burnout in medical students ranged between 7% and 75.2% according to the country, affecting personal accomplishment the most, followed by emotional exhaustion and depersonalisation (Erschens et al, 2019). Comparison with normative data (Year 12 students) showed that medical students demonstrated significantly higher rates of emotional exhaustion and depersonalisation. Rates related to the ethnicity of the medical student were mixed (Ishak et al, 2013).

Although the learning environment is believed to play a critical role, there is little detail provided (Dyrbye et al, 2009). Loss of connection with and detachment from self as well as a loss of meaning and a sense of irrelevancy in a technically oriented environment is thought to underlie burnout (Jennings, 2009). The exposure to death and human suffering without adequate preparation is believed to be another cause of student distress, as well as adjustment to the medical school environment, ethical conflicts, student abuse, personal life events and educational debt (Dyrbye et al, 2005). The fact that suffering seems to be rarely mentioned in the medical curriculum or in the literature is in itself a sign that students will not be prepared for encountering suffering. They also have little exposure to medical humanities and sociology, which leaves them without the resources to draw on when they do encounter suffering.

In other healthcare students, emotional vulnerability was highlighted in physiotherapy students with academic and personal issues being of greatest concern, with just over a quarter of students indicating stress and psychological morbidity (anxiety, depression, social dysfunction and loss of confidence) (Walsh et al, 2010). Pharmacy students have demonstrated a rate of depression of 60% in a study carried out in Pakistan (Khalid et al, 2017). The difference in rates of suicides across professions was believed to be due to work-related access to means of carrying out the act of suicide as a risk factor in the employed population, but this is associated with a greater risk for females than males. The findings of this study suggest the importance of controlling access to lethal methods in occupations where these are readily available (Milner et al, 2017).

The difficulty compiling data across countries that use different measurement instruments of depression and anxiety in medical students is clear yet does not detract from the fact that medical students and physicians continue to show much higher rates of depression and anxiety than the general population (Erschens et al, 2016). This has led to a call for a culture change in medical education and medicine (Ward & Outram, 2016). In part, the problem of burnout being at new highs amongst doctors and nurses at the front line of patient care is seen as a result of the continued exploitation of these professionals' sense of duty: "Healthcare is by no means perfect, but what good exists is because of individuals who strive to do the right thing" (Ofri, 2019). The moral ethic of not walking away from suffering is seen as both a strength and burden of healthcare workers.

Overall, there is a significant proportion of healthcare workers who suffer from clinician distress and burnout, and this proportion is believed to be increasing. Whilst most interventions are aimed at changing the workplace (National Academies of Sciences Engineering, and Medicine, 2019), there is significant impact on health professional relationships as well as a loss of attachment to self that need addressing. None of the studies looked at the type of relationships in the healthcare workforce according the models proposed by Fiske (1993) and Haslam (2012) and shown in relation to suffering in Table 1.1. Suffering of both clinician and patient, whilst a generic term, but one that encompasses wider human and existential issues, is generally not mentioned very much at all. This is a huge gap in the literature and could account for why students and graduates struggle with integrating suffering in themselves and in their work.

Interestingly, the escape through depersonalisation from exposure to intolerable patient suffering, and the personal contract which produces a high level of responsibility and personal culpability thinking, is worth exploring in greater depth. One has to wonder why there is such a silence on suffering:

> The expectation that we can be immersed in suffering and loss daily and not be touched by it is as unrealistic as expecting to be able to walk through water without getting wet. This sort of denial is no small matter. The way we deal with loss shapes our capacity to be present to life more than anything else. The way we protect ourselves from loss may be the way in which we distance ourselves from life and help. We burn out not because we don't care but because we don't grieve. We burn out because we've allowed our hearts to become so filled with loss that we have no room left to care.
>
> (Remen, 1996, p. 52)

Culturally, it seems as though the healthcare workforce prefers terms like burnout and moral injury to describe specific situations rather than exploring deeper meanings of life, loss, grief and death, even though these are the main concerns of their work.

However, it may be that under the onslaught of COVID-19, these terms will be severely tested during a pandemic of suffering. Evidence of the impact of the severe acute respiratory syndrome-related coronavirus (SARS) 2002–2004 epidemic on healthcare workers will now be reviewed, followed by a review of the impact of COVID-19. One year after the outbreak, when stress levels matched that of low risk healthcare workers, high risk healthcare workers reported elevated levels of stress, depression and anxiety in Hong Kong due to their increased risk of contracting SARS, post-traumatic stress owing to the impact of the SARS outbreak, mediated by contact with SARS, fatigue, sleep deprivation, worry about health and fear of social contract (McAlonan et al, 2007). Likewise, Toronto healthcare workers showed significantly higher levels of burnout, psychological distress and post-traumatic stress (Maunder et al, 2006; Nikell et al, 2004). Both systemic and personal variables were associated with prolonged distress: working in an emergency department or intensive care unit was associated with more adaptive coping (high intensity, high risk settings). It was recommended that effective support be put in place before an outbreak, when strong relationships had the time to develop.

In Taiwan, the fear of becoming victims to SARS themselves led healthcare workers experiencing an overwhelming level of fear, as well as fracturing of safety and trust in the hospital (Chong et al, 2004). Workers feared being stigmatised and rejected through being carriers of the disease. More than two-thirds experienced anxiety, worrying, depression, interpersonal difficulties as well as somatic problems. Feelings of extreme vulnerability, uncertainty and threat to life were significant, not surprisingly. Both micro and macro level interventions were believed to be necessary aimed at enhancing resilience of individuals and organisations (Maunder et al, 2008).

COVID-19 has brought a pandemic of suffering on populations globally due to a number of factors. From patients' and families' perspectives the uncertainty (Simpkin, 2020) in relation to transmission, diagnosis, treatment, recovery and death from COVID-19, as well as mitigation and containment strategies such as lockdown with the economic losses that entails, led to panic initially (Wang et al, 2020) followed by grief and loss (Nacoti et al, 2020; The King's Fund, 2020b). The burden of survivors in terms of long term rehabilitation required following intensive care treatment and associated delirium includes mental health issues such as anxiety and depression as well as PTSD (Servick, 2020). Death and dying have been profoundly altered as families are not able to say their last goodbyes face to face, as well as worrying that their loved one has died alone (Yardley & Rolph, 2020). The separation from families, rapid death and limited funerals means that often health professionals carry the emotional burden when bearing witness to a difficult death. Issues of basic humanity and what should be done arise and carry a poignancy like never before

(Yardley & Rolph, 2020). There are heightened disparities across ethnicity and socioeconomic status as those most vulnerable bear the greatest losses (Owen et al, 2020). Decades of adverse effects of the social determinants of health have been exacerbated, and some people have been referring to the systemic racism inherent in the higher proportion of deaths in ethnic minorities in both the UK and the US (Khunti et al, 2020).

Balancing up the personal risk with societal obligation has never been more prominent, especially amongst health professionals (Tsai, 2020). At the same time, there is a concern that if we cannot protect our healthcare workers, we will not be able to protect the patients (McCarthy & Rivolta, 2020). PPE has become a major issue and has dominated the coverage of the pandemic to the extent that this terminology is now being applied to psychological PPE, too (Hardacre & Margetts, 2020). The mental health of both the public and health professionals is a major concern, and there have been calls for research into this area as these are a major risk factor for suicide (Gunnell et al, 2020). Distress due to fear, self-isolation and physical distancing as well as the rise in domestic violence and worsening of pre-existing symptoms with little recourse to face-to-face treatment have added fuel to the growing concern (Holmes et al, 2020). Increased surveillance, monitoring and recording of mental ill-health have contributed to the feeling that we are in unprecedented times (Gunnell et al, 2020).

Health professionals are under pressure from the ever increasing numbers of the sick; overwhelming workload; lack of specific drugs; feeling inadequately supported; fear of contagion and death of family, friends and colleagues; uncertainty; stigmatisation; and high levels of stress, anxiety and depression, with over 71.5% of healthcare workers reporting distress in one study (Lai et al, 2020). The high volume of patients is related to capacity issues, with a rapid change around in availability of intensive care beds and a cancelling of £13.4 billion in NHS debt in order to fulfil the demand (ONS, 2020). The societal shifts and emotional stressors, extreme workloads, moral dilemmas and rapidly evolving practice environment have meant that now more than ever, health professionals feel the need to be heard and honoured (Shanafelt et al, 2020). Resources for health professionals have mushroomed as healthcare workers are seen as being in need of support like never before (Chau, 2020). The British government framed the lockdown strategies in terms of staying at home to protect the NHS, so that the system could cope with the tsunami of patients (Department of Health and Social Care, 2020). PTSD is believed to be the second tsunami of the COVID-19 pandemic as families, recovering patients and health professionals are all believed to be susceptible (Dutheil et al, 2020; Hill, 2020). There has been a fault line drawn – before and after COVID-19 – in the belief that life will not be the same again and that this situation has become the new normal (Brindley, 2020; McCartney, 2020).

All of these factors have brought a new urgency to the need to understand suffering as it has become more visible globally, over the last few months to the Western world at least. Culturally, geographically and racially, the Western world has not been that preoccupied with suffering perhaps because it was always perceived as something happening over there away from our front doorstep. However, now we can no longer turn away, and the evidence shows that suffering in healthcare inherently involves both patients and health professionals. Furthermore, there is a need to move beyond approaches that may suit a psychological isolate towards understanding the relational matrix we are in, and this necessitates drawing on both medical humanities and sociology.

2.3 Epistemology – ethics in the formation of how we know what we know

The previous two sections have shown that both health professionals and patients are inherently bound up with suffering and issues of social injustice. We operate in a world of inequities. Therefore we are required to make an ethical response based on how we know what we know. But the two are not separated; they are indistinguishable. Ethical responses are based on concepts, patterns and models of social order or disorder and have an instinctual component – a gut reaction, if you like. An individual's instincts do not necessarily coincide with social norms and proclivities. There is no direct social translation of government response to patterns of inequities – it is mediated by politics, beliefs, economies and bias. Individuals also have preferences and biases in their decision making. Therefore individuals may find themselves at odds with government policies and institutional guidelines as shown by the previous sections in terms of burnout. In addition, on further examination it may not always be possible to find conceptual clarity or even begin to make sense of what is happening in the latest reform measures within healthcare services. Some measures may decrease accessibility to services for certain groups of people more than others, thereby increasing suffering. Health professionals are caught up in this as much as patients; little progress has been made on this most fundamental aspect of public services.

Traditionally, hospitals were formed in order to keep the poor and the sick away from the healthier general (wealthier) population (Foucault, 1973). There were religious overtones to hospitals, often run by nuns and led by doctors who assumed the status of God. Transcendental religion played a large role in education and health and lent itself to consideration of suffering through the lenses of redemption and suffering. There were categorical imperatives as to what ought to be done from a moral perspective. However, the translation between a normative "ought" and a factual what "is" incurred a basic error of logic, a naturalistic fallacy (Walter, 2006). The separation between a normative "ought" of moral reasoning and a factual (biological scientific) "is" rests on beliefs, emotions and instinctual drives. The separation is dynamic, a process based on polarising forces of defection and co-operation in a social context (Wilson, 1998). Ethical beliefs cannot be separated from the social context in which they operate.

Ethical precepts struggle between beliefs embedded in subjective experience and those promoted by transcendent ethereal messages promoted by religion, which codifies rules and practices to ensure behavioural alignment of people with social edicts. This struggle can set people up against themselves as they experience an embodied reaction and lived reality versus what they sense are overruling "higher" laws. Health professional training has, in the past, been conducted more along the lines of a transcendent belief system than as a response to lived experience of patients. This produces a dilemma. Health professional practice necessitates an ethical response to patients but this is not necessarily facilitated by transcendent beliefs and values. What seems more pragmatic (Racine, 2008) is to understand human nature better and develop a response from there:

> *Ought* is not the translation of human nature but of the public will, which can be made increasingly wise and stable through the understanding of the needs and pitfalls of human nature.
>
> (Wilson, 1998, p. 280)

Empiricism used the "ought" to state what society chose first and then codified – "ought" is the product of a material process that discriminates and separates (Wilson, 1998).

Where this has application is understanding health promotion and health inequities (Guttman, 2017). If there is a social value that people need to be saved (from themselves) in order to protect their health – think bicycle helmets, seatbelts, banning of smoking in public venues, calorie labelling of food, speed limits, recent social isolation legislation – then these values are codified into law and prescriptive behaviours with associated stigma and discrimination if people do not comply. The increased taxes on certain goods such as sugar, tobacco and alcohol, however, affect some demographics more than others, and people who do not comply within these demographics are again more likely to be subject to stigma and discrimination (Guttman, 2017). What underlies these assumptions are perceptions about people and whether they exercise free will and choice. These perceptions form the basis of what is considered human. On that basis, decisions are made about the value of human life and whether or not it can be saved. These decisions can be compromised by beliefs in factual evidence from a group population level of statistical analysis in relation to social demographic measures such as age, gender, race, ethnicity, disability and socioeconomic status, for example. These populations' statistical measures are also reflective of suffering – they are perhaps proxies for suffering.

Suffering is implicit in statistical evidence that shows distinct disparities in health as has been shown recently in COVID-19 and detailed in the above section. Black and Asian minority ethnicities have been particularly affected. It is not yet known what causes the differential in deaths and prevalence of COVID-19, although some suggest biological markers such as a raised inflammatory response or the presence of co-morbidities such as diabetes, cardiovascular and chronic kidney disease; population density in geographical locations of deprivation; living arrangements and cultural values of close family contact; and language where healthcare services act as a barrier to accessibility. Others have suggested that the high death rates are from systemic racism and exclusion which can impact on all of the above. From a health promotion perspective, the ethical tailoring of responses would seem to be prudent.

Tailoring of responses is difficult when the concept of race is a contested term. Current health promotion guidelines are generally a one-size-fits-all approach not taking into account cultural diversity in beliefs, practices and cultural significance (Guttman, 2017). Health promotion guidelines do not generally consider ethical issues or the "is-ought" fallacy and how health professional practices can generate materialising processes of shaming and stigmatisation.

> The [moral] sentiments are thus derived from epigenetic rules, hereditary biases in mental development, usually conditioned by emotion, that influences concepts and decisions made from them. The primary origin of the moral instincts is the dynamic relation between co-operation and defection.
>
> The essential ingredient for the molding of the instincts during genetic evolution in any species is intelligence high enough to judge and manipulate the tension generated by the dynamism.
>
> (Wilson, 1998, p. 280)

Moral sentiments or instincts, in addition to gut feelings, also include conscience, self-respect, remorse, empathy, shame, humility and moral outrage. These affects and emotions bias people towards universal moral codes of honor, patriotism, altruism, empathy, justice, compassion, mercy and redemption (Wilson, 1998). However, colonialist ethical codes led to xenophobia and coercive regulations to the advantage of the ruling classes. There are major lacunae in understanding this, but there is no doubt that these moral instincts are in play in healthcare.

Ethical concepts must therefore be grounded on lived experience of human nature rather than just transcended notions of what it means to be a (colonialist) human. Wilson (1998) sees "melangés of moral reasoning" as a mess (p. 283). A chimera of odd parts stuck together – paleolithic egalitarian and tribalistic instincts – which seem to describe healthcare services as well as society generally. Whilst much works well in the health services on an individual patient level, in spite of insurmountable odds, there are still many disparities that need addressing at the population level.

Understanding that moral sentiments arose for survival is a key factor. Therefore empiricism of biological factors for survival seems to be pertinent if transcendentalism is to be relegated to a lesser force in the dynamism of co-operation and defection. This dynamic operates at both the patient and health professional level to produce effects of exclusion and manipulation.

Cognitive neuroscience that contributes to understanding personhood and how ethics arise has been called neuroethics (Racine, 2008). The two-way dialogue between life sciences and humanities focuses on moral reasoning, whilst responsibility and higher order cognition require inter-disciplinary analysis and synthesis of concepts. The "is-ought" distinction serves as a primary limit on how we know what we know. For example, managers of healthcare services are interested in employees' adherence to guidelines and performance:

> Mmm, I think you need to have a very good understanding of the bureaucracy because umm, when you work for the government, de-pending on the political party of the day or the government of the day, it may or may not be umm, ahh in line with your particular philosophy. However, if you're employed you are employed to do a job and so therefore you have to implement enthusiastically the whatever the will of the government of the day is. That sometimes creates inner conflict, but you, to get anywhere in a bureaucratic system you need to learn to cope with that and that, not personalize it, but well this is what has to be done and get on do it. I think resilience is something that's really important, because there's often not a lot of ahh constructive feedback or positive feedback, so you don't know whether you are necessarily performing well or where you fit in the organizational ahh structure and so therefore it's important that you have some mechanisms that you've set up yourself for assessing where you are at.
>
> (Ingrid) (Lowe, 2010)

This response speaks of the incitement to adhere to governmental norms with an expected corresponding slippage of self. The practice of the self is to understand the political will and to align oneself with that (enthusiastically). Further practices of the self include coping with inner conflict, not taking things personally and to get on and do tasks. Moreover, the practice of the self is to monitor how well you are fitting in as a worker, i.e., performing.

Here there is the intersection of the individual and the structural whereby the sharing of a truth occurs. The knowledge formed in the meeting place between the different workers and the hierarchy of the health service is about subjugation of the workers into a particular type of worker, one that will conform to norms and policies and procedures of a government bu-reaucracy. The workers are incited to perform as particular types of workers through control and supervision of each other and different levels within the hierarchy. The ideology of the training was that each worker graduated as competent to perform a particular role "to be able to do" and solve particular problems related to health. The institution then enacted its ideology by putting that task focused training into a context whereby fitting into the norms was most important and yet unspoken. The use of epistemology and concepts in that setting is perhaps less important than conforming to guidelines. There is a perhaps a line drawn between what is included and what is left out at this conceptual ethical level.

The line seems to indicate more than just who knows best how to "fix" problems of poverty and suffering. Stepping over the line to truly address issues of suffering and poverty can mean a de-institutionalisation, which could be perceived as threatening as institutions have invested so much in maintaining the way they work. There seems to be little interest in attending to the lived experience of poverty for that could perhaps mean coming undone (Butt, 2002).

Box 2.1 Reflection

The room is bright as sunlight floods in the wall-sized windows. There is a young man lying tidily in the bed, still, contained within the sheets which are almost like a shroud. He had been transferred to this hospital from another more acute one when it was decided that nothing more could be done for him following his motorbike accident. His level of consciousness had been determined as inactive through a diagnosis of brain death. Conversations with family had culminated in the decision to not actively treat any chest infection and to let him go in his own time. I was there to carry out passive movements with him to keep him mobile for care, to help ensure he didn't get pressure sores. I went over to the bed saying hello and stating my name and what I was there for. I was not expecting any response. As I continued on, I felt there was a charge in the room. I believed he was really angry as moving his limbs was proving impossible and I didn't think or feel it was all down to neurological reflexes. He seemed rigid with anger. For the time I was there on that ward, I carried on, speaking to him and letting him know what I was doing and why, but at the same time experiencing this discomfort about how conscious he really was. Talks with the nursing staff confirmed his neurological status as beyond any recovery.

I moved on to another placement in the community. One time I needed to return to that ward after a few months. I was surprised to find the young man sitting in a reclining chair at the nursing station having a conversation, albeit slow and laboured, with the nursing staff. He had recovered sufficiently to be able to communicate although was not yet able to walk and move independently.

I wondered whether the sense that I had picked up when seeing him previously had been an indication of his consciousness and yet this didn't fit with diagnostic criteria. There seemed to be no place for a discussion about the affect that I noticed and what this could mean for patient recovery and care.

Questions for reflection

1   How do you notice suffering? Do you have a predominate channel that you use such as emotions, affect, bodily felt sense, words, facial expressions?
2   How will you forgive yourself for not attending to suffering effectively at times?
3   What ethical dilemmas are there in healthcare practice constituted by the co-operation versus defection dilemma? How does this play out in real life?
4   Coming closer to the centre of the intersection of the social and individual may mean entering chaos and disorientation. How does the rigidity of healthcare services contain that chaos? How does it serve the chaos?
5   How can medical humanities work to reduce inequities in health outcomes?
6   What is your experience with notions of redemption and salvation in suffering?

Further Resources
Whyte D. 2014. *Solace–The Art of Asking the Beautiful Question.* Many Rivers Company: CD.
Whyte D. 2019. *Consolations: The Solace Nourishment and Underlying Meaning of Everyday Words.* Canongate Books: London.

References

Aldridge R. 2019. Homelessness: A barometer of social justice. *The Lancet Public Health*; S2468-2667(19):30240–30243.

Alimoradi Z., Golboni F., Griffiths M.D., Broström A., Lin C.Y., Pakpour A.H. 2019. Weight-related stigma and psychological distress: A systematic review and meta-analysis. *Clinical Nutrition*; pii: S0261–5614(19):33102–33104.

Alison L., Shortland N. 2019. Making life-or-death decisions is very hard – here's how we've taught people to do it better. https://theconversation.com/making-life-or-death-ddecisions-is-very-hard-heres-how-weve-taught-people-to-do-it-better-126249.

Amoafa E., Hanbali N., Patel A., Singh P. 2015. What are the significant factors associated with burnout in doctors? *Occupational Medicine*; 65:117–121.

Andrew L.B., Brenner B.E. 2018. Physician suicide. https://emedicine.medscape. com/article/806779-overview.

Annual Public Health Report of the Director of Public Health. 2018. *Healthy life expectancy in tower hamlets*. https://www.towerhamlets.gov.uk/Documents/ Public-Health/Tower_Hamlets_Public_Health_Report_2018.pdf.

Anonymous Doctor. 2016. By the end of my first year as a doctor, I was ready to kill myself. http://www.theguardian.com/healthcare-network/views-from-the-nhs-frontline/2016/jan/05/doctor-suicide-hospital-nhs.

Bendix J. 2019. The real reason docs burn out. 96(2). https://www.medicaleconomics. com/business/real-reason-docs-burn-out.

Bhui K., Halvorsrud K., Nazroo J. 2018. Making a difference: Ethnic inequality and severe mental illness. *The British Journal of Psychiatry*; 213:574–578.

Bodenheimer T., Sinsky C. 2014. From triple to quadruple aim: Care of the patient requires care of the provider. *Annals of Family Medicine*; 12(6):573–576.

Bowen, M., Marwick, S., Marshall, T., Saunders, K., Burwood, S., Yahyouche, A., Stewart, D., audyal, V. 2019. Multimorbidity and emergency department visits by a homeless population: A database study in specialist general practice. *British Journal of General Practice*; 69(685):e515–e525.

Brindley P. 2020. Opinion: Covid-19—Healthcare workers are scared but, in some ways, also lucky. *BMJ* 31 March. https://blogs.bmj.com/bmj/2020/03/31/peter-brindley-covid-19-healthcare-workers-are-scared-but-in-some-ways-also-lucky/.

British Medical Association (BMA) 2018a. Almost a fifth of EU doctors have made plans to leave UK following Brexit vote. https://archive.bma.org.uk/news/media-centre/press-releases/2017/november/almost-a-fifth-of-eu-doctors-have-made-plans-to-leave-uk-following-brexit-vote.

British Medical Association (BMA) 2018b. Bullying and harassment: How to address it and create a supportive and inclusive culture. https://archive.bma.org.uk/ collective-voice/policy-and-research/education-training-and-workforce/tackling-bullying-and-harassment-in-the-nhs/bullying-and-harassment-policy-recommendations.

Buchanan I. 2018. *A Dictionary of Critical Theory*. Second Edition. Oxford University Press: Oxford.

Butler, J. (1993). *Bodies that Matter*. Routledge: New York.

Butt, L. 2002. The suffering stranger. Medical anthropology and international morality. *Med Anthropol*; 21(1):1–24. Discussion 25–33. doi: https://doi.org/10. 1080/01459740210619.

Case A., Deaton A. 2020. *Deaths of Despair and the Future of Capitalism*. Princeton University Press: Princeton.

Chan L., Dennis A.A. 2019. Resilience: Insights form medical educators. *The Clinical Teacher*; 16:384–389.

Chau S. Who will heal the healers? The psychological aftermath of COVID-19. *BMJ*. https://blogs.bmj.com/bmj/2020/04/17/steven-chau-who-will-heal-the-healers-psychological-aftermath-covid-19/.

Chong M., Wang W., Hsieh W., Lee C., Chui N., Yeh W., Huang T., Wen J., Chen C. 2004. Psychological impact of sever acute respiratory syndrome on health workers in a tertiary hospital. *British Journal of Psychiatry*; 185:127–133.

Coggon J. 2018. *The Nanny State Debate: A Place Where Words Don't Do Justice*. Faculty of Public Health: London.

CSDH (2008). Closing the gap in a generation: Health equity through action on the social determinants of health. *Final Report of the Commission on Social Determinants of Health*. World Health Organisation: Geneva.

Dean W., Talbot S.G., Caplan A. 2020. Clarifying the language of clinician distress. *JAMA*; 323(10):923–924.

Dean W., Talbot S., Dean A. 2019. *Reframing clinician distress: Moral injury not burnout*. Federal Practitioner; 36(9):400–402.

Deleuze G., Guattari F. 2009. *What Is Philosophy?* Verso: London.

Department of Health and Social Care. 2020. Coronavirus: Stay at home, protect the NHS, save lives - web version. https://www.gov.uk/government/publications/coronavirus-covid-19-information-leaflet/coronavirus-stay-at-home-protect-the-nhs-save-lives-web-version.

Dutheil F., Aubert C., Pereira B., Dambrun M., Moustafa F., Mermillod M., Baker J.S., Trousselard M., Lesage X., Navel V. 2019. Suicide among physicians and health-care workers: A systematic review and meta-analysis. *PLoS One*; 14(12):e0226361. Doi: https://doi.org/10.1371/journal.pone.0226361.

Dutheil F., Mondillon L., Navel V. 2020. PTSD as the second tsunami of the SARS-Cov2 pandemic. *Psychological Medicine*. https://www.cambridge.org/core/journals/psychological-medicine/article/ptsd-as-the-second-tsunami-of-the-sarscov2-pandemic/4AE54B1B1A67988C721EF6634D064D62.

Dyrbye L.N., Thomas M.R., Harper W., Massie F.S., Power D.V., Eacker A., Szydlo D.W., Novotny P.J., Sloan J.A., Shanafelt T.D. 2009. The learning environment and medical student burnout: A multicentre study. *Medical Education*; 43:274–282.

Dyrbye L.N., Thomas M.R., Shanafelt T.D. 2005. Medical student distress: Causes, consequences and proposed solutions. *Mayo Clinic Proceedings*; 80(12):1613–1622.

Eichbaum Q.G. 2014. Thinking about thinking and emotion: The metacognitive approach to the medical humanities that integrates the humanities with the basic and clinical sciences. *Permanente Journal*; 18(4):64–75.

Eisenstein L. 2018. To fight burnout, organize. *The New England Journal of Medicine*; 379(6):509–511.

Epstein E.G., Hamric A.B. 2009. Moral distress, moral residue, and the crescendo effect. *Journal of Clinical Ethics*; 20(4):330–342.

Erschens R., Herrmann-Werner A., Bugaj T.J., Nikendei C., Zipfel S., Junne F. 2016. Methodological aspects of international research on the burden of anxiety and depression in medical students. *Mental Health and Prevention*; 4:31–35.

Erschens R., Keifenheim K.E., Herrmann-Werner A., Loda T., Schwille-Kiuntke J., Bugaj T.J., Nikendei C., Huhn D., Zipfel S., Junne F. 2019. Professional burnout among medical students: Systematic literature review and meta-analysis. *Medical Teacher*; 41(2):172–183. doi: https://doi.org/10.1080/0142159X.2018.1457213.

Firth-Cozens J. 2020. What I learnt from studying doctors' mental health over 20 years – An essay by Jenny Firth-Cozens. *BMJ*; 369:m1374. doi: 10.1136/bmj.m1374.

Fiske A.P. 1993. *Structures of Social Life: The Four Elementary Forms of Human Relations*. The Free Press: New York.

Foucault M. 1973. *Birth of the Clinic: An Archeology of Medical Knowledge*. Vintage Books: New York.

Francis R. 2013 Report of the mid staffordshire NHS foundation trust public inquiry executive summary. *The Mid Staffordshire NHS Foundation Trust Public Inquiry.* https://www.gov.uk/government/publications/report-of-the-mid-staffordshire-nhs-foundation-trust-public-inquiry.

Fransham M., Dorling D. 2018. Homelessness and public health. *British Medical Journal; 360*: k214.

Gastaldo D. (1997). Is health education good for you? Re-thinking health education through the concept of bio-power. Chapter 6 in *Foucault – Health and Medicine.* Petersen A., Bunton R. (eds). Routledge: New York.

Gerada C. 2019. The making of a doctor: The matrix and self. *Group Analysis;* *52*(3):350–361. Doi: https://doi.org/10.1177/0533316418823117.

Gillepsie, G.L., Grubb, P.L., Brown K., Boesch M.C., Ulrich D. 2017. "Nurses eat their young": A novel bullying educational program for student nurses. *Journal of Nurses Educational Practice;* 7(7):11–21.

Gunnell D., Appleby L., Arensman E. Hawton K., John A., Kapur N., Khan M., O'Connor R.C., Pirkis J. 2020. Suicide risk and prevention during the COVID-19 pandemic. *The Lancet.* https://www.thelancet.com/journals/lanpsy/article/PIIS2215-0366(20)30171-1/fulltext.

Guttman N. 2017. Ethical Issues in Health Promotion and Communication Interventions. Oxford Research Encyclopedia, *Communication (oxfordre.com/communication).* Oxford University Press: USA.

Hardacre J., Margetts A. 2020. Psychological PPE: Survival kit for creating a safer culture in the Covid-19 context by Dr Jeanne Hardacre & Dr Alexander Margetts. *BMJ.* https://blogs.bmj.com/bmjleader/2020/04/15/psychological-ppe-survival-kit-for-creating-a-safer-culture-in-the-covid-19-context/.

Haslam N. (Ed). 2012. *Relational Models Theory: A Contemporary Overview.* Routledge: London.

Hassanally K., Asaeia, M. 2018. Homelessness mortality data from East London. *London Journal of Primary Care; 10*(4):99–102.

Hawton K., Clements A., Sakarovitch C., Simkin S., Deeks J.J. 2001. Suicide in doctors: A study of risk according to gender, seniority and specialty in medical practitioners in England and Wales, 1979–1995. *Journal of Epidemiology Community Health; 55*:296–300.

Hill A. 2020. NHS staff to be offered mental health support for COVID-19 'shell shock'. https://www.theguardian.com/society/2020/apr/08/nhs-staff-mental-health-shell-shock-tackling-covid-19-coronavirus.

Holmes E.A., O'Connor R.C., Perry V.H. et al. 2020. *Multidisciplinary research priorities for the COVID-19 pandemic: A call for action for mental health science. The Lancet Psychiatry.* doi: 10.1016/S2215-0366(20)30168-1.

Hutton P.H. (1988). *Ch2 in Technologies of Self.* Martin L.H., Gutman H., Hutton P.H. (eds). The University of Massachusetts Press: Amherst.

IPSOS MORI Social research Institute (2009, August). Fitness to practise: The health of healthcare professionals. http://webarchive.nationalarchives.gov.uk/+/www.dh.gov.uk/prod_consum_dh/groups/dh_digitalassets/@dh/@en/@ps/documents/digitalasset/dh_113549.pdf downloaded 26th January 2016.

Ishak W., Nikravesh R., Lederer S., Perry R., Ogunyemi D., Bernstein C. 2013. Burnout in medical students: A systematic review. *The Clinical Teacher; 10*:242–245.

Jennings M.L. 2009. Medical student burnout: Interdisciplinary exploration and analysis. *Journal Medical Humanities*; *30*:253–269.

Johnston N.E. 2013. Strengthening a praxis of suffering: Teaching-learning practices. *Nursing Science Quarterly*; *26*(3):230–235.

Joyce R., Xu X. 2019. Are the inequalities seen today a sign of a broken system? Launch of the IFS Deaton Review of inequalities. *Nuffield Foundation & Institute for Fiscal Studies*. https://www.ifs.org.uk/publications/14109.

Kamel N.F., Hashish E.A.A. 2015. The relationship between psychological need satisfaction, job affective well-being and work uncertainty among the academic nursing educators. *Journal of Nursing Education and Practice*; *5*(8): 99–108.

Khalid S., Bukhari A., Azhar S., Saeed N., Manzoor S., Syed H, Khan F.M., Syed A., Ali S.A., Ali M., Kamboh M.S. 2017. Incidence of depression and the coping styles used for it by undergraduate and postgraduate pharmacy students: A comparison. *Journal of human Virology and Retrovirology*; *5*(2):00146.

Khunti K., Singh A.K., Pareek M., Hanif W. 2020. Is ethnicity linked to incidence or outcomes of COVID-19? *BMJ*; *369*:m1548. doi: 10.1136/bmj.m1548.

Kristeva, J. 1982. *Powers of Horror – An Essay on Abjection*. Columbia University Press: New York.

Kristeva J., Moro M.R., Ødemark J., Engebretsen E. 2018. Cultural crossings of care: An appeal to the medical humanities. *BMJ Medical Humanities*; *44*:55–58.

Kuehn B.M. 2020. Trauma-Informed Care may ease patient fear, clinician burnout. *JAMA*; *323*(7):595–597.

Lai J., Ma S., Wang Y., Cai Z., Hu J., Wei N., Wu J., Du H., Chen T., Li R., Tan H., Kang L., Yao L., Huang M., Wang H., Wang G., Liu Z., Hu S. 2020. Factors associated with mental health outcomes among health care workers exposed to coronavirus disease 2019. *JAMA Network Open*; *3*(3):e203976.

Leung J., Rioseco P. 2017. Burnout, stress and satisfaction among Australian and New Zealand radiation oncology trainees. *Journal of Medical Imaging and Radiation Oncology*; *61*.146–155.

Levin D. M. 1991. Visions of narcissism: Intersubjectivity and the reversals of reflection. Chapter 3 in *Merleau Ponty Vivant*. Dillon M.C. (ed). State University of New York Press: Albany.

Lowe W.A. 2014. Complexity or meaning in health professional education and practice? *Health Education Journal*; *73*(1):3–8.

Lowe W.A. 2010. Health and 'I': An analysis of curricular phenomena in health professional education through the focus of critical pedagogy. *Unpublished Thesis. School of Education*, Murdoch University: Western Australia.

Marmot M., Allen J., Boyce T., Goldblatt P., Morrison J. 2020. *Health Equity in England: The Marmot Review 10 Years on*. Institute of Health Equity: London.

Mars S. 2012. *The Politics of Addiction: Medical Conflict and Drug Dependence in England since the 1960s*. Palgrave Macmillan: Basingstoke.

Martinek N. 2017. Burnout culture and disconnected medicine. https://www.gatheringofkindness.org/post/burnout-culture-and-disconnected-medicine.

Matthews-King A. 2017. NHS makes undisclosed settlement to Richard Branson's Virgin Care after legal dispute. https://www.independent.co.uk/news/health/nhs-richard-branson-virgin-care-legal-settlement-tendering-contract-a8080961.html.

Maunder R.G., Lancee W.J., Balderson K.E., Bennett J.P., Borgundvaag B., Evans S., Fernandes C.M.B., Goldbloom D.S., Gupta M., Hunter J.J., McGillis Hall L. Nagle L.M., Pain C., Peczeniuk S.S., Raymond G., Read N., Rourke S.B., Steinberg R.J., Stewart T.E., VenDeVelde-Coke S., Veldhorst G.G., Wasylenki D.A. 2006. Long-term psychological and occupational effects of providing hospital healthcare during SARS outbreak. *Emerging Infectious Diseases*; 12(12):1924–1932.

Maunder R.G., Peladeau N., Leszcz M., Romano D., Savage D., Rose M., Adam M.A., Schulman R.B. 2008. Applying the lessons of SARS to pandemic influenza. *Canadian Journal of Public Health*; 99(6):486–488.

McAlonan G.M., Lee A.M., Cheung V., Cheung C., Tsang K.W.T., Sham P.C., Chua S.E., Wong J.G.W.S. 2007. Immediate and sustained psychological impact of an emerging infectious disease outbreak on health care workers. *The Canadian Journal of Psychiatry*; 52(4):241–247.

McCarthy M., Rivolta G. 2020. COVID-19: If we can't protect our workers, we can't protect our patients. *BMJ*. https://blogs.bmj.com/bmj/2020/04/17/covid-19-if-we-cant-protect-our-workers-we-cant-protect-our-patients/.

McCartney M. 2020. The art of medicine. Perspectives. Medicine: Before COVID-19, and after. *The Lancet*; 395:1248–1249. https://doi.org/10.1016/S0140-6736(20)30756-X.

McCartney M. 2016. *The State of Medicine: Keeping the Promise of the NHS*. Pinter & Martin: London.

McManus C. 2007. Stress in Health Professionals. Chapter in *Cambridge Handbook of Psychology, Health and Medicine*. Second Edition. Ayers S., Baum A., McManus C., Newman S., Wallston K., Weinman J., West R. (eds). Cambridge University Press: Cambridge. pp. 500–505.

Medisauskaite A., Kamau C. 2019. Does occupational distress raise the risk of alcohol use, binge-eating, ill health and sleep problems among medical doctors? A UK cross-sectional study. *BMJ Open*; 9:e027362.

Miller M.N., Mcgowan R., Quillen J.H. 2000. The painful truth: Physicians are not invincible. *Southern Medical Journal*; 93(10):966–973.

Milner A.J., Maheen H., Bismark M.M., Spittal M.J. 2016. Suicide by health professionals: A retrospective mortality study in Australia, 2001–2012. *Medical Journal of Australia*; 205(6):260–265.

Milner A., Witt K., Maheen H., LaMontage A.D. 2017, Apr 4. Access to means of suicide, occupation and the risk of suicide: A national study over 12 years of coronial data. *BMC Psychiatry*; 17(1):125. doi: 10.1186/s12888-017-1288-0.

Moberly T. 2017. UK has fewer doctors per person than most other OECD countries. *BMJ*; 357:j2940.

Monrouxe L.V, Rees CE. 2012. "It's just a clash of cultures": Emotional talk within medical students' narratives of professionalism dilemmas. *Advances in Health Sciences Education*; 17:671–701.

Montgomery A., Panagopoulou E., Esmail A., Richards T., Maslach C. 2019. Burnout in healthcare: The case for organisational change; *BMJ*; 366:l4774.

Nacoti M., Ciocca A., Giupponi A., Brambillasca P., Lussana F., Pisano M., Goisis G., Bonacina D., Fazzi F., Naspro R., Longi L., Cereda M., Montaguti C. 2020. At the epicentre of the COVID-19 pandemic and humanitarian crises in Italy: Changing perspectives on preparation and mitigation. *NEJM Catalyst*; 1–5, doi: 10.1056/CAT.20.0080.

Nagington M., Sandset T. 2020. Putting the NHS England on trial: Uncertainty-as-power, evidence and the controversy of PrEP in England. *Medical Humanities*; 46:176–179.

National Academies of Sciences Engineering, and Medicine. 2019. *Taking Action Against Clinician Burnout: A Systems Approach to Professional Well-Being.* The National Academies Press: Washington, DC.

NHS England. 2016. NHS Five Year Forward View: Recap briefing for the Health Select Committee on technical modelling and scenarios. www.england.nhs.uk.

Needle J.J., Petchey R.P., Benson J., Scriven A., Lawrenson J., Hilari K. 2011. *The allied health professions and health promotion: A systematic literature review and narrative synthesis. Final report. NIHR Service Delivery and Organisation programme.*

Nikell L.A., Crighton E.J., Tracy C.S., Al-Enazy H., Bolaji Y., Hanjrah S., Hussain A., Makhlouf S., Upshur R.E.G. 2004. Psychosocial effects of SARS on hospital staff: Survey of a large tertiary care institution. *CMAJ*; *170*(5):793–798. doi: 10.1503/cmaj.1031077.

Office for National Statistics (ONS). 2019. How does UK healthcare spending compare with other countries? https://www.ons.gov.uk/peoplepopulationandcommunity/healthandsocialcare/healthcaresystem/articles/howdoesukhealthcarespendingcompar-ewithothercountries/2019-08-29.

Office for National Statistics (ONS). 2020. NHS to benefit from £13.4 billion debt write-off. https://www.gov.uk/government/news/nhs-to-benefit-from-13-4-billion-debt-write-off.

Ofri D. 2019. The business of healthcare depends on exploiting doctors and nurses. https://www.nytimes.com/2019/06/08/opinion/sunday/hospitals-doctors-nurses-burnout.html.

Ogden J. 2001. *Health and the Construction of the Individual: A Social Study of Social Science.* Routledge: London.

Olasoji H.O. 2018. Broadening conceptions of medical student mistreatment during clinical teaching: Message from a study of "toxic" phenomenon during bedside teaching. *Advances in Medical Education and Practice*; 9:483–494.

Orange, D.M. 2011. *The Suffering Stranger: Hermeneutics for Everyday Clinical Practice.* Routledge: New York.

Owen W.F., Carmona R., Pomeroy C. 2020. Failing another national stress test on health disparities. *JAMA*; *323*(19):1905–1906, doi:10.1001/jama.2020.6547.

Papanicolas I., Mossialos E., Abel-Smith B., Gundersen A., Woskie L., Jha A.K. 2019. Performance of UK National Health Service compared with other high income countries: Observational study. *BMJ*; *367*:l6326.

Petersen A., Lupton D. (2000). *The New Public Health – Health and Self in the Age of Risk.* Sage Publications: London.

Phelan S.M., Burgess D.J., Hellerstedt W.L., Griffin J.M., van Ryn M. 2015. Impact of weight bias and stigma on quality of care and outcomes for patients with obesity. *Obesity Reviews*; 16:319–326.

Public Health England [PHE]. 2018. *Homelessness: Applying all our health.* Available at: https://www.gov.uk/government/publications/homelessness-applying-all-our-health/homelessness-applying-all-our-health.

Racine E. 2008. Which naturalism for bioethics? A defense of moderate (pragmatic) naturalism. *Bioethics*; 22(2):92–100.

Rahman T. 2016. The negative culture of medical school. https://medium.com/@tarun_rahman/the-negative-culture-of-medical-school-2e02cfa6f438.

Remen R.N. 1996. *Kitchen Table Wisdom: Stories that Heal*. Penguin: New York.

Reynolds L. 2018. *Research: Homelessness in Great Britain–The numbers behind the story*. https://england.shelter.org.uk/__data/assets/pdf_file/0020/1620236/Homelessness_in_Great_Britain_-_the_numbers_behind_the_story_V2.pdf.

Rich A., Viney R., Needleman S., Griffin A., Woolf K. 2016. 'You can't be a person and a doctor': The work-life balance of doctors in training – A qualitative study. *BMJ Open*; 6:e013897.

Rios I.C. 2016. The contemporary culture in medical school and its influence on training doctors in ethics and humanistic attitude to the clinical practice. *International Journal of Ethics Education*; 1:173–182.

Saxena A., Meschino D., Hazelton L., Chan M.K., Benrimoh D.A., Matlow A., Dath D., Busari J. 2019. Power and Physician Leadership. *BMJ Leader*; 3:92–98.

Schwenk T.L., Davis L., Wimsatt L.A. 2010. Depression, stigma and suicidal ideation in medical students. *JAMA*; 304(11):1181–1190.

Servick K. 2020. Survivors' burden. *Science*; 368(6489):359.

Shanafelt T., Hasan O., Dyrbye L.N., Sinsky C., Satele D., Sloan J., West C.P. 2015. Changes in burnout and satisfaction with work-life balance in physicians and the general US working population between 2011 and 2014. *Mayo Clinic Proceedings*; 90(12):1600–1613.

Shanafelt T., Ripp J., Trockel M. 2020. Understanding and addressing sources of anxiety among health care professionals during the COVID-19 pandemic. *JAMA*; 323(21):2133–2134. Published online April 7, 2020. doi: 10.1001/jama.2020.5893.

Simpkin A.L. 2020. Embracing uncertainty: Could there be a blueprint from COVID-19. *BMJ*. https://blogs.bmj.com/bmj/2020/04/16/embracing-uncertainty-could-there-be-a-blueprint-from-covid-19/.

Sinclair S. 1997. *Making Doctors: An Institutional Apprenticeship*. Bloomsbury Publishing: London.

Squiers J.J., Lobdell K.W., Fann J.I., DiMaio J.M. 2017 Oct 31. Physician burnout: Are we treating the symptoms instead of the disease? *The Annals of Thoracic Surgery*; 104(4):1117–1122.

Srinivasa S., Gurney J., Koea J. 2019. Potential consequences of patient complications for surgeon well-being: A systematic review. *JAMA Surgery*; E1–E7. doi: 10.1001/Jamasurg.2018.5640.

The King's Fund. 2015. Ten priorities for commissioners: Transforming our health care system summary. https://www.kingsfund.org.uk/publications/articles/transforming-our-health-care-system-ten-priorities-commissioners/summary.

The King's Fund. 2019a. NHS waiting times: Our position. https://www.kingsfund.org.uk/projects/positions/nhs-waiting-times.

The King's Fund. 2019b. The King's Fund position: What do we think about key health and care issues? https://www.kingsfund.org.uk/projects/positions.

The King's Fund. 2020a. NHS hospital bed numbers: Past, present, future. https://www.kingsfund.org.uk/publications/nhs-hospital-bed-numbers.

The King's Fund. 2020b. Responding to stress experienced by hospital staff working with COVID-19: Guidance for planning early interventions. *COVID Trauma Response Working Group Rapid Guidance*. https://www.kingsfund.org.uk/audio-video/stress-hospital-staff-covid-19.

Thomas F., Hansford L., Ford J., Hughes S., Wyatt K., McCabe R., Byng B. 2019. *Poverty, Pathology and Pills: Final Report of the DeStress Project*. University of Exeter Medical School.

Tower Hamlets Health and Well-being Board. 2017. *Tower hamlets together: Tower hamlets health and wellbeing strategy 2017–2020*. https://www. towerhamlets.gov.uk/Documents/Public-Health/Health_Wellbeing_Strategy.pdf.

Townsend P., Davidson N. (Eds). 1982. Inequalities in Health: The *Black Report*. Penguin: London.

Tsai C. 2020. Personal risk and societal obligation amidst COVID-19. *JAMA*; 323:1555–1556, doi:10.1001/jama.2020.5450.

Wadhera R.K., Khatana S.A.M., Choi E., Jiang G., Shen C., Yeh R.W., Maddox K.E.J. 2019. Disparities in Care and Mortality Among Homeless Adults Hospitalized for Cardiovascular Conditions. *JAMA Internal Medicine*; 180(3):357–366.

Walsh D., McCartney G., Collins C., Taulbut M., Batty G.D. 2016. History, politics and vulnerability: Explaining excess mortality in Scotland and Glasgow. *Glasgow Centre for Population Health*. Glasgow Centre for Population Health: Glasgow.

Walsh J.M., Feeney C., Hussey J., Donnellan C. 2010. Sources of stress and psychological morbidity among undergraduate physiotherapy students. *Physiotherapy*; 96:206–212.

Walton M., Murray E., Christian M.D. 2020. Mental health care for medical staff and affiliated healthcare workers during the COVID-19 pandemic. *Acute Cardiovascular Care*; 9(3):241–247.

Wang W., He Q., Liu M., Wang M., Sun X. Covid-19: Lack of knowledge is driving public panic. *BMJ*. https://blogs.bmj.com/bmj/2020/02/28/communicating-research-evidence-about-covid-19-to-reduce-public-panic/.

Ward S., Outram S. 2016. Medicine: In need of culture change. *Internal Medicine Journal*; 46:112–116.

Warraich H. 2017. *Modern Death: How Medicine Changed the End of Life*. Duckworth Overlook: London.

Walter A. 2006. The anti-naturalistic fallacy: Evolutionary moral psychology and the insistence of brute facts. Evolutionary *Psychology*; 4:33–48.

Watton R., Gallivan C. (2013). The challenge of providing medical care to homeless men. *British Journal of General Practice*; 63(617):659–660.

Wilson E.O. 1998. *Consilience: The Unity of Knowledge*. Abacus: London.

World Health Organisation. 2003. *Adherence to long-term therapies: Evidence for action. Global Adherence Interdisciplinary Network*. Geneva. https://www.who.int/chp/knowledge/publications/adherence_report/en/.

World Health Organisation. 2020. Controlling the global obesity epidemic. https://www.who.int/nutrition/topics/obesity/en/.

Yardley S., Rolph M. 2020. Death and dying during the pandemic. *BMJ*; 369:m1472.

Zembylas M. 2019. "Shame at being human" as a transformative political concept and praxis: Pedagogical possibilities. *Feminism & Psychology*; 29(2):303–321.

3 Suffering as foundational to health professional education

3.1 Introduction

Understanding suffering seems to be a difficult lifelong task. Rilke is often quoted to provide solace for the task ahead: "Nearby there is the country they call life. You will know it by its seriousness. Give me your hand" (2005, p. 59). There are many different perspectives from which to view suffering in healthcare, including philosophy, spirituality, sociology, the humanities and science. However, the challenge is, rather than viewing suffering from a lofty academic perspective, to keep the experience of suffering at the forefront of our minds, lest the text becomes abstract prose and therefore, perhaps, less meaningful. This act of keeping the experience of suffering at the forefront is important because part of the experience of suffering means a loss of the (experiencing) self. Frank (2001) speaks eloquently of the need to keep the particularity of suffering, with its difficult lacunae of absence, loss and muteness:

> Such research organises suffering by making it reappear as categories that may all be valid enough for what can be spoken, but they refuse to acknowledge that aspects of suffering remain unspeakable. Suffering, the mute embodied sense of absence, both eludes extralocal categories and threatens the standpoint of discourse that supports those categories. Suffering threatens discourse because discourse cannot assimilate it to extralocal demands. When expressions of suffering break into discourse, the reader is returned to his or her own contingent embodiment in all its locality. When one's own body is attended to, the textual spell of the extralocal is broken.
>
> (Frank, 2001, p. 358–9)

Suffering by its very nature means that words and texts break down and seem alien, or extralocal, and unable to be incorporated into the body of work in healthcare. Therefore to write a text on suffering, one of the key questions is how to enter into suffering without making of it an alienated and alienating experience for the reader and sufferer? This book attempts to write about suffering in a way that will not add to the suffering.

Frank advocates paying attention to the particular over the universal ob-servations and categories of suffering. This paying attention is inspired by the need to avoid objectification of people who suffer since the perceived objec-tification only adds to the sense of the sufferer "becoming other to the person I had been and to those who knew that person" (Frank, 2001, p. 354). The management of those who suffer can add to suffering unnecessarily as people fight to be recognised in their suffering rather than reduced to a category (Orange, 2011; Waldman et al, 2011). Yet there is a requirement within academia and healthcare that discussions such as these provide guidelines and structure to understanding for professionals. This book attempts to provide structure to understanding suffering within the context of medical humanities and social science without losing the contingent (concrete influences of) embodiment of suffering.

Whether or not healthcare workers have suffered themselves, there seems to be an underlying difficulty in assimilating suffering into the work we do because of the work we do. I say this because while it may seem obvious that hospitals, GP surgeries and pre-hospital environments can be places where suffering is most manifest, oftentimes this is not spoken about nor is there room always to process the suffering that goes on between four walls or on the roadside in pre-hospital care, for example. Perhaps this is out of respect for the stoicism on the part of the sufferer, or perhaps it is borne out of a culture that cannot speak of suffering for fear of opening a Pandora's box of/for all the suffering in the world.

However, not speaking about suffering can contribute to a feeling of alienation that is at the root of suffering. Suffering involves a loss of the intactness of the self, an absence, that we are required to encounter (Frank, 2001). By not speaking about suffering, we are carrying on while the ele-phant in the room only looms larger. Yet it is difficult to talk about suf-fering for fear of being detached and abstract through categorisation of experiences best left in their particularity (Frank, 2001) or fear of becoming mired in an engulfing helplessness from which health professionals fear they could not recover or be able to function (Orange, 2011). There is a balance required between providing structured guiding rails to hold onto before letting go and fully immersing oneself in the experience of suffering.

In a recent workshop, a group of doctors identified that suffering was a part of life characterised by isolation, loneliness, helplessness on the part of both patient and doctor; physical, mental and emotional pain; fear and guilt on the part of the doctor when treatment did not work or there was an unexpected death; overwhelm in medical students when left on their own to deal with circumstances that were well beyond their capacity; and that sometimes there was just too much protracted pain and suffering, which could end in suicide. That part of the "too much" pain and suffering came from the impoverishment and numbing accompanying prolonged exposure to multiple causes of suffering. Acting as an advocate for patients in order to provide/facilitate social justice was one way in which doctors thought they could attend to suffering. Being on the front line of service provision and experiencing the high level of suffering without having recourse to do much about it was excruciating. The participants clearly identified that while no-one was immune to suffering, there were constraints in attending to this suffering.

Some of the constraints included compassion fatigue, where Mid-Staffordshire was cited as an example where this had occurred (Francis, 2013), and limits to understanding the social/economic factors, distributive justice whilst recognising the reach of medicine. Questions were asked such as

Is medical school a constraint?

Is being a doctor a constraint?

What happens when defences are too much?

Is medical school doing enough teaching on social justice?

While participants clearly recognised the suffering that is present, what was not so clear was how to attend to and encounter the suffering. Discussion of suffering in medical education is minimal (Cassell, 2004), and one can assume fairly safely that this is the case for all health professionals. Therefore this book aims to introduce different concepts and theories related to suffering drawing on medical humanities and sociology to demonstrate how they can be used to attend to and encounter suffering. There are both individual and social components of suffering as will be shown in the following sections. These components will necessarily draw on individual and social theories from different disciplines. Mostly different disciplines do not communicate with one another, so suffering is viewed from within academic silos.

Encountering suffering is a complex, nuanced matter – a matter that requires an understanding of different disciplines such as humanities, social sciences, as well as the natural and applied sciences of medicine and healthcare. Yet mostly these different disciplines are not integrated into one text to support the exploration of suffering. This books aims to draw on the different disciplines of humanities, social sciences and applied sciences to explore suffering from different perspectives in order to facilitate nuanced conversations about suffering. This is necessary because of the different forms of and responses to suffering. Mostly, suffering is written about as an individual phenomenon, yet now more than ever, there is a global awareness of suffering of populations, religious groups, people from different ethnicities and genders and displaced people, for example. Whilst suffering is an individual experience, there are social aspects of how suffering is made and seen that need to be integrated into any consideration of suffering.

However, writing about suffering on a larger scale risks objectifying in-dividuals (Frank, 2001). Categories of bodily, mental, social and existential suffering (Hofmann, 2015) may provide a piecemeal approach to individual suffering when the context is not considered. That is, the individual is seen to suffer separately from and is not shaped by their environment, including healthcare. That being said, there are ways to explore suffering that take on board the context of definitions and categorisation whilst always keeping an eye on who is best served by these definitions and categories.

3.2 Definitions and categories of suffering

3.2.1 *Definitions*

Definitions of suffering refer to the idea of a loss of a self-contained in-dividual, one who is usually able to navigate the vagaries of life, either implicitly or by default, as when this sense of the individual is missing in action. The distress of suffering in response to events beyond a person's control leads to a loss of intactness of the self (Cassell, 2004). Part of the loss of the intactness of the self is the inability to speak of the suffering: "Our suffering was why we could not talk. Our suffering was what we could not say" (p. 354). The unspeakable, experiencing yourself on the other side of life as it should be and the distress that threatens the intactness of the self by making that self absent, also contributes to the hole in what clinicians can say and do (Frank, 2001). There is an embodied absence along with the unknowable, unspeakable and incomprehensible that puts us on the wrong side of the fault line (Frank, 2001). There is an inner sense of chaos and disintegration with the lived flow of experience being stopped (Frank, 2013). There can be a threat to human agency, loss or threat to an individual's value system or an experienced negative feeling (Hofmann, 2015). There is a "before" and "after" sense, on either side of the fault line, when the lived flow of experience was disrupted, so that individuals are no longer recognizable as their former self or no longer recognise their life in its previous form.

This biographical break means that suffering makes people different – different from what they were before and different in their self-perception compared to other people (Hofmann, 2015). They cannot be as they were before, both morally and in terms of character traits. They cannot do as they did before either – they cannot wish and aspire or even hope as before (Hofmann, 2015). This profound disruption in being and doing gives a sense of uncanniness, loss of joy and meaning, as well as a change in per-ception and action around control and balance.

These living experiences of suffering are thought to be common to all human beings and are made explicit through phenomenological studies, although more will be discussed in relation to theories at a later section. Such studies aim to determine the essential properties and structures of humans' experience of suffering through systematic reflection (Hofmann, 2015). One of the essential turns in suffering is the turn to introspection (looking into themselves) and empathy (experiencing another's suffering as our own). Thus while previous ways of being and doing may be lost through biographical disruption, there is also the essential emergence of the person through capacities of introspection, empathy and compassion.

If these turns are an essential part of suffering, and suffering itself is thought to be a basic human experience, then we have to consider why the experience of suffering is not reflected in any of the frameworks of human nature and development. Why has such a significant part of the human experience not been included in health professional curricula, particularly when the majority of health professional work will be involved with some form of suffering or other? There is a cultural silence about suffering that affects us all; the hole is not just located in the individual – there is a cultural hole, too. Cultural values extol the upbeat extrovert individual; there is little value attributed to those who reflect and bear out suffering in solitude (Cain, 2012).

Wilkinson (2005) believes that the silence about suffering may be due to the limited amount of words we have, that suffering itself resists articulation, especially because of what suffering does to people individually and socially. The questions of whether suffering is comprehensible to others and how much other people can alleviate suffering seem to relate to the experience of the sufferers as being different to what they were before. However, when texts are explored for their discussion of suffering and what this may amount to, there are different cultural factors that need bearing in mind. For example, Victor Frankl, over 70 years ago, talked about the existential vacuum of private and personal forms of nihilism, relating this to the way people were taught:

> First of all, there is a danger inherent in the teaching of man's "nothingness," the theory that man is nothing but the result of biological, psychological and sociological conditions, or the product of hereditary and environment. ... "But in addition to being a professor in two fields I am a survivor of four camps – concentration camps, that is – and as such I also bear witness to the unexpected extent to which man is capable of defying and braving even the worst conditions conceivable."
>
> (Frankl, 1997, p. 132)

Therefore, perhaps some of the collective silence towards personal suffering is more a matter of the way we have been taught to think about ourselves as human beings. In addition, Frankl (1997) also seems to be saying that there is something more beyond the disciplinary ideas about humans, and this something more may be what gets us over the fault line. Arendt (1971) discussed how, with increasing capability through technology, we seem less able to be responsible for our actions and show less human agency and political freedom. These are important issues that seem not to be able to be addressed while definitions of suffering remain at the individual level.

The hole in what health professionals can say or do in relation to suffering can lead to a person's fear of being objectivised (Frank, 2001), which can widen the gulf between the sayer and the doer. Staff can feel lost and so ignore or minimise the suffering through distancing, walling off, avoidance and disconnection (Hofmann, 2015). These defences on the part of health professionals are an attempt to not address the vulnerability of both themselves and patients. With these defences firmly in place, the silence around suffering unfortunately only grows louder.

The silence around suffering in health professional education is astonishing given the amount of suffering at both a collective and individual level. Table 3.1 draws together the range of possible experiences under the umbrella of suffering. Whilst so far, the above definitions have focused on individual suffering and its relevance to the context of healthcare and health professional education; it can be seen that, as stated above, suffering is a basic human experience. Perhaps if suffering were made the foundation of health professional education, then not only could this keep the human at the core of healthcare, but we may also find a way to address one of the features of suffering as the person being on the wrong side of the fault line (Frank, 2001). Perceiving oneself to be on the wrong side of the fault line can lead to existential suffering.

So far, suffering has not been examined in relation to categories of race, ethnicity, gender, sexuality, disability, socioeconomic status or class, what I have included in institutional categories of suffering in the spirit of structural inequalities. But clearly these categories intersect with personal, interpersonal, family, professional and ideological suffering, too. Institutional here can mean broad ideas of organisations or social networks implicit in effect including educational colonialist dominance of the curriculum, for example. Structural stigma refers to the pathologies of the social systems that impact the material realities of patients' lives (Metzl & Hansen, 2014). I am reluctant to reinforce categories as a form of violence yet there is value in knowing the breadth and depth of suffering attributable to inequalities in health, for example (Marmot, 2020). As a manifestation of the inequalities and how this relates to suffering, Jermaine Singleton (2015) provides an analysis that goes more than skin deep in *Cultural Melancholy*. This analysis will be discussed in depth in the theory section. In some ways, though, cultural melancholy is not so far from existential suffering.

Existential suffering is typically understood as a psychological or spiritual condition that robs individuals of their capacity for peace in their present state of being (in Boston et al, 2011; Williams, 2004). There is a sense of annihilation and impending separation, from the self, others and life itself. There is also a search for meaning or purpose in life and an ultimate sense of wanting to find an answer to questions such as "Why am I here?",

Table 3.1 Range of experiences of suffering

Range	Examples
Personal	Physical – pain, loss of function, loss of limb, damage, trauma
	Emotional – sadness, anguish
	Grief – loss of person, physical, emotional, relationships
	Loss of self – depersonalisation, dehumanisation
	Tragedy – events, accidents, illness, disease
	Trauma – overwhelming event, helplessness
	Isolation – lack of support or networks
	Existential – fear of death, loss of meaning and hope, futility and pointlessness of life
Family	Loss of attachment – bereavement, divorce, separation, migration
	Domestic violence, abuse, neglect
	Poverty, deprivation
Interpersonal	Bullying, victim blaming, harassment
	Punishment, withdrawal, isolation
Institutional	Racial, ethnicity, gender, sexuality, disability, socioeconomic status or class
	Injustice
	Bureaucratic dehumanisation
	Discrimination
	Prejudice
Professional	Events – iatrogenic, exposure to trauma
	Carrying out techniques that inflict harm
	Bearing witness to other's suffering without acknowledgement
	Silence – holes in what to say or do
Ideology	Political, religious, economic – austerity, educational, capitalism, etc.
	Colonialism – stigma, exclusion, marginalisation
	Terrorism
Community	War – displacement, refugees
	Poverty, deprivation, homelessness
	Disasters – plane crashes, dams bursting
Natural disasters	Earthquakes, floods, tsunamis, climate change, volcanic eruption
National and global	Climate change, pandemics, Holocaust, racism, white supremacy, genocide

"What is the purpose of my life?" and "What will happen to me after I die?" (Boston et al, 2011). There is also an intense fear or terror of dying, emerging helplessness and the likelihood that this situation will endure (Kissane, 2012). Distress, grief, loneliness and powerlessness also hallmark existential suffering (Kissane, 2012).

Existential suffering has an established important place in the literature on palliative care (Boston et al, 2011). Yet even though patients' will to live has been highly correlated with their satisfaction in their relationship with their health professional, existential suffering is rarely the focus of care planning (Boston et al, 2011). Moreover, physicians' vulnerability in facing life and death issues has been underestimated, and the need to belong to a community that understands the loneliness and powerlessness of the physicians' position is of paramount importance, just as it is for the patient. Understanding the caregivers' perspective in terms of their vulnerability is important; the lack of understanding may account for the defences mentioned above. Knowing how to engage with and manage existential suffering seems to be a core competency for health professionals (Williams, 2004).

Suffering could be said to be one of the core competencies of health professionals and human beings, yet it is rarely mentioned. In the muteness about suffering, an understorey is formed whose parameters are scientific progress and social justice (Phillips, 1999). Who could have thought that in this world, there could be created such a system that manifested the split between self and other so perfectly as the division between science and social justice, pitting people unwittingly against each other? Is there any other thing we could have chosen that would have so beautifully polarised people and disciplines whilst at the same time burying completely the whole experience of suffering? The understorey of suffering is hidden by more explicit dialogues on scientific progress and social justice in order to implicitly reduce suffering. However, the relationship between suffering, scientific progress and social justice is not linear in an inverted form or otherwise. Suffering itself gets lost. But when this happens, theories can become even more abstracted and rhetorical, such as those in behavioural change or public health. Perhaps the only way to mitigate against abstraction and rhetoric is to make suffering foundational in health professional education (Figure 3.1).

Suffering as a foundation for health professional practice and education keeps the patient explicitly at the core. Knowing as a basic premise that not only do health professionals cause suffering as part of an intervention (Ferrell & Coyle, 2008) but the very nature of disease – being in hospital, traumatic events – induces suffering therefore means that the way healthcare is taught must change. Taking suffering as the understorey of healthcare provides guide rails that could otherwise be missed by stories of scientific progress and social justice. Guide rails of indeterminacy, precarity and a life without stability that

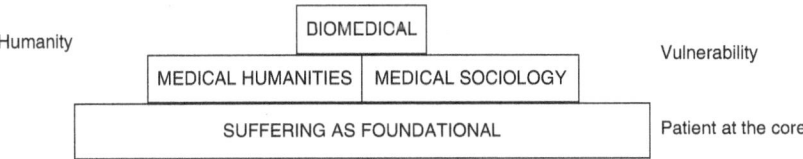

Figure 3.1 Suffering as foundational in health professional education.

as humans we presupposed and dreamed of through the Industrial Revolution and modernisation (Tsing, 2015). When life seems to fail, we can turn to patchiness, "a mosaic of open-ended assemblages of entangled ways of life, with each further opening into a mosaic of temporal rhythms and spatial arcs" (Tsing, 2015, p. 4). These sorts of notions are new to healthcare and health professional education but show the shift that may be necessary to reduce the sense of alienation over suffering.

Suffering is an understorey to the larger story of life as we know it; how we undergo, engage and respond to suffering are determined in large part by how we define suffering and the sorts of categories we use to try and gain some traction on the experience and notion of suffering. Definitions and categories of suffering in turn determine the theories we use in suffering. How these theories intersect with medical humanities and medical sociology will be explored in the following sections.

3.2.2 Categories or types of suffering

Table 3.1 shows a range of suffering experiences from the individual to the collective. There is no doubt that suffering has preoccupied humans throughout the ages; it is just that little of this preoccupation has formally concerned health professionals since it is not included in their education. Suffering is considered a spiritual, philosophical, psychological and socio-logical concern. As an example, Buddhists' primary concern is with suffering – there are three main types according to Ekman and Ekman (2016, p. 4):

1   Explicit suffering – due to injury or disease – pain sensations and mental anguish are included here, real or imagined. This is known as the "suffering of suffering."
2   The suffering of change – everything is impermanent and our failure to accept this is what causes suffering. The reification (reinforcement and celebration) of the self's independent and unchanging existence is a false premise upon which we base our lives, according to Buddhist philosophy. Cravings – the discomfort and unease of not getting what we want – and aversion – getting what we do not want –apparently come from not accepting the ever changing nature of things, people or situations.
3   All-pervasive suffering – basically conceived of as the unsatisfactory nature of all forms of existence. This is a feeling that nothing is quite the way we want it, ennui, with a habitual mental habit of wanting things to be different. The authors identified what type of suffering they were encountering in order to determine what type of compassion to cultivate. There was also the notion that some people have the suffering of all people in their emotional database (Ekman & Ekman, 2016, p. 48).

The Buddhist ideas on suffering centre on the illusory nature of the self, with a view to transcending the self. Briefly, this transcendence of self could be seen as an expression of suffering, rather than its antidote. Still heavily based on masculinist assumptions of autonomy and individualism, this kind of transcendence has the propensity to allow more suffering through making a part of ourselves wrong. Thankfully there are more ways than this of regarding suffering.

Regarding suffering as a basic part of human life means accepting that all consciousness is consciousness of death and suffering (Unamuno, 2013). Turning towards suffering and embracing it adds substance to our lives since we are embracing all that consciousness perceives. Turning towards and entering suffering means having different tools at our disposal than just transcendence. Nietzsche wrote of the creative function of suffering (Nietzsche, 2013). The Islamic Sufi poet Rumi wrote in "Choose a suffering": "Everyone chooses a suffering that will change him or her to a well-baked loaf" (Barks, 2001, p. 25). Rumi noted that suffering could be pragmatic and practical as much as esoteric and existential (stories, searching for evidence, soul work). He emphasises the concrete and also includes narrative, abstract conceptualisations and the process of suffering as something akin to baking – a transformative process.

The spiritual legacy that goes with suffering cannot be denied. Categories of purpose and meaning of suffering include purifying the soul, ennobling the person and a path to spiritual growth through moral challenges (Hofmann, 2015). The boundary between hospital and religion has not always been clear, so there may be leakage in meaning between the two. This can be the case in palliative care, for example, where existential suffering is seen as a psychological or spiritual condition that robs individuals of their capacity for peace in that present state of being (in Boston et al, 2011; Williams, 2004). The difference between psychological or spiritual seems to be a moot point when one clearly relates to the other.

Further categories of existential suffering in psychotherapy, for example, include death anxiety; freedom as it provides the opportunity for choice, responsibility and guilt; isolation or the unbridgeable gulf between people and meaninglessness (Yalom, 1980). Whilst it is not always clear what is meant by suffering, and that perhaps a decided absence of any fixed definition may be preferable, there is a prevailing theme of the notion of suffering as a personal, dynamic, moving and emergent process rather than a fixed entity of suffering (Yalom, 1980). Yalom draws on theories of existentialism as propounded by Kierkegaard, Frankl, Sartre, de Beauvoir and Heidegger. The theme across these theorists is that human existence is the starting point for everything we do, and this existence is seen as concrete, personal, individual, riven with choices and concomitant anxiety, as well as ambiguous to the core – we have to do two near-impossible things at once – understand ourselves as limited by circumstances and yet continue to pursue our projects as though we were truly in control. This freedom alongside contingency exerts a psychological pull, and it is this perceived notion of freedom that could be seen as being at the root of existential suffering. That is, everything that impinges on our entitlement to freedom could be seen as a source of suffering. Categories of suffering tend to determine the type of response to suffering that is seen as beneficial (Kissane, 2012). Table 3.2 shows a range of possible responses to different categories of suffering.

These categories and responses are by no means intended as a recipe for attending to suffering. Rather, they are meant to demonstrate the limited means we have for speaking about suffering, even though that suffering is perhaps becoming more visible.

Iris Murdoch noted many years ago (1997) that suffering has become more visible through technology – "we are not only coming into possession of the means to cure ills, we are in the position of not being able to avoid quite literally seeing them" (p. 230). From a sociological perspective, the suffering society has more means to record and monitor suffering than ever and yet the means to address this seem to be ever receding:

> [W]e see that we are still even now patently unable to set things to rights, unable to stop famine in India or war in Africa. I think this is fundamentally the situation which drives young people into a kind of frenzy.
>
> (Murdoch, 1997, p. 230)

It could be said that each cohort has its own form of generational suffering. Perhaps this generation of young people may achieve more than their predecessors, seeing as suffering is perhaps more visible than previously. The different generational suffering is another category of individual and social suffering.

The different categories of suffering have so far not mentioned suffering by race, gender, ethnicity, family status, religion, sexual orientation and disability – all of which have been sources of tremendous suffering from a

Table 3.2 Possible responses to suffering

Art	Spiritual	Social Justice	Science
Sublimation	Transcendence	Restoration	Transcendence
Catharsis	Salvation	Activism	Prevention
Transform to a purer form	Redemption		Denial
Transcendence	Compassion		Avoidance
Dissociation	Purifying		Distancing
Self-regulation			Ignore
Introspection			Disconnect
Protection			Walling off
Haptic			Surgery
			Medication
			Treatments

socialised perspective. This absence has the potential to make suffering appear decontextualised and abstract, distanced from the lived experience. The experience of suffering can become the abstract touchlessness when people are seen without the context or concrete social influences. Statistical summaries of suffering have their place in governance and planning but sight should never be lost of the lived experience, the particularities and detail of suffering (Nussbaum, 1986).

One last challenge to categories of suffering between the individual and social is in the difficulty of separating out suffering from patients and that of the observing health professional, or witness (Behar, 1997; Ferrell & Coyle, 2008). What seems to happen is that the shared human experience of suffering seems to cross diversity and boundaries of patients, professionals, contexts and disciplines – "We are all, at the core, human beings experiencing illness or responding to suffering. The human suffering is more similar than different" (Ferrell & Coyle, 2008, p. 19).

> There is often an inseparable relationship between the suffering person and the suffering of those professionals who witness suffering whilst providing care. This relationship can be close and intense, and each party is vulnerable to the other.
>
> (Ferrell & Coyle, 2008, p. 87)

Whilst culture may well influence the acceptance, expression, perception, interpretation and response to suffering, the embodied experience of human suffering can be shared. This mutability of suffering as cultural, shared yet also individual, perhaps provides opportunities as well as challenges in how to respond in healthcare and the kinds of theories useful in understanding suffering.

3.3 Methodological plurality and theories – increasing the granularity

Having laid out the field of suffering and the notions associated with it, the next section lays out the linguistic veil of different disciplines drawn on to provide theoretical background. The point of this section is to describe the different way that phenomena can be explained or modelled. Both the sciences and medical humanities use various forms or models to describe suffering and produce challenges and dilemmas as a result. Each is trying to describe reality in its own ways and here there is a sense of unity at the highest order of explanation (Carusi, 2016). This section is crucial to foreground the kinds of dilemmas in integrating medical humanities and sociology into an understanding of suffering. Various ways of working with medical humanities and medicine have been suggested with the most recent proposing medical humanities has a role to play in cultural crossings of care, that is, in a bidirectional negotiation of the gap between objective biomedical science and subjective relativism of the humanities (Engebretsen et al, 2020; Kristeva et al, 2018).

However, critically interrogating both biomedicine (simplistic reductions to biology) and the humanities (simplistic reductions of suffering and health injustice to cultural relativism; Kristeva et al, 2018) means coming up against issues of representationalism and cognitive solipsism as outlined in Chapter 1, Section 1.8.3. The point is to embrace methodological plurality without reinscribing false dichotomies that only perpetuate exclusionary practices.

Nearly a century ago, Bernard wrote on the role of feeling, and hence subjectivity, in experimental method in medicine, including different forms of knowing:

> Feeling, from which everything emanates, must keep its complete spontaneity and all its freedom for putting forth experimental ideas; reason also must preserve that freedom to doubt, which forces it always to submit ideas to the test of experiment. Just as, in other human actions, feeling releases an act by putting forth the idea which gives a motive to action, so in the experimental method feeling takes the initiative through the idea. Feeling alone guides the mind and constitutes the *primaum movens* of science ... but we must never forget, that correctness of feeling and fertility of idea can be established and proved only by experiment.
>
> (Bernard, 1957, p. 43)

Slightly more recently, Van der Schaaf et al (2019) discuss the role of embodied cognition, clearly demonstrating the interrelationship between mind, body and the environment. "'Knowing how' is the ability to co-ordinate mind, body and tools in an environment into a dynamic system geared to a specific purpose" (p. 219). Embodied cognition uses the range of ideas from cognitive internal representations with a bodily origin to a radical enactivist view that avoids assumptions about internal representations (Van der Schaaf et al, 2019). The authors' assumption rests on the view that cognition sparks from stimulating a motor-action neural circuit during bodily interactions with the physical environment (Van der Schaaf et al, 2019). Action and perception are bound by purpose, which means that in a consideration of suffering, where the purpose is to understand and respond to suffering, there are many lacunae around notions of reality.

In order to work from a place of unity rather than adversity, that is, where both objectivity (external reality processed through perception and nervous system) and subjectivity in cognitive solipsistic (external reality all in inner landscape) models of evidence can complement each other, an assumption is required that neither on their own will be able to provide a complete understanding or knowledge of suffering (Carusi, 2016). Both medical humanities and biomedical science, as well as sociology, offer partial perspectives, so these disciplines are more united by the spaces, gaps and lacunae.

Both science and medical humanities from a modernist perspective are defined by the reality they cannot grasp, as much as they are defined by what they can grasp. In other words, and this has been particularly relevant over the last few months in relation to COVID-19, it is a case of all hands to the pump in an effort at combined critical scholarship. Thinking about how we think about suffering in terms of the theoretically different standpoints of psychology, psychoanalytic, hermeneutics, phenomenology, critical race studies, sociology, biomedical and philosophical existential issues means having a wide range of tools at our disposal that are focused on the particularities of suffering and how we stitch that understanding together.

A combined approach requires a critical analysis of language, meaning signifiers, historical colonial constructions, etc., as well as accepting and building on materiality and embodiment:

> The material and semiotic aspects of things and processes are complementary to one another. They describe two different systems of relationships that we can construct among objects and processes. One of these is the familiar system of material, physical, chemical, thermodynamic, ecological relations webs of material interaction. The other is the semiotic system of relationships of meaning: similarity, difference, categorization, ordering and association etc.
>
> (Lemke, 1994, p. 6)

> Paradigmatic relations define contrasting alternatives, meaningful differences within similarity. Syntagmatic relations tell us what parts make up some whole. ... Intertextual, or indexical, relations tell us in a broader sense what goes with what. (p. 7)

> You can continue to believe that there is an objective external reality out there somewhere, and that truth is the common quality of propositions that correctly describe it, so long as you do not use these assumptions to try and gain power over your opponents in intellectual debate. (p. 7)

A combined approach means therefore that science and medical humanities work together with multimodal representations to learn about suffering. In this case, there is movement between and within both modernist and postmodernist ideologies on the basis that there is unity at the level of attempting to model or represent reality (Table 3.3).

3.4 Theories of suffering

There are three main theories or bodies of work that pertain to suffering that will be explored here: cultural melancholy (Singleton, 2015), the suffering stranger (Orange, 2011) and phenomenology as it relates to social justice (Levin, 1991). Each draws on theories within different disciplines to

Table 3.3 Multimodal representations when learning about suffering

Mode	Concrete	Conceptual	Narrative	Symbolic	Abstract
Epistemology (nature of knowledge)	Embodied cognition Phenomenological Materialism	Biomedical Modernism	Stories Interpretive Meaning	Metaphors	Deconstruction
Pedagogical aspects (organisational meanings)		Split into different disciplines Behaviourist Theories of motivation Social cognitive theory Cognitive theories Affective theories	Hermeneutics	Sociocultural theories of learning Relational pedagogy	Analysis of binaries e.g. subject-object
Orientational meanings (social aspects)			Sociocultural theories of learning Relational pedagogy	Bridging gap	Governmentality Differend Nomadology Intertextuality
Theories on suffering	Psychoanalytic Cultural melancholy	Social Determinants of Health Health inequities	Critical Pedagogy Critical race theories		Will to abstraction
Epistemological ⟶					Ontological

enrich understanding of suffering, and therefore the theories are not limited to the ones above. However, they are the main ones described here. Part of the difficulty in explaining this section is that there is overlap between different areas of study and gaps in others such as sociology and medical humanities. This will become apparent as the following will show.

Cultural melancholy draws on interdisciplinary theories of psychoanalysis, critical race studies and socioeconomic history to make visible the hole at the centre of suffering. This suffering, whilst always individual, is contextualised by a particular history. Thus a sociology of suffering is necessary that can take into account both the individual and social nature of suffering. However, social sciences in general have not integrated cultural melancholy into their thinking and so have floundered in their progress to address suffering.

The social sciences are concerned with society, organisations and the relationships among individuals within society. Sociology could be seen as always having been concerned with suffering, yet a sociological theory of suffering remains elusive (Wilkinson, 2005). In part, the frustration of a cohesive sociological analysis of suffering could be due to the inadequacies of categories of thinking about suffering; it "falters upon the intrigue of its own making" (Wilkinson, 2005; p. 37). In order to understand more about the frustration at the heart of exploring suffering, it seems necessary to make explicit the conundrum between the social and individual perspectives on suffering.

The crucial understanding required to progress is that suffering is socially constructed and personally experienced. Therefore theories of suffering must encompass macro social theories as well as micro embodied individual theories and the relationship between the two. Both socially and personally, suffering comes up against limits:

- Language
- Disciplinary
- Analytical
- Visual
- Emotional
- Cognitive (Wilkinson, 2005)

Coming up against these limits can provide a compulsion to keep trying to explain, frustration, struggle and a war against the paradox of suffering – making itself known whilst at the same time obscuring itself from ever being fully realised (Wilkinson, 2005). He suggests we generate styles of writing that involve:

> readers as much as possible in experiencing the moral confusion and intellectual frustration of attempting to make sense of suffering, on the understanding that, within this struggle, we are made to address

fundamental questions of human value, origins and purpose; associated with political risks and ethical dilemmas.

(Wilkinson, 2005, p. 14)

In short, we are expected to come undone.

To return to theories of suffering, then, we must know how to cross the bridge between social and individual perspectives on suffering and the relationship between them. Singleton has accomplished this elegantly with his interdisciplinary cultural melancholy work on critical race studies, psychoanalysis and socioeconomic history. Melancholy is a psychic state wherein losses of self are retained and at the same time barred from conscious recognition – "a loss that claims yet cannot be claimed" (Singleton, 2015, p. 4). This loss of self seems to be similar to the hole described in suffering. Cultural melancholy uncovers a host of hidden dialogues – the understorey – hidden affects (emotions) and disavowed social loss of cultural practices of racialisation. Singleton (2015) refers to Freud's idea on melancholy as a loss that is unmourned and barred from recognition, which is then unconsciously displaced discreetly on to the subject's sense of self, or ego, thereby enacting an unconscionable loss of self, similar to the hole experienced in suffering in healthcare. The sense of inexplicable loss means that words are lost. The loss of words to describe emotions hidden from view by cultural forces means there is a hole in the experience of the self.

The trinity of impossible mourning of cultural melancholy are avowed affect, hidden affect and the disavowed loss of self (Singleton, 2015). This trinity is inherently bound up with the white mainstream Other through the means of social crisis, ritual and process of subject formation. This means that the hidden understorey is maintained through re-enactment, which produces a stable coherent person who is also insecure and torn with contradictions (Singleton, 2015). There is always a dialogic inherent in the loss or hole at the centre of the self, between self and other. This hole is reinforced by repetitive rituals between persons in an unconscious racialised manner. Self and other are both involved in the introjection of loss; the racialised subject through a lost, never possible social perfection, an inarticulable loss that informs a sense of subjectivity to white people (Singleton, 2015). White people secure their authority and identity through melancholic introjection of racial others (objects) "that it can neither fully relinquish nor accommodate and whose ghostly presence nonetheless guarantees its centrality" (Cheng Xi quoted by Singleton, 2015, p. 9). Thus both are implicated by one another.

Being hidden, this loss at the heart of the sense of self underscores, circumvents and obstructs the process of working through the legacy of racial slavery: "At ease with grievances but not with grief" (Singleton, 2015, p. 10). The melancholy takes a particular form because the ego can't see or claim loss – there are multiple and contradictory emotions which are high maintenance in their unassimilability, which wrestle with one another for attention, where affective states smoulder under the surface of personality, blocking one another from getting the upper hand (Singleton, 2015). The ego demands to see itself through difference whilst struggling to bar loss of self from recognition.

Cultural melancholy is a particular type of suffering that produces both stability and insecurity. The materialisation of this type of suffering renders visible the understorey of the loss of self in relation with others. The lacunae reaches across horizontal and vertical connections, whilst the substrate or understorey is always one of suffering producing a visual crisis whereby whiteness is invisible and blackness is visible. Singleton (2015) shows the extraordinary power of an interdisciplinary work that deepens our understanding through an exploration that both challenges as well as draws on at the same time categories of race in the service of suffering.

Singleton (2015) calls for interdisciplinary surmounting of the clinical separation of ethnic studies, psychoanalysis and socioeconomic history because doing so is essential to re-engage and resolve racial grievances. The interdisciplinarity requires that we work across theories as well as disciplines to put words to the understorey of suffering and melancholy. There are a host of hidden dialogues – "psychic, social, personal and political, individual and collective, past and present" (Singleton, 2015, p. 2) that continue to contribute to racial subjugation and inequality. Inherent in the experience of cultural melancholy is the dialogic between self and other, not unlike that between health professional and patient. Theories relating to the therapeutic relationship will now be reviewed.

Orange (2011) proposes drawing on hermeneutics or understanding and interpreting itself as a way of making sense of what happens between two people when one is trying to understand another's suffering. Implicit in Orange's (2011) proposal are philosophy, phenomenology and existentialism. Again there is the idea of putting ourselves at risk as we leave aside our competence and work in the dark in a dialogic process that tries to understand the other. There is acknowledgment of various embodied entities – face, hands, voice, the gaze – in relation with the other, where suffering is palpable yet ungraspable, an infinite demand of the-one-for-the-other (Orange, 2011). The assumptions underpinning understanding are that this is hard, incomplete and disruptive, and we can expect to be affected. Yet this work is built on principles of hospitality, trust, radical finitude, relational – nonjudgmental, nonviolence, gentleness and an infinite responsibility. She draws on phenomenology, the study of human experience; the structures of consciousness from the perspective of "I" where "'I' am I insofar as I am affected" and "Who am I, so inconstant, that not withstanding, you count on me?" (Orange, 2011, pp. 48, 51).

The tension in suffering between inconstancy and constancy, becoming undone and providing a constancy that can be relied on tears at the fabric of what and how we know ourselves to be. Therefore, at the heart of theories of suffering there is a rending of ideas, perceptions and judgments about self. At the time when one must stand firm with courage in the face of suffering, the very ground on which we stand can feel as if it is collapsing underneath us. Yet there is a propulsion to keep moving forward, to skip lightly over intransigent mobile suspended stepping stones, to get to the other side. Making these characteristics of suffering explicit, to encompass both the process, tension, conflict and embodied sense, seems a big ask but one that is necessary.

In some ways, Levin (1991) suggests that this task of living with suffering is something that we are primed to do just from the fact of being embodied, in terms of Merleau Ponty's phenomenological conception of body-subject. Recognising our deeply intersubjective nature means that we are inherently tied up together as Singleton (2015) suggests in the inherent dialogic and the introjection of loss between both self and other. The body of experience senses injustice and the absence of reciprocity when it occurs. This seems to have direct relevance to the understanding of suffering, or not, that occurs between health professional and patient. That perhaps when the words are lost to signify suffering, then the body can become the vehicle of expression.

3.5 How does this all fit together?

Drawing on the lacunae metaphor described in the first chapter, the different theories in use such as cultural melancholy, suffering stranger and the phenomenological body subject work to represent the cell body of the osteocyte in the lacunae, the processes and structures that reach out to the surrounding social matrix and other cell bodies in their lacunae as well as the materiality of the body in the spaces. In Chapter Four, theories and perspectives on the self will be explored in greater detail since they impact how we perceive and respond to suffering. Suffice to say at this time, some of the social and cultural ideas there are about the self can impact on an embodied subjective level so that while our bodies and self may feel like the psychological isolate that Gerada (2019) described rattling around alone in the social matrix, partly this is because of the way we look at life. There is much more to explore here on the social constructedness of self and body and how we represent these to ourselves.

This is the very point at which critical medical humanities and sociology have much to contribute, albeit in a different form than currently, and this will be explored further in Chapter Four. The gaps currently in these disciplines is that they do not acknowledge the key features and definitions of suffering, especially in the construction of self. These gaps occur along fault lines (Mendenhall, 2019), as exemplified by the lacunae metaphor. Therefore, as emphasised in Chapter One, a different way of thinking about suffering is required which critical medical humanities can facilitate if it can move beyond the false dichotomy of subjectivity and objectivity. Before moving on to Chapter Four, a brief recap of Chapters One and Two will be provided in order to show the groundwork of suffering upon which any new medical humanities scholarly activity must be based.

Given that suffering is such an embodied response, albeit with lacunae – the hole and speechlessness – then a phenomenological account is necessary. The embodied experiential account of suffering also relates to social norms – being on the wrong side of the fault line (Frank, 2001) – and is mediated by and through relationships, both between and within health professional and patient and society. Therefore relational accounts are also necessary, such as those suggested by Fiske (1993) which take into account the relationship with religious authority and preferences in attitudes towards suffering, such as transcendence, redemption and salvation. Science, art, spirituality and social justice also exhibit attitudes towards suffering that construct the experience of suffering, often out of conscious awareness. This can also be reflected in the individual forms of avowed and disavowed grief, and the displacement or loss of the self. Health professionals are implicated in this since there tends to be silence in their training in relation to suffering, even though this can form a large part of their workload and to which they themselves are not immune. The silence in training on suffering can result in a curious state of affairs whereby whilst working alongside suffering, health professionals focus on tasks to get them through, perhaps as a protection of place and space, and so may appear as if they are denying that suffering exists.

This curious state of affairs is mediated by reversals, absences of self and metaphors cropping up in texts and speech. Therefore a plurality of approaches is required – embodied experiential, relational and linguistic – with each having reference to pedagogy that is concrete, conceptual, narrative, symbolic and abstract. The materiality of the body is tied up with issues of self and identity – I felt I was not who I used to be (Frank, 2001) – and so suffering is less about causality and more about response and meaning, in the context of writing about medical humanities and sociology. Until we can understand suffering as a foundational experience, one replete with reversals, absences, disavowed grief and an unconscionable loss of self (Singleton, 2015), then I don't see how progress can be made whilst working solely from the basis of an autonomous psychological isolate (Gerada, 2019) who exerts control and agency. Humans are all these things and more. The time has come though to acknowledge suffering and situational patterns of working with it, or denying it, to see how suffering is.

Part of seeing through the eyes of an observer is the notion that health professionals may feel complicit in perpetuating suffering because they carry large levels of responsibility and have been able to do little to change the suffering in the world (Zembylas, 2019). They may engage more in culpable thinking and this could account for some of the high rates of burnout of health professionals, especially since workplace conditions associated with burnout seem entrenched. Including shame as a relational solidarity with the Other may bridge the epistemic gap between health professionals and patients in order to be able to understand both.

Perhaps, overall, the following chapters will demonstrate how we are all implicated in suffering as a reflection of our basic humanness. At present, suffering tends to be a decontextualised embodied experience, individualised and yet generally unnameable, whilst a certain section of the community are able to focus on doing in a mainstream cognitive capacity. Yet the implication of suffering still exists no matter how busy we become. These two extremes – individualised suffering versus a focus on cognitive competency – provide a tension in healthcare. The challenge is to work with both and find a way through by stitching together what we know about suffering.

The following suffering framework aims to do so by resting on these underpinning assumptions:

1   People may not know cognitively the experience of suffering; it may be outside their awareness or consciousness because of the speechlessness that accompanies suffering.
2   Both health professionals and patients are involved, intersubjectively, with/in suffering.
3   Any works on the self have to take into account the hole in the self. Therefore previous assumptions that prevail in mainstream about the self do not apply in the experience of suffering. Yet both suffering and not suffering belong to the self.
4   Critical race theory must be included in any exposition on suffering in order to counter knowledge and attitudes built upon colonialist projects of the self.
5   Given all the above assumptions, compassion is necessary to move beyond exclusionary practices and epistemic injustice. The epistemic gap is between suffering and mainstream practices.

Therefore, the suffering framework explored in this book has three main areas of activity to address the epistemic gap between suffering and mainstream practices – stitching across the social matrix, deconstruction through questions and containing as a metaphor for surviving suffering. These activities work with the vertical and horizontal axes of languishing-acting and self-other (Devisch et al, 2017). Implicit in these activities and dimensions are theories relating to the holy trinity of cultural melancholy (Singleton, 2015); relational models (Fiske, 1993) and properties including transcendence, salvation and redemption; and phenomenology to explore the embodied experience of suffering further in the sense of embodied cognition (see Figure 3.2).

Clearly medical humanities has a role to play in developing and using this framework. This role will be explored further in the next chapter. At this stage, it is clear that the awareness of suffering from an observer's point of view shows patterns of denial and nothingness in relation to the social construction and individual experience of suffering. Yet that same awareness can also identify more – the real something under the nothing (Whyte, 2018) – that critical medical humanities can contribute to if it so chooses.

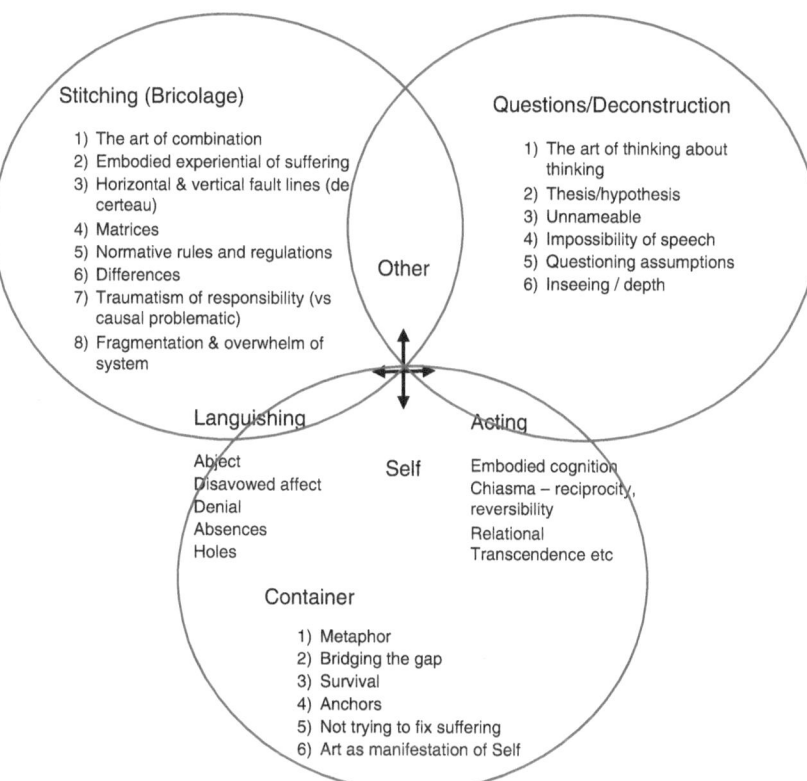

Stitching (Bricolage)

1) The art of combination
2) Embodied experiential of suffering
3) Horizontal & vertical fault lines (de certeau)
4) Matrices
5) Normative rules and regulations
6) Differences
7) Traumatism of responsibility (vs causal problematic)
8) Fragmentation & overwhelm of system

Other

Questions/Deconstruction

1) The art of thinking about thinking
2) Thesis/hypothesis
3) Unnameable
4) Impossibility of speech
5) Questioning assumptions
6) Inseeing / depth

Languishing

Abject
Disavowed affect
Denial
Absences
Holes

Self

Acting

Embodied cognition
Chiasma – reciprocity, reversibility
Relational
Transcendence etc

Container

1) Metaphor
2) Bridging the gap
3) Survival
4) Anchors
5) Not trying to fix suffering
6) Art as manifestation of Self

Figure 3.2 Framework of suffering.

Box 3.1   Reflection

Aspects of suffering remain unspeakable. Aspects may remain at the level of bodily experience for which there are no words and so it is the body that needs attending to. This is a very strange paradox in healthcare. As shown in the preface, health professionals want to attend to suffering and do so fervently by their attention to the body in terms of measurements of blood pressure, heart rate and rhythm, blood gases and so on. Health professionals believe they are attending to suffering by watching over these concrete objective signs and symptoms and thereby making a correct course of action for treatment and diagnosis. Emotions and feelings seem somewhat more nebulous and abstract as implied through their absence in training. And it would seem somewhat mealy mouthed of patients to complain about the lack of embodied experiential attention to emotions and feelings when they have survived a life-threatening experience through the care of their health professionals.

However, the paradox is that through this process, patients feel objectified and alienated from themselves and their families – their experiential embodied reality is what seems more real and concrete to them. Health professionals respond to overt suffering through compassionate care, yet there is much to explore with this term. For example, at a recent forum, when asked what constitutes compassionate care, the idea that knowing about suffering was seen as interesting but not concrete enough or compulsory for delivering compassionate care. What seems to get us over the fault line is the sense of our shared humanity, as Victor Frankl noted.

However, even the concept of shared humanity is not straightforward. Health professionals may draw the line at sharing their own feelings with patients or debate when or how much to empathise with patients and to what purpose. From their own experience of being patients, the last thing health professionals want is an emotionally overwrought worker, and sometimes they prefer not to state their own profession in order to remain anonymous from that perspective. Yet there are subtleties; when dying, patients and families appreciate knowing they have connected and moved health professionals. The question seems to be more about what are some of the consequences of our shared humanity in the clinical situation and how much of these are influenced by the culture around suffering. How can we know this?

Questions for reflection

1   How do you see concrete experiences of suffering? How do these experiences relate to concepts about suffering?
2   Think about an example of suffering in your own life and the narratives, symbols and abstract ideas about that. Which was easier for you to consider? What preference do you have for thinking about suffering and how does this influence how you see suffering in other people?
3   What concepts and narratives can you think of that relate to the idea of shared humanity?
4   Reflect on Orange's (2011) words: "Who am I, so inconstant, that notwithstanding, you can count on me?" What does this mean to you in terms of your own identity and sense of self in the face of suffering?
5   What does "becoming undone" mean to you and how do you feel about that notion?

Further Resources
Frankl V.E. 1997. *Man's Search for Ultimate Meaning*. Plenum Press: New York.

References

Arendt H. 1971. Thinking and moral considerations: A lecture. *Social Research*; 38(3):417–446.

Barks C. 2001. *The Soul of Rumi – A New Collection of Ecstatic Poems*. Translation, Introduction and notes by Coleman Barks. Harper San Francisco: New York.

Behar R. 1997. The vulnerable observer. *Anthropology that Breaks Your Heart*. Penguin Random House: New York.

Bernard C. 1957. *An Introduction to the Study of Experimental Medicine*. Dover Publications: New York.

Boston P., Bruce A., Schreiber R. 2011. Existential suffering in the palliative care setting: An integrated literature review. *Journal of Pain and Symptom Management*; 41(3):604–618.

Cain S. 2012. *Quiet: The Power of Introverts in a World That Can't Stop Talking*. Crown Publishing Group.

Carusi A. 2016. Modelling systems biomedicine: Intertwinement and the 'real'. Chapter 2 in *Edinburgh Handbook of Medical Humanities*. Whitehead A., Woods A (eds). Edinburgh University Press: Edinburgh.

Cassell E.J. 2004. *The Nature of Suffering and the Goals of Medicine*. Oxford University Press: Oxford.

Devisch I., Vanheule S., Deveugele M. Nola I., Civaner M., Pype P. 2017. Victims of disaster: Can ethical debriefings be of help to care for their suffering? *Medical Health Care and Philosophy*; 20:257–267.

Ekman P., Ekman E. 2016. Is Global compassion achievable? Chapter 4, in *The Oxford Handbook of Compassion Science*. Seppälä E.M., Simon-Thomas E., Brown S.L., Worline M.C., Cameron C.D., Doty J.R. (eds). Oxford University Press: New York.

Engebretsen E., Fraas Henrichsen G., Ødemark J. 2020. Towards a translational medical humanities: Introducing the cultural crossings of care [published online ahead of print, 2020 Apr 27]. *Medical Humanities*. doi: 10.1136/medhum 2019-011751.

Ferrell B.R., Coyle N. 2008. The nature of suffering and the goals of nursing. *Oncology Nursing Forum*; 35(2):241–247.

Fiske A.P. 1993. *Structures of Social Life: The Four Elementary Forms of Human Relations*. The Free Press: New York.

Francis R. 2013. Report of the Mid Staffordshire NHS Foundation Trust Public Inquiry. https://www.gov.uk/government/publications/report-of-the-mid-staffordshire-nhs-foundation-trust-public-inquiry.

Frank A.W. 2001. Can we research suffering? *Qualitative Health Research*; 11(3):353–362.

Frank A.W. 2013. *The Wounded Storyteller: Body, Illness, and Ethics*, Second Edition. The University of Chicago Press: London.

Gerada C. 2019. The making of a doctor: The matrix and self. *Group Analysis*; 52(3):350–361. doi:10.1177/0533316418823117.

Hofmann, B. 2015. Suffering: Harm to bodies, minds, and persons. In: Edwards S., Schramme T. (eds.) *Handbook of Concepts in the Philosophy of Medicine*. Springer: Berlin.

Kissane D.W. 2012. The relief of existential suffering. *Archives of Internal Medicine*; 172(19):1501–1505.

Kristeva J., Moro M.R., Ødemark J., Engebretsen E. 2018. Cultural crossings of care: An appeal to the medical humanities. *BMJ Medical Humanities*; 44:55–58.

Lemke J.L. 1994. Semiotics and the deconstruction of conceptual learning. *Journal of the Society for Accelerative Learning and Teaching*. http://academic.brooklyn.cuny.edu/education/jlemke/papers/jsalt.htm.

Levin D.M. 1991. Visions of narcissism: Intersubjectivity and the reversals of reflection. Chapter 3, in *Merleau Ponty Vivant*. Dillon M.C (ed). State University of New York Press: Albany.

Marmot M., Allen J., Boyce T., Goldblatt P., Morrison J. 2020. *Health Equity in England: The Marmot Review 10 Years on*. Institute of Health Equity: London.

Mendenhall E. 2019. *Rethinking Diabetes: Entanglement with Trauma, Poverty and HIV*. Cornell University Press: London.

Metzl J.M., Hansen H. 2014. Structural competency: Theorizing a new medical engagement with stigma and inequality. *Social Science & Medicine*; 103:126–133.

Murdoch I. 1997. *Existentialists and Mystics: Writings on Philosophy and Literature*. Penguin Books: London.

Nietzsche F. 2013. *On the Genealogy of Morals*. Penguin Putnam Inc: New York.

Nussbaum M.C. 1986 *The Fragility of Goodness: Luck and Ethics in Greek Tragedy and Philosophy*. Cambridge University Press: Cambridge.

Orange D.M. 2011. *The Suffering Stranger: Hermeneutics for Everyday Clinical Practice*. Routledge: New York.

Phillips, A. 1999. *Darwin's Worms. On Life Stories and Death Stories*. Faber & Faber: London.

Rilke R.M. 2005. *The Book of Hours: Love Poems to God*. Penguin Putnam Inc: New York.

Singleton J. 2015. *Cultural Melancholy: Readings of Race, Impossible Mourning, and African American Ritual*. University of Illinois Press: Champaign, IL.

Tsing A.L. 2015. *The Mushroom at the End of the World: On the Possibility of life in Capitalist Ruins*. Princeton University Press: New Jersey.

Unamuno M.D. 2013. It is only suffering that makes us persons. *The Philosophy Book*. Penguin Random House: London. p. 233.

Van der Schaaf M., Bakker A., Cate O.T. 2019. When I say ... embodied cognition. *Medical Education*; 53:219–220.

Waldman D.A., Carmeli A., Halevi M.Y. 2011. Beyond the red tape: How victims of terrorism perceive and react to organizational responses to their suffering. *Journal of Organizational Behavior*; 32:938–954.

Whyte D. 2018. *Compass points: Setting direction for a future life: A week in the English Lake District*, June 29, 2018–July 6, 2018.

Wilkinson I. 2005. *Suffering: A Sociological Introduction*. Polity Press: Cambridge.

Williams B. 2004. Dying young, dying poor: A sociological examination of existential suffering among low socio-economic status patients. *Journal of Palliative Medicine*; 7:27–37

Yalom I. 1980. *Existential Psychotherapy*. Basic Books: New York.

Zembylas M. 2019. "Shame at being human" as a transformative political concept and praxis: Pedagogical possibilities. *Feminism & Psychology*; 29(2):303–321.

4 Sorting the wood from the trees

Challenges integrating medical humanities and sociology into a medical curriculum

4.1 Introduction

Medical humanities provides a deepening of observation and perception when reflecting on a subject which is not often available through biomedical science:

> Each discipline or art invoked the powers of observation to intuit living action beneath the surface of natural form; each excited a more intense perception of truth through penetrating glance and comparative vision; each achieved through comprehension of the pain of truth a parallel satisfaction and calm wonder.
>
> (de Almeida, 1991, p. 48)

However, this deepening of reflection does not come without a conflict between what medical students, for example, feel they should be doing in relation to their learning.

Often when supervising medical students on a critical medical humanities project, we have a conversation around the fear of being allowed to study a topic in medical humanities and what would happen if anyone (peers, clinicians, lecturers) found out. Such is their concern, they question their decision and doubt themselves as they know this is not mainstream medicine, and yet they are also driven by a usually compelling desire to learn more and are completely engaged in the process. The stigma associated with studying medical humanities in medical school is about the perception that medical humanities and sociology are not seen as "proper" sciences and therefore not useful. Part of this perception must come from the way medical humanities is presented as well as a cultivated prejudice from competitive medical schools intent on developing scientific prize scholars, research funding bodies that prize the latest biochemical findings and public demand for cures for diseases. The sense of having to choose one form of learning over another (Greenhalgh et al., 2016), and then condemning the rejected one into the academic wastebasket, seems to add to the confusion surrounding medical humanities, especially when medical students have been selected on their ability to be an all-round student who may well have studied art, music, history or the social sciences before coming to medical school.

By learning to feel ashamed perhaps about these subjects as a focus of study (as opposed to a "hobby") at medical school, medical students may be learning to distance themselves from resources which may help them in times of distress (Hardacre & Margetts, 2020). The confusion surrounding the value of medical humanities and sociology in medical school is also a temporal phenomenon since in the past earlier forms of medicine promoted the use of poetry and creativity (de Almeida, 1991). Partly, the subsequent distancing from art and poetry was to ensure the robustness of medical practice and to protect the public from charlatans. "Not getting lost in the underbrush of psychology and sociology" was another reason why clinicians were reluctant to engage (Herman, 2001). In addition, reasons for not engaging could be that students can get lost when going down deeply into matters, as they have stated, so there is a valid concern that must be addressed on a pedagogical level through providing appropriate scaffolding when teaching and learning about medical humanities and sociology. Above all, there seems to be a yearning for clarity about these subjects, which is not always addressed. In fact, the clarity is at times eschewed since clarity itself is seen as a problem manifest in objective science (Lather, 1991).

In this chapter, I will review my experience at medical humanities conferences and forums in the UK and internationally in order to provide a flavour of current activity in the field that is not always captured in the literature, as well as providing key themes from the literature about the art and science of medicine, and the value of medical humanities and sociology generally. As stated previously, my academic journey from a clinical physiotherapist, to a scientific researcher, then turning to the medical humanities through art therapy, training courses on embodied psychotherapy, public health and then sociology and pedagogy, in order to fill in what I believed were the gaps in my undergraduate training has influenced my perception and underlined my need for clarity in the healthcare field. Part of the way I have addressed this is by exploring assumptions underpinning statements and content of the different subjects. Interestingly one of the essays we were asked to write all those years ago was about the art and science of physiotherapy. Finally, in line with multimodal representations of learning about suffering in Chapter Three, I will draw on pedagogical aspects of teaching and learning about medical humanities and science from the fundamental aspects of observation as highlighted in the quote at the start of this chapter, in the hope that this will provide some clarity as to the unity that the level of observation provides and the intersections with suffering that become apparent.

4.2 Background

Chapter One emphasised the importance of how we stitch knowledge together, at one point drawing on the metaphor of a forest to state that "A forest is not ordered according to clear binary disjunctions; instead it is a labyrinth" (Eco, 2014, p. 36). The metaphor of being lost in the woods, or not being able to see the wood for the trees (Figure 4.1), is one I will draw on for exploring current thinking in medical humanities. Bleakley (2015) provides a comprehensive account of the development of medical humanities in both the UK and the US, so that will not be repeated here. However, I think he would concur that at times medical humanities appears to have been lost in the woods and at times seems to obscure its own value. There almost seems to be an unspoken sense of despair about not being drawn on more, when medical humanities has so much to offer in terms of understanding. At the same time, there seems to be an unspoken fear that perhaps medical humanities doesn't have much to offer to the mainstream scientific evidence based medicine and that literally all the work is in their imagination.

For example, at a fairly recent forum for medical humanities (Birckbeck College Medical Humanities, 2017), discussion took place on the role of medical humanities in medicine. Various roles were suggested aimed

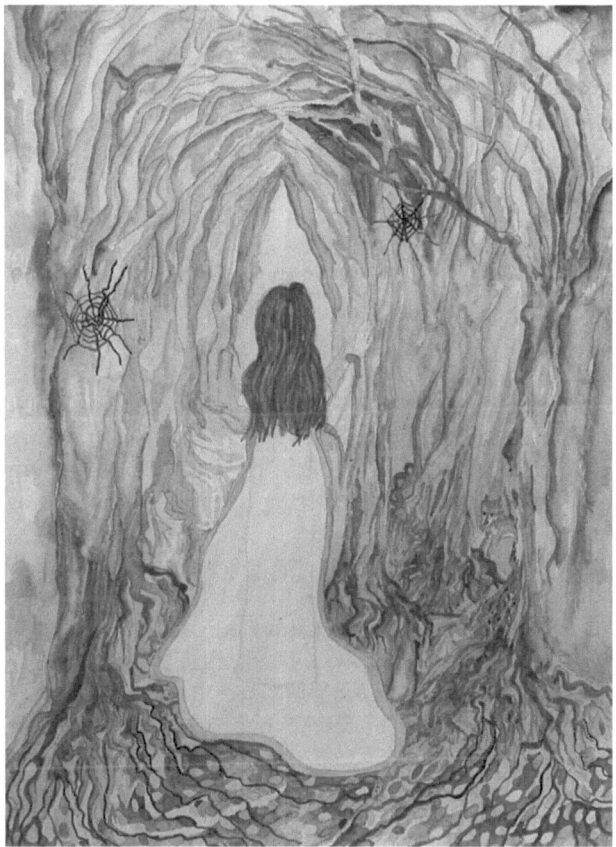

Figure 4.1 Lost in the woods.

primarily at addressing the perceived tunnel vision of medical training, such as reducing the objectification of the patient by a medical humanities practitioner being present with the trainee at the beside and reflecting afterwards on language, nonverbal gestures, approach and holding binary oppositions on what it means to be a doctor and a human in healthcare, in order for fixed professional identities to be challenged if required. A major line of discussion was around dehumanisation by training which impacts on patient centred care and the illness experience. Providing a model of reflective practice through conceptual analysis to see situations differently, drawing on different theoretical lenses, was considered paramount, rather than the predominantly banal tick box exercise currently.

In addition, addressing the problem of attrition of doctors, particularly in their foundational year (Buchen et al., 2019; UK Foundational Programme, 2017), was seen as urgent. The attrition was framed as an outcome of students having learnt certainty throughout their undergraduate years, then experiencing uncertainty once qualified and being responsible for making decisions in much more precarious circumstances. Such things as diagnostic uncertainty for complex patients with multi-morbidities, capacity to perform procedures especially with the risk of deterioration, or ambiguity over decisions and outcomes, complexity and incomprehensibility of what is happening all add to the potential level of overwhelm, financial cost including cognitive overload, followed by physician stress and burnout (Milne, 2019). Different specialities use different techniques to reduce uncertainty and deal with it, but some strategies included eliminating life threatening conditions, lowering cognitive load and optimising clinical decision making. References were made to internal cognitive biases, pattern recognition (system 1) and interpretation of physiology (system 2), where system 1 and 2 referred to fast and slow thinking (Kahneman, 2012) respectively, with the integration of both where needed. System 1 predominated and system 2 was recruited when encountering ill-fitting features (Kahneman, 2012). I include these details because it is clear that clinicians are thinking along different lines when considering uncertainty in contrast to medical humanities scholars.

Healthcare is an organisation of uncertainty that paradoxically draws on hierarchies of power/knowledge (Foucault, 1980) to perhaps contain this uncertainty. Clinicians' responses to uncertainty varies (George & Lowe, 2019). The participants in the forum (Birckbeck College Medical Humanities, 2017) believed that medical humanities can support with interpretation of that response, methodological agility, to think creatively and obtain multiple perspectives on an issue. Yet the response is context dependent, and clearly medical humanities' response must be appropriate to the context along with showing situational awareness. There is a place and time for medical humanities interventions and during the acute phase of a patient's illness may not be the best time. This paragraph highlights that there is a place for everything and that a more nuanced approach is required to thinking about when or where or how medical humanities may be helpful.

During the forum, participants discussed how the medical humanities' narrative could be just as problematic as the biomedical narrative, with some parts of biomedicine being completely out of reach. The different approaches to uncertainty highlight a different purpose for medical humanities and medicine. For example, one person stated, "Sometimes I want them just to fix it (like a plumber), and sometimes I want discussion (like an architect)." There was seen to be a necessity to fit the approach to the purpose – "to render unto Caesar what is Caesar's." There was the belief that medical humanities takes people further in their thought process although evidence is required to substantiate claims that medical humanities improves the ability to tolerate uncertainty and professional identity.

Evidence was also required to suggest that when clinicians do engage, medical humanities improves patient safety (because clinicians see more), improves communication (because clinicians write more and because of reflective practice), improves adaptability and flexibility of the workforce (because clinicians look at things differently), which in turn was believed to decrease burnout and absenteeism due to facilitating change to meet demand. Whilst there is some evidence for the role of art in improving health and well-being (World Health Organization [WHO], 2019), medical humanities has a long way to go before it can claim these as rightful territory.

However, the theme that kept coming up was that in real life clinical practice, what was needed was a look at how clinicians deal with uncertainty and learn how to survive in the healthcare environment. This means adjusting practices, thoughts, beliefs and behaviour to the location and task at hand. Whilst medical humanities can be seen as a bridge between biomedicine and sociology, without going deeply into either, there is a clear adjustment to be made as to the time, place and purpose. Likewise, delving into the patient-clinician encounter also requires subtlety and awareness. I am reminded of Foucault's (1973) acerbic remark:

> Our contemporaries see in this accession to the individual the establishment of a 'unique dialogue', the most concentrated formulation of an old medical humanism, as old as man's compassion. The mindless phenomenologies of understanding mingle the sand of their conceptual desert with this half-baked notion; the feebly eroticized vocabulary of 'encounter' and of the 'doctor/patient relationship' (*le couple medecin-malade*) exhausts itself in trying to communicate the pale powers of matrimonial fantasies to so much non-thought.
>
> (Foucault, 1973, p. xiv)

Medical humanities must keep its feet firmly on the ground when considering its role and purpose. Clinicians may well look askance at medical humanities for a reason.

At times in the forum, the subtext seemed to be one of medical humanities disciplining medicine, which could account for some of the resistance in the field. The stitching together of knowledge in this instance seems to be about problem solving – seeing what was potentially a problem in medicine and trying to fix it through creative means. The clinical environment was seen as one that must be survived from both the clinician and patient perspective. There was a subtle disciplinary jostling over whose voice would be heard and in what sort of capacity. The lack of evidence for medical humanities tends to lend a kind of whimsical wish-list approach to its integration with medicine.

In contrast, the Personification Across Disciplines Conference, held by the Medical Humanities department of Durham University in September 2018, showcased an interdisciplinary host of speakers ranging from patient voices, cognitive scientists, neuroscience researchers, social and narrative researchers as well as psychological, psychiatric and anthropological disciplines. The varied platform encouraged inclusion of a wide range of knowledge making which explored in depth issues around the individual – social interface through the use of symbolic, interactional, narrative, conceptual and person centred processes. The semiotic model of the self – personhood, mind, psyche, personality – was seen as a Cartesian theatre – that no matter how materialist researchers tried to be, they came up against infinite regress – the head within the head within the head, leading to the idea of the ghost in the machine. Phenomenological selfhood (individual agency or doing, shared, relational, material, independent) moved towards otherness, or external agency, whereby personification was more a reflection of being or a laying of a consciousness frame. These and many other ideas were related to clinical situations where reciprocal gazes between patients and clinicians informed each other's actions. There was the notion that we are always thinking through other people's minds. This conference explored the groundwork of concepts, symbols and personifications in use between clinicians and patients, never losing sight of the people at the centre of these interactions.

The conference never lost sight of the relationships either. Yet rather than be preoccupied with relationships between disciplines, between medical humanities and medicine, the content of the conference seemed more interested in carving out bodies of work about the person to person relations and what that may mean in terms of personification, narrative capacity and social rehearsing. Perhaps the depth and breadth of knowledge displayed was more of a function of confidence in their own right to exist as a discipline separate from but related to medicine. There didn't seem to be a concern with disciplining medicine; rather, the focus was on participant researchers finding their own voice.

The flavour of the third conference I will describe, "Cultural Crossings of Care" in Oslo University (2018), was different again. Here the focus was on the gap between medicine and the medical humanities, between presumed objectivity and subjectivity, and drawing on critical dialogue to analyse that gap as well as translating knowledge (Engebretsen, 2020; Kristeva et al., 2018). A wide variety of researchers lamented the gap and spent time researching focused on the dissonance between medicine and medical humanities whilst at the same time suggesting strategies to reduce the dissonance and justifying medical humanities' role from outside the medical academy. Others saw the dichotomy as false, preferring instead to emphasise methodological plurality from within medicine of which medical humanities was inherently a part.

The tension in medical humanities – between the perception of medical humanities as being on the "outside" trying to "get in" and the perception of medical humanities as already within medicine providing a resource for clinicians to enhance their critical thinking skills and practice evidently – produces a different climate at such medical humanities conferences. This tension is reflective or figurative of a type of wounding from a perceived rejection or exclusion and is emblematic of some parts of medical humanities. Drawing on Fiske (1993), the discourse in medical humanities, from the perspective of "being outside" at times seems fixated on the authoritarian relationship and not able to move between different types of relationship such as democratic, equality or collaborative.

Conversely, from the perspective of working transculturally within psychiatry, Moro (2018) demonstrated understanding and practice working across cultures. Basing the work on the two principles of universality in psychological functioning whilst also acknowledging cultural coding in individuals, she managed to walk the thin line between social and individual influences on health. Drawing on the work of Devereaux, the clinic mandatorily but never simultaneously uses multiple methodologies such as cultures, psychiatry, anthropology, history, etc. The point is that at least two disciplines are taught as well as the interaction between them. Clarity on the inside-outside nexus, subjectivity and narrativity, and the Other meant an awareness of contradictory tensions and working with them; that alterity was to assist rather than discriminate, holding and protecting participants whilst providing a passage between two worlds or cultures.

Providing a passage between two worlds also seemed to be a medical humanities theme in a recent Medical Education Conference (AMEE, 2019). Issues of liminality, threshold concepts (Ray Land) and knotworking were introduced by Engeström; democracy in learning between two worlds of biomedical and clinical communication skills curricula, artefacts of subjects and objects, with medical humanities and ethics as metaphor or a third thing to ward off insensitivity and insensibility in medical students, along with concomitant symptoms of anxiety, depression, alcohol and drug abuse, and burnout (Alan Bleakley) were the main conference proceedings that gained attention on social media. Medical education is a third thing between medical humanities and medicine where the key concepts in use in medical humanities can be integrated by observing how medical students and clinicians are socialised and professionalised as well as being complicit with these social influences in order to belong and identify with medicine.

Identity and belonging with undertones of shame were associated with the medical humanities' epistemic function of the following:

- Art as expertise: mastering skills
- Art as dialogue: interaction, perspective taking, relational aims
- Art as expression and transformation: personal growth and activism

Pedagogy as a way of navigating evidence based medicine on the one hand, and medical humanities on the other hand, is a further turn in the discourse about medical humanities' place in medical education. The different flavours of recent conferences give a sense of what medical humanities is currently grappling with in the field.

At this point, it seems worth thinking about medical education in relation to medical humanities and biomedicine. Medical education could be a third mediating middle ground between the two disciplines, or it could be seen as a third dimension in relation to the biomedical disciplines and medical humanities in order to form a more three-dimensional picture. The difficulty in thinking about the combination of these approaches is that both the individual level and social level of teaching and learning must be thought of at the same time. That is, both the individual learning of facts, experience and attitudes, as well as the contextual nature in which this occurs and to which the learning, is applied.

But this three-dimensional structure is the nature of a bricolage. For better or worse, both medical humanities and sociology connect to biomedicine, with its focus on a rational approach in molecular, cell and integrative biology as well as evolving treatments for disease of patients and promoting human health in the general population. There are core knowledge and skills required as well as understanding and communicating in the social situation. That seems fairly straightforward yet translating these into straightforward teaching and learning in medical education is not so obvious – knowledge (analysis down to the smallest part) does not always equate to understanding (synthesis into the larger picture). There is a disconnect between learning outcomes and practice: the so-called theory-practice gap. It is this gap that medical humanities and social sciences have tried to bridge. And this also seems to be where controversy and contention abound. Yet in medical education, there is little robust evidence on what makes a good teacher – a scientist, a medical humanist or a pedagogist? – certainly in relation to the use of medical humanities and sociology and how we teach medicine beyond good content knowledge and strong teaching practices such as demonstrating and questioning, etc. Here is where there is a major gap in knowledge and understanding and perhaps why medical humanities has not been taken up as much as it would have liked.

Perhaps the medical humanities approach has been going about its integration in an inverted way. Rather than solely trying to examine and analyse doctors' practice, which goes straight to higher order learning outcomes, perhaps there is a stronger case to look at the micro learning processes and see how anchor points can be inserted in the process. Perhaps if we went back to the basic learning processes – experience, interpretation, perception, concepts, frameworks – then medical humanities could offer its expertise in those domains which gives biomedicine something concrete to work with. At the same time, medical humanities must keep the bigger contextualised picture in mind as situational awareness and accept that biomedicine is what it is at that level of conceptualisation. Part of the debate is around what medical students are being educated for and therefore what is the best way to learn, within the current constraints.

Techniques and knowledge are embodied in a relational context of biomedicine as well as the larger picture of potential suffering. Techniques and knowledge can help clinicians cross a gap of uncertainty and potential terror, whilst sometimes anatomical and clinical language can help overcome potential embarrassment and shame in the clinical situation. Knowing what types of relationships exist in the organisational structure is crucial and how they govern practice is paramount to surviving the landscape, yet the individual and social are inseparable. The basic cognitive, sensorimotor and affective knowledge and skills are the building blocks of learning within situationally aware relational contexts with particular rules and regulations. Students are keen to have scaffolding at their level of understanding which takes them a bit beyond, but they do not tolerate well knowledge which seems out of their depth. It takes time to build what seems to be a dual awareness of both the individual and social level of influences on learning and practice, and there are multiple external and internal influences on this process.

Closer to home, a new initiative with medical students and clinicians focuses on collaborative enquiry to facilitate the articulation of voice, expression of personal situated ways of seeing and reflecting lived experiences in medical education (Younie, 2019):

> The emphasis on the human self of the medical student, practitioner and patient provides meaning; for opportunities of unique creative expression to making sense and seeing; using different lenses and perspectives through the creative arts; to connect with the ineffable, emotional, and intuitive dimensions of practice and experience; exploration of interior landscapes; metaphor, image, colour and silence to engage with the complexity and messiness of what it means to be human and learn from each other, share, see and interpret lived experiences.
>
> (Younie, 2019)

Various workshops and student courses have been run to provide an outlet for student and practitioner expression which, according to feedback, they would otherwise not have had. Providing a space for passage between the worlds of learning and practice that is collaborative is an inspiring example of medical humanities locally and one that takes place in various forms in other medical schools across the UK.

Having provided a flavour of different expressions and applications of medical humanities currently in order to show what this looks like from an academic and practice perspective, there is a sense that medical humanities is on the move. There are at least two different streams of medical humanities, from the scholarly analytic focus drawing on a long tradition of theoretical work and the practical pragmatic application of medical humanities as part of a multimodal means of learning about patients, healthcare and medicine as well as the practitioners or clinicians themselves. From disciplining medicine to inspiring a new wave of students and practice, there are some flavours discussed here that are not always apparent in the literature. The medical humanities literature will be reviewed after exploring on a broad level the debates in relation to whether medicine is an art or science in order to provide the context for following sections and how this relates to suffering.

4.3 The art and science of medicine – missing the point

4.3.1 Introduction

Debates about the relative value of and relationship between the art and science of medicine seem to be missing the point despite their longevity and, at times, passionate insistence. At times, art and science are both treated as objects for dissection rather than the dynamic processes they predominantly are. Historically, creative processes were actively encouraged in medicine; it is only relatively recently that the emphasis on evidence based medicine has excluded certain forms of knowledge for fear of loss of credibility, inexact science and treatment, as well as inadequate understanding of disease processes (Altschuler, 2018). The exclusion ignores the fact that many aspects of modern medicine developed out of this creative period:

> As a fertile period of transition between the birth of the clinic and the discovery of the cell, as an era of speculative insight between the imaginative reaching of life signs and the visual knowledge of bacterial life, Romantic medicine engendered biology, zoology, immunology, clinical diagnoses and evolution theory.
>
> (de Almeida, 1991, p. 3).

Thus rather than distancing itself from its epistemological past, medicine may perhaps be better served by understanding better what is involved in how we know what we know.

Epistemology, the study of how we know what we know, is the focus of this section. This is important because in relation to suffering, with its muteness and loss of self, different ways of knowing are required, apparent and necessary. In fact, with the advent of COVID-19 pandemic, ways of knowing have been thrown into the spotlight and perhaps been scrutinised more than ever before. Altschuler (2018) suggest that moments of crises – epistemic crises – are both rich for opening up knowledge production and the complexity of knowing through the creative imagination as well as revelatory in showing the limitations of epistemological objectivity and empiricism alone.

However, in order to not go around in circles in debates about integration of or differentiation between art and science, a deep dive is necessary into what is actually meant by epistemology in this context. Clarifying an imperative before reviewing any of the literature on critical medical humanities provides an anchor: an antidote to becoming lost in the woods. A dual awareness of the value of art and science is necessary. Therefore this section will review debates on the art and science of medicine, followed by an analysis of how we know what we know, before moving on to a critical review of medical humanities and sociology. There is a necessity to look at how perceptions, interpretations, concepts and judgments are formed in a metacognition of both art and science.

4.3.2 Epistemology of art and science

As mentioned above, the literature ties itself in knots trying to decide whether art and science are a part of medicine, yet independent of each other – which therefore requires further delineation in order to see what each one does and is – or whether they form integrated knowledge bases within medicine as a whole and therefore a process of integration is more important than differentiation. The inside-outside mindset plays a deterministic function in role allocation.

Part of the difficulty is that there is believed to be no direct access to the epistemological process itself by simply observing doctors; therefore any account has to be based on a conceptual analysis (Bærøe, 2015). Moreover, as in quantum physics and observation of electrons, any observation of the process will change the process – the path taken can only be seen by the outcome or behaviour of the entity under study. This means that accounts of the epistemological process tend to fall into two main threads of description (a representation of what is believed to be going on in the clinician's mind) or normative guidelines (what should be going on or what is aimed for – an ideal) (Bærøe, 2015). When each of these threads is described, there is an assumption that the conceptual description provides an understanding of the essence of medical practice, which in itself is a contested notion.

For example, in the past, the four primary concerns, or essence, of romantic medicine were thought to be the physician's task, the meaning of life, the prescription of disease and health and the evolution of matter and mind (De, 1991). In contrast, Bærøe (2015) suggests that a conceptual understanding of medicine includes the following:

- Interpretation of the medical role and how to effectuate it in practice
- Help societies regulate and organise adequate provision of healthcare
- Enable critique of ongoing practice
- Identify improved solutions for the future
- Distinguish medical practice from other healthcare practise as a way of supporting medical professionalism
- Providing accountability for privileged locations (Bærøe, 2015)

The latter conception of medical essence can be thought of as more regulatory and disciplinary in its practice in contrast to the more philosophical approaches in the past suggested by de Almeida (1991). The key difference is that the latter is more reproducible than the former; a key requirement for establishing knowledge in science.

The reproducibility criterion of knowledge in science means a focus on empirical data collection. However, there is an argument for considering the importance of medicine as an applied science – that of translating the reproducible knowledge to the individual person or patient. Medicine is not seen as a science in this case in itself; medicine is seen rather as an activity based on the translation of scientific knowledge into practice (Bærøe, 2015). There are nuances within this perception in that Bærøe (2015) suggests the closer to the treatment of the bodily malfunction the medicine is practised, the more the focus of knowledge production has to be on explainable relations between the interventions and expected outcomes (Bærøe, 2015). In other words, the relationship between epistemology and medicine depends on the empirical observation in the first place. When a medical issue is deemed to be less of a physiological, anatomical or biochemical matter, then the focus shifts to obtaining knowledge to understand the person more.

> Art understood in the broad sense of representing a kind of translational judgment is also considered a crucial condition for adequately realizing science in successful evidence-based practice.
>
> (Bærøe, 2015, p. 6)

Art comes into play in clinical practice through both a (1) judgment in translating general knowledge into particular cases by practical reasoning and (2) specifically involving and combining both non-medical and biomedical knowledge in clinical care in order to bring about health (Bærøe, 2015). Translation and combining knowledges is deemed to be an art that includes moral, ethical, values, intuition, affections and interpretive listening.

The paradox in this form of epistemology is that the art of translation is not objectively controllable the way empirical scientific processes are required to be, precisely because humans are involved (Bærøe, 2015). Therefore the associations to uncontrollable, unforeseen reasoning processes, such as values, ethics and moral judgments, can be seen as representatives of another kind of emergent rationality, the art of making clinical judgments. The trouble with these kinds of epistemological relationships is that they tend to go round in circles because art is considered a process, perhaps a translation, and an outcome as well as an overall perspective on a clinical encounter between human beings that is context driven, both personal and political.

The alternative perspective means seeing art and science as inseparable – knowing is an art, and science requires personal participation in knowledge (Saunders, 2000). Some people believe that "without understanding people as objects in this way, there can be no such thing as a medical science" (Pearl, 2014, p. 18). That knowledge can only be accumulated by objectification, and scientific thinking must be insulated from all kinds of psychological, sociological, economic, political, moral and ideological factors that could bias or prejudice that thinking and knowledge (Pearl, 2014). Reductionists have urged doctors not to get lost in the psycho-sociological underbrush, put down hermeneutic exploration as "pastoral skills" and focus themselves on concentrating on "real" diseases (Herman, 2001).

Herman (2001) hypothesises that "the close connection between scientific and artistic activity, if demonstrated with sufficient authority, might break down the supposed dichotomy between art and science in medicine" (p. 42). The dichotomy is manifest in the dissonance between "the science of objective measurement" and the "art" of clinical proficiency and judgment. Saunders (2000) suggests that for medicine to be seen as an art, its chief and characteristic instrument must be human faculty. It is this faculty that provides coherence to the perceptions, interpretations, translations and judgments of phenomena that must be taken into account.

Providing cohesion to this debate means delving down further into human faculty. It is hard to see how progress could be made without doing so even though progress is seen as such an imperative. Altschuler (2018) suggests that the medical imagination has much to contribute epistemologically yet stops short of describing how this may be so beyond epistemic humility and humanistic competencies. Humanistic competencies include narrative, attention, observation, historical perspective, ethics, judgment, performance and creative imagination. She suggests these practical competencies as part of a pedagogical tool kit, yet, again, there is a lack of explanation of how exactly they interconnect from an epistemological perspective: "Creativity, we hope, will teach us new ways of seeing and knowing that can reveal more about health and human suffering (Altschuler, 2018, p. 202)." Reassembling knowledge, experience and observation towards new discovery at times of epistemic crises means stitching together narratives about art and science to form new meta cognitive strategies and processes. It is to this that we now turn.

4.3.3 Breaking out of circular thinking

The above section shows that much of the thinking about medicine as art and science tends to go around in circles with concepts, perceptions and interpretations calling for either further differentiation or integration, depending on the empirical (observation or experience) theoretical logic of the narrator. To explore this further we return to the first chapter and our network of knowledge through the technique of bricolage (see Section 1.5).

We have explored the idea of an anchor when piecing together a quilt. An anchor in this instance is a stitch through the fabric or field of inquiry about suffering. One such stitch is understanding how we know what we know as this directly impacts on how we respond to suffering as clinicians. Seeing medicine as an applied science based on observation of empirical data means that generally clinicians are seen as objective and detached from the person who becomes objectified. Seeing medicine as an art means that clinicians are seen as more empathic and subjective. Thus a dichotomy is introduced into how we know what we know and one term or position is more valued over the other. This dichotomy has pre-occupied medical humanities a long time and will be discussed further in Section 4.4.

If we were to see the art and science as inseparable, we may draw on a network of knowledge which consists of various elements such as pre-cognitive pre-categorical recognition or intuition, or observation, perception, interpretation, categorisation, concepts, schemata, and judgment or beliefs, whereby the entire embodied cognitive process comes down to inference:

> Sensations appear as interpretations of stimuli; perceptions as interpretations of sensations; judgments of perceptions as the interpretations of perceptions; particular and general propositions as interpretations of perceptual judgments; and scientific theories as interpretations of propositions.
>
> (Eco, 2014, p. 486)

There is interplay between these various components since reflective judgment can be seen as more than observing (and subsequently producing schemata) and actually produces schemata to observe and test (Eco, 2014). This schematism is of the imagination, without concepts, as the primary capacity to organise perceptions.

A gap can remain between schemata and symbols; there is intuition but not yet a concept. A pre-categorical perception exists that precedes conceptual categorisation. When conceptual categorisation coincides with a schema of the empirical concept, the schema, concept and meaning coincide with one another and speech is possible, for example. The unity of the act is where there is coincidence of linguistic meaning and perceptual meaning which gives a sense of internal symmetry, when possible. "The schematism of our intellect which also concerns the simple form of appearances, is an art hidden in the depths of the human soul. Schematism is an art, a procedure, a task, a construction, but we know very little about how it works" (Eco, 2014, p. 475). Perhaps the word "soul" is used here to indicate awareness and consciousness of a more subtle yet inclusive nature.

Imagination, the capacity to represent an object even without its being present in the intuition, provides a schema to the intellect so that this can be applied to the intuition. Imagining can be an evocation of an image as well as knowing from sensible impressions – or figuring (Eco, 2014). This figuring for understanding is crucial for the so-called transcendental grounding of empirical concepts and for allowing perceptual judgments that are implicit and nonverbalised. These in turn create the subjective world of personal consciousness. There is an interweaving of imagination, schema, intellect and judgment which shows that art and science are inseparable and part of the same process of coming to know. Where they become separated is at the stage of the "legislative intellect" (Eco, 2014).

The movement from concrete experience, through symbolic representation to linguistic/narratives, to abstract categories and concepts, patterns or models or schemata, and finally to judgment involves a process of comparison, reflection and abstraction:

> In order to make our presentations into concepts, one must be able to compare, reflect and abstract, for these three logical operations of the understanding are the essential and general conditions of generating any concept whatsoever.
>
> (Eco, 2014, p. 465)

Comparing by noticing objects are different from one another, reflecting on what they have in common, abstracting size and shape of objects means that concepts are gained. This arrival at formulations of empirical concepts in ways that have nothing to do with the legislative activity of the intellect (i.e., obeying rules and regulations) rescues the matter of the intellect from our own blindness and moreover provides the same ground for both art and science. The places where they differ is in producing judgment of perception, whereby we "understand perception as a complex act, an interpretation of sensible data that involves memory and culture and that results in our grasping the nature of the object" (Eco, 2014, p. 466).

> By reflecting on the data form the sensible intuition, by comparing it and evaluating it, by activating an arcane and inborn art hidden in the depths of the human soul (and therefore existing within our own transcendental apparatus), we do not abstract but rather we construct the schemata.
>
> (Eco, 2014, p. 478)

The construction happens quickly, without necessarily aforethought, from a process of enculturation or education, but works because we believe we are seeing what we are seeing because we are receiving sensations. The point in going through these details of how we know what we know is to demonstrate the inseparability of art and science at a fundamental level of recognition of sensible intuition, which has implications for the speechlessness of suffering, how learning is written up in medical curricula as well as for the role of medical humanities.

The inseparability is also demonstrated at the level of logical and empirical statements (Ney, 2019). Synthetic statements are verified through empirical (experience and observational) means whereas analytical statements are verified by logical rational means. However, Ney (2019) suggests that nothing we believe is really confirmed by empirical observation or logic alone; there is an intertextual reality which is more likely to be settled by pragmatic practical choices about which overall systems of belief we want to adopt. These beliefs form a web in which

> The totality of our so-called knowledge or beliefs ... is a man made fabric which impinges on experience only along the edges. Or, to change the figure, total science is like a field force whose boundary conditions are experience. A conflict with experience at the periphery occasions readjustments in the interior of the field .... But the total field is so undetermined by its boundary conditions, experience, that there is much latitude of choice as to what statements to re-evaluate in the light of any single contrary experience.
>
> (Quine in Ney, 2019, p. 129)

This means a rejection of a chain of verification, leading back to a basic set of beliefs directly verifiable by experience. Rather, the picture is one where there is no ultimate belief, just a web of knots of beliefs, connected through supporting relations to a periphery of sense experience, a bit like the picture of the lacunae in Chapter One. Some beliefs in the web lie closer to the outside, the periphery of sensory experience; others lie closer to the centre where they are more insulated from what we observe and are therefore not directly supported or undermined by empirical evidence. This quilt or bricolage of beliefs shows the inseparability of synthesis, analysis and imagination, all of which come into play when understanding suffering in healthcare practice and in the elucidation of the role of medical humanities.

I believe we must be very clear on this epistemological process, since suffering with its muteness and perceived loss of self returns us to a pre-categorical state. Therefore we are compelled to understand this since part of the anguish of suffering is the hole in what we can say and, by inference, in what we can know. As health professionals, we can unwittingly contribute to that hole by objectifying patients. But perhaps more damaging is the lacunae in acknowledging that this pre-categorical or pre-objectifying knowledge even exists yet it is perhaps the closest state to that of someone suffering.

It's strange because in health professional and social work curriculum just about all students cover human development with its stages of cognitive development from Piaget of sensorimotor, pre-operational, concrete operational and formal operational periods. Yet there is little application of the process of cognitive development to how we know what we know, and how this impacts on the patient, in the healthcare field. We have an understanding of the learning process at this basic level, even without being able to look inside our heads – an understanding which has been around for centuries (Eco, 2014) – yet we still insist on creating dichotomies or gaps in knowledge which were never there in the first place.

These lacunae in what we perceive we know and understand can directly impact on patient suffering. In terms of why this state of affairs has persisted for so long, and resisted any forays into its basis, over the last century, the question must be asked what is there to be gained, apart from power/knowledge which Foucault has elegantly and comprehensively described over many volumes (Foucault, 1980). One can only imagine that a reason for the complicity in this arrangement is because there is a fear that if we drop below the dichotomising debates, there will be nothing else there. Part of the reason for structuring debates in a dichotomising nature historically was more about whose reality was right, rather than what that process actually achieved and meant. However, from the above we can at least imagine that this art hidden in our depths is still there, in spite of a century or more of obfuscation by discourses on science and whose reality gets to be right.

Foucault (1973) seems to write from this place, hidden depth, when he demonstrates how the texts on medicine changed to reflect the shift in structure of relation between the visible and invisible, and the sayable. From an epistemological sense, the relation between what we can see or sense is a relation of power, according to Foucault (1973). Power/knowledge does not reside solely in medicine and doctors, however; it is also enacted through varying levels within and outside the healthcare service, through rules and regulations and what is considered normal and right, for example. These practices can constrain what is observed and said. But most importantly, an epistemological relation that governs knowledge is that between life and death (de Certeau, 1984) as stated in Chapter One.

Death as an organising principle has also been written about at length by Becker (1961) as well as Foucault (1973). And so by minimising the sayable about death in life and healthcare, the epistemological constraint is exercised with hidden associations of shame and guilt. The secret was invented by knowledge:

> Knowledge *develops* in accordance with a whole display of *envelopes*; the hidden element takes on the form and rhythm of the hidden content, which means that, like a *veil*, it is *transparent*.
>
> (Foucault, 1973, p. 166; emphasis original)

That which hides and envelopes is life and the practices we engage in to obscure the knowledge of death as the ultimate alterity; it is death that opens up the body to the anatomists. Thus as we move on to the next section, reviewing medical humanities and sociology, the Gaze (Foucault, 1973) of the text, or narrator, will be turned to practices that obscure this epistemology of the inseparability of the art and science of medicine.

4.4 Medical humanities and sociology in medical education

Medical humanities has as its focus scholarly activities centred on medicine and includes patient centred practice, medical practitioners, professionalism, identity, the body, self and ways of thinking differently. Medical humanities is an interdisciplinary approach to exploring and understanding medicine, both from within and without, drawing on multiple modalities of art, literature, history, anthropology, critical studies, feminism, performance, theatre and music. This shouldn't be taken as a bucket of leftovers from medicine, though – everything medicine doesn't address – rather, medical humanities draws on a multiplicity of ways of thinking about medicine. Whilst there is general agreement on these sorts of topics of focus, there are also controversies, contradictions and fault lines within the UK (Bleakley, 2015).

Thinking with an arts and humanities perspective therefore means embracing ambiguity within the field of medical humanities itself since the term means different things to different people (McFarlane et al., 2018); this is not always comfortable. Bleakley (2015) identifies three disparate medical humanities groups in the UK:

- Arts in health practitioners who align with psychological views of health and illness and who refuse to be medicalised
- Humanities scholars who took medicine as their topic and were not necessarily interested in medical education
- Medical educators, often clinicians, who were interested in how medical practice could be humanised, but were not interested in either psychological therapies or academic scholarship (Bleakley, 2015, p. 32).

In addition, institutions like the Wellcome Trust are keen to develop a new vision that explicitly embraces critical conversations between artists, academics and practitioners (Bleakley, 2015). These three main groups are motivated differently and want different outcomes, even though these outcomes are not able to be (e.g., overall psychological health, inclusion into mainstream medicine and completely humane medical treatment), and such notions are usually rejected anyway as too aspirational and unable to be evidenced quantitatively as to their effectiveness in the short term. Schwartz et al., (2009) suggest a long term approach to medical humanities evaluation while admitting there are many confounders to this idea.

The difference between medical humanities as an intervention, a critical thought process and a tool for medical education becomes clearer when the evidence is considered. In a review of the literature, Taylor et al., (2018) found that most (69%) publications on medical humanities were commentaries, reflections or opinions. These commentaries tended to discuss the relationship between medical humanities and medicine, arguing for greater inclusion. Only 22 of the articles included any outcome measures on trainee knowledge, attitudes or behaviours. The lack of consideration of the pedagogy is surprising given that out of 156 journal articles, 31% were curricular interventions and only 10 out of 156 evaluated the impact beyond learner satisfaction (Taylor et al., 2018). The main focus of work was on empathy, reflection and bridging the gap between science and the humanities. The main challenges were a lack of funding and difficulty scheduling these topics into the medical curriculum. The rationale for the review seems to be to provide a holistic approach for patient care, yet very few studies were found to include patients.

In this way, much work on medical humanities tends to read as a wish list with all the right sort of rhetoric to suggest a progressive approach yet fails to deliver any granularity (e.g., Jones et al., 2019; Lechopier et al., 2018). By this lack of granularity, I mean an understanding of the types of suffering, relational contexts and patterns of behaviour being engaged with. Jones et al., (2019) see medical humanities as experiential, emotional and existential reflections for both patients and doctors through literature, narratives, creative art and theatre to increase empathy and openness to others. This stance could be problematic depending on the context – not all situations are safe for students and clinicians to show empathy and openness – so much more nuance is necessary. The study found that communication and interpersonal skills improved in graduate medical trainees but these improvements could have been confounded by the older age and longer life experience of the graduates. The sorts of concepts and models in use require thinking through much more deeply.

Lechopier et al., (2018) saw medical humanities as having a role in preparing health professionals for a transforming and largely unpredictable workplace. The authors identified four crucial issues that need to be addressed such as changes in medical roles from carer to co-ordinator with a need to document these changes, new biomedical concepts and innovations including personalised medicine and a need to critically analyse these concepts, analysis of long term consequences on health social contract in relation to genetic profiling and implications for health risk and lifestyle behaviour and ethical issues in health care daily settings such as donors, patient-doctor relationships, expensive treatments, care organisation and management. The resources were organised around transformatory connections to patient experiences, social and cultural constructions of these experiences, social responsibility and critical reflexivity of medical doctors, demographic, epistemic and technological changes in today's medicine, as well as independence of professional judgment mediated by medical education yet central to public debate about health ethics and society (Lechopier et al., 2018). Whilst there was some granularity in these proposals, the main emphasis was on a plea for reflexivity and critical thought, even though there was no mention of health inequalities.

Bleakley (2015) argues for medical humanities as a democratising and politicising medical culture in medical education. To him, this means moving clear of art therapy, where art is a medium for working with patients and not primarily a cultural object or artefact that has independent impetus to challenge the "health" of medical culture (Bleakley, 2015). However, this could be contentious in itself seeing as this is the area that has the most evidence base for its success (Wald et al., 2018; World Health Organization WHO, 2019). Wald et al., (2018) suggest that medical humanities is education for the heart and mind, where core elements of physicianship are "anchored" in the arts and humanities (p. 1). Evidence exists for the effectiveness of medical humanities in dealing with burnout and related issues of professionalism to promote well-being and resilience (Wald et al., 2016, 2018). There is an uneasy relationship between the individual practitioner and social workplace constraints in these initiatives.

Counteracting burnout, emotional exhaustion and depersonalisation through a counterbalance to relentless reductionism, othering and asking "What kind of curriculum could offer the best preparation for times of psychological and moral duress?" is the approach advocated by Gordon (2005) which has particular prescience for these times (p. 6). Gordon (2005) sees imagination as key: "students who, in the hours outside the classroom, manage disease, pain, suffering and loss move into a classroom where they may feel overwhelmed or deficient" (p. 7). She turns this situation around by the use of imagination to draw on the situation of overwhelm as providing food for thought: "An excess of imagination is sometimes too painful in clinical practice, but the arts, humanities and social sciences thrive on imagination and on new interpretation of old ideas" (p. 7). Gordon (2005) identified that in the heat of the clinical moment, it is not always possible to process experience. Processing may need to be left to a more removed location in time, space and psychological resourcefulness. Campo (2005) also sees the role of medical humanities as providing renewal, reconnection and meaning.

Reconnecting to one's meaning is a pre-requisite for thinking differently. Yet some say "the practice of medicine thus permits, provokes, inspires, and rebuffs the very ideas that the humanities affords" (Schlozman, 2017, p. 703). Art doesn't have to be useful nor does it have to be in the service of medicine or, ironically, participate in the further alienation of the self from the self. There can be truth in both subjectivity and objectivity; what is perhaps more important is one receiving acknowledgment and validation from the other. This notion seems a requisite for connecting to meaning and for taking on existential challenges. Such challenges include self-other dichotomies, self-alienation and concrete-abstract dichotomies which could all benefit from disciplined thinking of the ways in which one studies the humanities (Schlozman, 2017). Granularity is supplied by Patel (2018) who suggests asking "How best to support a patient who is dying? Do you cry with the patient? Is it acceptable to be detached? Is it OK to resume your life and laugh a few hours later? How, where and from whom do you learn these skills?" Granularity of meaning seems vital to a profession engaged with these matters on a daily basis in order to be relevant.

Meaning seems inherent in thinking differently about how one studies medical humanities. Various approaches have been proposed such as entanglement (Fitzgerald & Callard, 2016; Slaby, 2015; Viney et al., 2015), a renewed praxis developing understanding of binaries (Wear, 2009) and a conceptual framework encompassing qualities of the arts (representational, metaphorical, subjective, ambiguous/complex, universal); engagement with the arts (reflection, interpretation, imagination, embodiment, aesthetic, affective/emotional); construction of new meanings (self-awareness, openness to alternate perspectives, enhanced ability to cope with ambiguity, more nuanced and deep understandings) and translation to medical practice (increased empathy, increased skills in communication, observation and ethical reasoning) in group engagement and processing (Haidet et al., 2016). These three arts based pedagogical strategies of engagement, meaning making and translation were devised from a review and meta synthesis of 49 medical humanities journal articles.

However well-intentioned these reviews are, the fact remains that there is little venturing "beyond a neoliberal, humanist notion of the individual body-subject and associated conceptualisations of responsibility, rights and risk management to really explore alternative "collective" and "relational" approaches to "flourishing"" (Atkinson et al., 2015, p. 77). Even using terms like entanglement, borrowed from quantum physics, is to not be explicitly cognisant of racial disparities and inequalities in health. This seems to be a key issue – that whilst acknowledging humanities entanglement, how do we not lose sight of the fault lines along which some lives are perhaps more entangled than others, and this produces inequalities. A prime example of this was during the COVID-19 pandemic lockdown where people were advised to socially distance themselves and isolate at home. This clearly had greater consequence for people who could not afford to stop work as they would not be able to put food on the table and yet they were scapegoated because of their lack of adherence to the government's advice. These people will also be the first to suffer the economic consequences of the pandemic. It is much easier for people who are from privileged locations and have safe and secure housing to self-isolate amongst decent surroundings, with little overcrowding in the home, and thereby abide by the rules, perhaps sanctimoniously.

There are many methodological and theoretical issues as well as lacunae apparent in the literature, not the least of which is the persistence of the ideal normative reference point of what it means to be a human.

Under medical humanities rhetoric, Bleakley (2015) suggests that if you scratch the surface, you will still find a white cis heteronormative male. Puustinen et al., (2003) suggest viewing medical practice as an activity that enforces the joint consideration of the object and subject – who is doing what to whom – that requires many tools. A semiotic focus on concepts, signs and symptoms enables thinking differently, where the humanities are both theoretically and methodologically internal to the analysis itself (Puustinen et al., 2003). This seems useful when thinking about the relational aspects of suffering beyond the normative ideal of humanity.

Blease (2016) provides a useful analysis of the thinking about instrumentality versus intrinsic value of medical humanities in a medical education curriculum. She explores the false dichotomy and suggests that "the task of articulating *strictly* intrinsic justifications for the humanities is thorny and intricate – and arguably elusive" (Blease, 2016, p. 104; emphasis original). In her view of a broad education as one that encompasses both sciences and humanities she suggests we are missing the point and risk embracing hobbyism if we suggest that the pursuit of knowledge in the medical humanities is worth doing in itself:

> Arguments about content versus application suggest that one can straightforwardly divest *understanding* of the *vehicles* of that understanding – namely, that one can easily differentiate propositional knowledge from the meta-cognitive appreciation of that knowledge (in other words, from 'insight').
>
> (Blease, 2016, p. 107; emphasis original)

Blease's (2016) point is that studying the humanities is a meta-cognitive enterprise, asking a variety of questions about the nature of ideas and concepts. These intellectual tools about how we think about thinking may not have any products as such but they are still a useful, moral, ethical task (Arendt, 1971). Issues on the utility of curriculum as preparation for life versus carrying out a task have been around forever (Benjamin, 1939).

Rather than perpetuating and staying stuck in old dichotomies and the "defensive silos that they burrow" she suggests focusing on the following:

> How do different levels of analysis fit together: how does a psychological level of explanation fit with neuroscientific levels of analysis? In short, a raft of philosophical and historical questions can open up to the student upon contemplation of just one key theory from the history of medicine.
>
> (Blease, 2016, p. 107)

She proposes that medical humanities do more of the heavy lifting by getting down to the workmanship of application and by being intellectually honest about subtexts of improving medicine, working out in a straightforward instrumental proposition how this may be so.

Unearthing fallacies within medical humanities means theorising through the disciplined process of analysis of common assumptions. Bleakley (2017) identify six common fallacies of medical humanities in medical education:

1 Arts produce health – utilitarian fallacy and normalising of absolute health
2 "Fun" and creativity fallacy – trivialises medicine, shows shallow optimism where creativity is a weasel word
3 Fallacy of personal expressions – art speaks for itself, doesn't need to interpret or confess
4 Artistic production is narrative based – not everything is narrativizable
5 Error of excluding artists from judging artwork or including them in conversation
6 Fallacy that interpretation is necessary (Bleakley, 2017)

The author resists the civilising of art. Perhaps he is referring to a sense that medical humanities is in danger of being co-opted by practices that seek to normalise what is human. There is also the issue that medical humanities could become another technology of self (Hutton, 1988) or a disciplinary technique of both medicine and the professional self.

In a guide that provides granularity, Wu (2018) suggests six domains to develop critical medical humanities with medical students and stimulate deeper thinking and reflection: identity, Gaze, stories, context, citizenship and uncertainty. In a critical review he includes the usual suspects of observation, pattern recognition, empathy and narrative medicine but also goes beyond these to consider suffering and healing in general, as citizens:

> Modern health professionals face the inconvenient truth that they are no longer powerful interveners in diseases, but merely companions of suffering individuals or communities in the enterprise of risk management.
>
> (Wu, 2018, p. 94)

The work, by explicitly mentioning suffering, brings a more grounded approach that eschews the two culture approach to science and humanities which he sees as having been discredited. Any gap seems to be perpetuated by the way we think about these matters and upon the criteria we use for decision making. Including suffering in an approach seems to pull the different threads together and provide the type of application that Blease (2016) recommends.

There is a sense that unless suffering is made explicit, medical humanities can become just another tool in a normative self-disciplining toolbox. Pickersgill et al., (2018) provide examples of how the social sciences and humanities have had a positive influence on self-management of diabetes, provision of psychological therapy, handwashing, hospital checklists, stroke guidelines, tobacco control and in responses to Ebola and Zika, but it is not clear what criteria the authors are using to include these as humanities interventions. Some sound like public health interventions more than critical medical humanities. In 2018, these disciplines received a cut in funding from Theresa May's government as they were seen as poor value for money (Pickersgill et al., 2018). This sort of undermining may explain some of the persistence of the utilitarian fallacy and value for money as "arts produces health" gestalt.

Likewise, Slaby (2015) advocates that medical humanities works on scholarship and analysis of concepts in general about life, risk, health, well-being, mental capital, empathy and resilience to counter one-sided narratives about empathy and emotionality. The brain and neuroscience are seen as particular sites of application for a critical medical humanities to critique the conceptually confusing character of the mind/brain relationship, operational logic, responsibility and associated identity:

> There is no other scientific domain where 'promise' could be housed in a comparably murky conceptual impasse that is at the same time so close to the very core of human self-understanding while the health industry has learned to turn human mortality into an inexhaustible profit formula, neuroscience has settled in a lacuna of human self-understanding, in a riddlesome material pinnacle of who we are.
>
> (Slaby, 2015, p. 20)

The brain's presumed functioning is therefore used to invoke normative demands on the individual and how we should live according to what the brain apparently demands, otherwise known as neuronormativity. We need to be wary of invoking the brain as justification for empathy and sociality and instead look for relationality in which subjectivity is embedded, strategic positioning and ideology to counter neoliberal individualism (Slaby, 2015).

For example, if we take as a point of departure from neuronormative beliefs Slaby's statement about the conceptually confusing character of the mind/brain relationship, then we have to examine the nature of the context in which that character is embedded:

> Appeared on the scene is the sad figure of a self-possessed consumer, absorbed entirely within its homely sphere of somatic well-being, wrapped securely in a techno habitat, constantly anxious about the inevitable prospect of fleshly peril. We are left with a fearful, risk obsessed health consumer whose ethical horizon rarely exceeds the bounds of the individual's somatic experience. Agency gets more and more narrowed down to consumer choices and to "pro-active" behaviours in line with the recommendations of expert bodies.
>
> (Slaby, 2015, p. 20)

This situation, Slaby suggests, has created a profound dependence in core dimensions of human existence. The confusion arises because the mind/brain is primed to see itself through a neo-liberal lens, is complicit with social cultures of consumerism and therefore cannot see itself outside of that lens. This is the confusion that arises when the instrument of analysis (the mind/brain) tries to analyse the object (the mind/brain). The confusion is shown in another paper by Stuckey and Nobel (2010) who state that "we often find ourselves struggling with the 'fundamentals' of art and health and their meaning in society. We make no attempt to clarify or resolves these fundamental issues" (p. 254). Instead they go on to perform a narrative review of public health interventions using four genres of art that reinforces the ideal of the neo-liberal human subject. This ideal is critiqued because it is seen as the site of injustice, and therefore suffering, from a colonial project that sought to achieve economic and social advantage over disenfranchised others through emphasising difference and therefore sub-human-ness (Desal & Sanya, 2016). Paradoxically, by promoting this consumer ideal, medical humanities reinforces "the sad figure of a self-possessed consumer" (Slaby, 2015) that also disadvantages some groups of people over others.

Therefore what is in the curriculum matters. Culturally, the neo-liberal brain is trained through neo-liberal curricula so that the very knowledge we create is culturally and biologically located in and of the Western brain. Further, skins and masks inform our self-understanding through the enculturation of the dominant Western ways of seeing ourselves, thereby sharing group identity and providing a sense of belonging to place and community (Desal & Sanya, 2016). The way we see the brain, skin and masks leads us to make assumptions about ourselves. Micro injustices are seen in assumptions about what is knowledge, who can and does produce knowledge and how the human is conceptualised, as explained in Section 1.3 on epistemic injustice. This knowledge inscribes normative rules and standards about rationality and the self which thereby discipline and regulate people. Desal and Sanya (2016) argue that until we can question and bring about changes in how we see ourselves, beyond the reference point of the Western man, we will continue to be the effect of these cultural practices. Thus medical humanities will continue to be the effect of these cultural whitewashed practices until we can scratch below the surface and see beyond shallow multicultural referent-we understandings of humanity to explore the cultural melancholy and suffering below that (Singleton, 2015).

Therefore, medical humanities is implicated in perpetuating this mono-understanding until the field critically examines the social relationship between knowledge, curricula and personhood. By focusing on epistemology and micro matters such as concepts of the mind/brain, medical humanities is being asked to work the minor in order to decompose the major from within (Cerecer et al., 2019). Working from the inside out means working through everyday contradictions of neoliberalism by attending to experience:

Collective creative inquiry affords us the space for creating a world within a world where we are thinking through, undoing and redoing theoretical propositions together as a way of knowing and being in the world.

(Cerecer et al., 2019, p. 220)

More specifically, walking through these portals means seeing the epistemic gaps and links between clinical knowledge, broader cultural knowledge and idiosyncratic personal experience (MacNaughton & Carel, 2015). The idea is that by continually critiquing what it means to be a neo-liberal con-sumerist human, more doors may be opened in the mind/brain and that by stepping through these portals we will find something else on the other side.

This is a difficult path to tread since on the one hand there is emerging evidence that engaging with art helps to make sense (Kaptein et al., 2018). Yet on the other hand, theories such as psychoneuroimmunology, Theory of Mind and the Common Sense Model of Self-Regulation re-inforce the neuronormative ideal of sociality and empathy (Slaby, 2015) without questioning who is served by these models and who is dis-advantaged by them. Unless medical humanities fully critiques who it is speaking with, to, and for – for whom does medical humanities stand? – then it seems as though it will remain lost in the dark woods (Frank, 2017; Altschuler, 2018).

In order to explore these sorts of questions in relation to the experiential side of suffering, a different order or knowledge is required, specifically, the mythopoetic curriculum (Leonard & Willis, 2010). The mythopoetic cur-riculum could sit eminently well within medical humanities yet has not been included in the medical humanities literature; instead it is situated within the literature on pedagogy. As stated above, how we know what we know through medical humanities, sociology or biomedicine is rooted in as-sumptions which then go on to shape behaviour and character through various types of curricula. The mythopoetic curriculum is a "meta-discourse about curriculum that infiltrates the current horizon of expecta-tions to expose deeply archetypal individual and cultural elements that shape understanding of curriculum" (Holland & Garman, 2010, p. 12). These deeply archetypal elements are explored through insight, visualisa-tion and imagination – "myth" – as a source of knowledge with the lan-guage of "poetics" as a means of expression. Driven by two major value themes, McDonald describes these as follows:

One has been expressed in a desire to construct intellectually satisfying conceptual maps of the human condition which were educationally meaningful and personally satisfying. The second has been expressed in a utopian hope that somehow people could improve the quality of their existence specifically through educational processes and generally through broader social policy.

(Pinar, 1975, p. 3 cited in Holland & Garman, 2010, p. 14)

These two driving forces of accounting for "what is" as well as striving for an ideal may perhaps explain why progress has not been made in understanding suffering more. Critical theory and social justice are embedded in a mythopoetic curriculum that seeks to both demystify (through critical theories) and demythologise (through the use of interpretive theories) through both reduction of illusion and restoration of meaning.

The mythopoetic curriculum sits well within an exploration of suffering and medical humanities. "If science is the language of detachment, mythology is the language of concern" (Holland & Garman, 2010, p. 19). Since the concern with suffering in medicine is also a medical education curriculum issue, with medical humanities and sociology being prime means for exploring the individual and social as well as the relationship between them. Between different traditions, interpretivists "use the mythopoetic as strong warp threads to shape the phenomenological fabric of their writing. Writers within the critical tradition more often use the mythopoetic in subtle ways, like weft threads that give pattern and texture to the fabric of their work" (Holland & Garman, 2010, p. 23). Both the individual phenomenological and social critical approaches are necessary to understand the interweaving between them. The warp and weft fit well within the metaphor of a bricolage and show how to combine medical humanities and sociology to understand suffering.

4.5 Medical sociology

Sociology of health and illness questions how we conceive health and why people consult their doctors. A prevalent theme is to explore social structures such as practices around gender, age, race and ethnicity and socioeconomic status and how these stratify health outcomes (Scambler, 2008). Whereas medicine is interested in causes of ill-health and risk factors, sociology tends to focus on outcomes in terms of patterns of ill-health and death and accessibility to healthcare services. The nature of medical problems and the medicalisation of social problems, the stigma and labelling associated with those, disability and rehabilitation, delivery of healthcare, health policy and the structure and function of the NHS in the UK, evaluation of healthcare and health as a social value are all grist for the mill in sociology (Scambler, 2008). Professional medical identity and medical school culture has also been explored (Armstrong, 2002; Becker, 1961; Sinclair, 1977). However, as Wilkinson (2005) points out, there has yet to be developed a sociological theory of suffering.

Numerous topics, too many to mention here, have been developed from a sociological imagination perspective – stepping back to see the wider perspective (Wright Mills, 2000). The focus on socialisation has preoccupied studies on medical education through a rational lens. Yet as Scambler states, this has not impacted a great deal on medical students:

Even in the lively innovative phase it is questionable to what extent London's medical students came to think sociologically, that is, to see beyond the world of events to their patterning and to the manner in which social structures like class, gender, and ethnicity underpin this pattern.

(Scambler, 2008, p. 198)

Medical students are trained to think of causes from a biological chemical perspective and so have trouble thinking about social determinants of health, valuing these ideas and have even greater trouble imagining what they could do about these when in a clinical situation.

The "new" model of social medicine – considering the social determinants of health – has been around since the 1950s. Yet the medical curriculum is still structured around pathology, lifestyle behaviours and risk factors, with the rise of chronic ill-health and deteriorating living conditions for some segments of the population yet to make an impact. Health inequalities (Commission on Social Determinants of Health [CSDH], 2008; Institute of Health Inequalities, 2020) and vulnerability to social destabilisation, displacement and deindustrialisation have been suggested as mediators of these inequalities (Walsh et al., 2016), and still this knowledge has made little difference since the inequalities keeping increasing. Public health academics have worked hard to understand this issue but must feel as if they are fighting an uphill battle at times when government policies such as austerity only increase disadvantage experienced by the most vulnerable in society.

Gaps in medical sociology and medical education include the influence of the political economy, post-structuralism and post-modernism, as well as feminisation of the profession, all of which have been largely ignored by faculty (Bleakley et al., 2011). Challenges with the growth in numbers of medical students, particularly through widening participation, and what this means in the context of a business model of higher education have received little attention. The perceived erosion of medicine's knowledge base and professional autonomy, decrease in medical status, as well as the knowledge explosion and flattening of the medical hierarchy have all impacted professional identity and possibly burnout through the loss of the social matrix (Gerada, 2019). Whilst there may be a need for democracy in medical education (Bleakley et al., 2011), doctors themselves seem to find political activism difficult perhaps as it could be perceived as threatening by professional regulatory bodies such as the British Medical Association (BMA) and General Medical Council (GMC). Issues concerned with identity, location of healthcare and power are thought to be the future concerns of the medical profession (Bleakley et al., 2011).

At the centre of these debates are questions about the character of medical knowledge:

- What types of knowledge distinguishes the medical professional from other groups?

- What sorts of knowledge are needed to produce a competent but caring doctor?
- What counts as legitimate knowledge within a medical curricula? (Bleakley et al., 2011)

Bleakley et al., (2011) ponder the crisis in medical education and suggest that this is perhaps a symptom of current educational practice. There are fundamental epistemological and social struggles in medicine as medical schools adapt to changing circumstances of practice. Yet the tools necessary to inform responses are not always available, appreciated or acknowledged, and this could be due to the current higher education climate as well as how sociology is perceived within that climate. The character of medical knowledge is so different from sociological knowledge that it is difficult to know how to approach this thorny persistent issue. And yet doctors are embedded in working with people who suffer the worst health and worst living conditions; they are surrounded by suffering and perhaps focus on the techno-rational curriculum in order to survive and help patients to survive.

But perhaps because suffering is not generally considered explicitly as part of the medical curriculum, issues around the history of colonialism, medical professional identity and the culture of difference (Seth, 2018) are rarely discussed, as explained in Chapter One. These gaps and lack of understanding of the epistemological process in both medical humanities and sociology, as explained in Section 4.4, means that these disciplines could unwittingly be obscuring knowledge and learning, contributing to epistemic injustice about suffering. Since there is a lack of understanding about embodied experiential cognition, relational processes and transcendental learning outcomes abstracted from context, both medical humanities and sociology continue to tread well-worn paths on empathy and communication skills without thinking differently about specific issues characteristic of suffering. These lacunae are magnified during epistemic crises such as that of the current pandemic.

4.6 Where do medical humanities and sociology stand during the current COVID-19 pandemic?

There are two main concerns during this current pandemic evident from the literature that relate to the disciplines of medical humanities and sociology. Perhaps predictably medical humanities and sociology have renewed their call for being part of a response to address mental health issues for the public and health care workers (Peckham, 2020). The second major cause for concern is the disparity in infection and death rates by race and poverty in both the UK (Aldridge et al., 2020) and US. Both concerns are related to each other and to suffering.

As stated in Chapter One, the connection here between health professionals and patients is the crossover point where much can be learned with thinking about how we think about suffering. In particular, how we understand ourselves as humans seems to be a vital underpinning, as well as how we conceive the learning and knowledge process. Human being as praxis means walking along wandering lines within, yet also in order to go beyond, current institutional understandings. Yet currently there are no clear understandings of the interrelationship between health professional and patients from a sociology or medical humanities perspective, and certainly not from the perspective of the current pandemic.

Health professionals are the meat in the sandwich, between social policies on the one hand and providing lifestyle advice for individual risk factors on the other hand. This has become more apparent during COVID-19, as well as the additional risk of themselves turning into patients due to the nature of their work. These circumstances have resulted in impassioned pleas on social media of "I'm staying at work for you; please stay at home for me." Mixed in with this confusion of boundaries, there has been a resurgence of messages about fighting a war against COVID-19 with debates as to whether this metaphor is useful or not. Making the body a battle field depersonalises and positions people as warriors that have to combat with their strengths and knowledge as an "assault weapon" (Bleakley, 2017). Health professionals are in an invidious position, caught between risk rhetoric and war metaphors in order to preserve life and place: "I want to make it out of the next 18 months alive without crippling guilt about ethical judgment calls I had to make during a global pandemic."[1] Sociology has typically focused on the rhetoric of risk and the good citizen through a process of analysis of power. This may not be enough in the face of such suffering.

4.7 Moving forward

In the next two chapters, issues will be explored around the concept of the self and the potential depersonalisation and burnout that both patients and health professionals suffer in healthcare. It has been clear from this chapter that the main trends in medical humanities and sociology bring into question the use of arts and humanities in service of what is considered the self in medicine. Both medical humanities and sociology are at risk of staying at the level of disciplining medicine and the self with exclusion of knowledge that does not fit with the rational socialised individual. This seems to be where the confusion arises and where subjects can find themselves lost in the woods, not being able to see the woods for the trees. If someone can't see the woods for the trees, they are so involved in the details of something that they do not understand or pay attention to the most important parts of it. Medical humanities seems so lost in the idea of whether it is in or out, of instrumental or intrinsic value, subjectivity and objectivity – caught up in dichotomies – that sight is lost of art at the pre-categorical pre-cognitive level way of knowing. How cognition is defined is an effect and a cause of some of these difficulties.

Pedagogical aspects of operational logic such as concrete, conceptual, narrative, symbolic, schemata and abstract modes seem to provide a way forward, as long as they are embedded in a relational context that acknowledges suffering.

Suffering requires that we use multimodal representations of both individual and social suffering embedded within relational constructs drawing on a dual awareness of each. This is in essence the dialogic that occurs between self and other. At the moment there is little dialogue between medicine, medical humanities, sociology and medical education. Most of the curriculum is centred around the autonomous individual – the psychological isolate (Gerada, 2019) – which may be contributing to issues of burnout and depersonalisation. Taking into account the core characteristics and properties of suffering – the loss of intactness of self, hole in what can be said, distress, finding oneself on the wrong side of a fault line, languishing versus agency, self versus other – then this dialogue starts with the place where knowledge and experience has been racialised under a colonial project of differentiation and othering. The medical imagination is a necessity at this level of curriculum from a metacognitive perspective such as that offered by the mythopoetic curriculum.

Box 4.1   Reflection

Getting lost in the woods and not being able to see the woods for the trees means that from a medical humanities perspective, we have become lost in conceptual detail and remain stuck in narratives about dichotomies, making us spin our wheels further and further in the mud, trying to find a way out, perhaps as a way of avoiding suffering. This seems to create a lot of noise around the experience of suffering. When faced with profound suffering in the moment, there is a sense of wanting – yearning – to be real and yet what does that really mean? There is a power in being real, which requires us to stay in the unknown, yet so often health professionals have been taught and encouraged to hide behind symbols of authority and imaginaries of power. And at the same time, patients know we are human, can see beyond the white coat and the stethoscope and often want to connect with us there.

At times of profound suffering we often want to hide behind symbols, imaginaries and abstractions, which also then feels like a betrayal of the social contract we have with each other and with ourselves. Besides, there are so many competing demands on what seems real that it is difficult to know which to choose in the moment. So how do we choose? What moral authority do we rely on? In hindsight, it is always easier to judge ourselves for seemingly false consciousness and to feel culpable for not choosing the right path through the woods. The important aspect seems to be to recognise these moments of crisis for what they are: ruptures in how we know what we know. There is a finiteness to knowing what we can know in any moment. Part of our shared humanity is in knowing that, knowing that we did not come into this world with a pre-set manual for how we should be and what we should know, and to proceed from there.

Imagination and intuition may be useful at these times; images help us through as ways of putting into speech what we are experiencing. The places where we come up against the boundaries of our experience are places where we learn about who we think we are and where we may well come undone.

Questions for reflection

1   What images have you drawn on to carry you through difficult times? How have they worked for you?
2   How have these images been influenced by the social and cultural milieu in which you were?
3   How do you see the relationship between the social and the individual in forming these images?
4   Have you ever brought the images into the relational realm? What do you consider private and personal or shareable and public?

Further Resources
Popova M. 2019. *Figuring*. Canongate: Edinburgh.

References

Aldridge R.W., Lewer D., Katikireddi S.V., Mathur R., Pathak N., Burns R., Fragaszy E.B, Johnson A.B., Devakumar D., Abubakar I., Haywar A. 2020. Black, Asian and Minority Ethnic groups in England are at increased risk of death from COVID-19: Indirect standardisation of NHS mortality data [version 1; peer review: Awaiting peer review]. *Wellcome Open Research*; 5:88, doi: 10.12688/wellcomeopenres.15922.1.

Altschuler S. 2018. *The Medical Imagination: Literature and Health in the Early United States*. University of Pennsylvania Press: Philadelphia.

AMEE. 2019. AMEE Annual Conference, Vienna, Austria. 24–28th August 2019. www.AMEE.org.

Arendt H. 1971. Thinking and moral considerations: A lecture. *Social Research*; 38(3):417–446.

Armstrong D. 2002. *A New History of Identity: A Sociology of Medical Knowledge*. Palgrave: Basingstoke.

Atkinson S., Evans B., Woods A., Kearns R. 2015. 'The medical' and 'health' in a critical medical humanities. *Journal Medical Humanities*; 36:71–81.

Bærøe K. 2015. Medicine as art and science. *Handbook of the Philosophy of Medicine* In Schramme T., Edwards S. (eds). Springer: Dordrecht.

Becker E. 1973. *The Denial of Death*. Souvenir Press: London.

Becker H.S. 1961. *Boys in White: Student Culture in Medical School*. University of Chicago Press: Chicago.

Benjamin H.R.W. 1939. *Saber-Tooth Curriculum, Including Other Lectures in the History of Paleolithic Education*. McGraw-Hill: New York.

Birckbeck College Medical Humanities. 2017. *Informal Discussion with Various Interested Parties*. Birkbeck, University of London: London.

Bleakley A. 2015. *Medical Humanities and Medical Education: How the Medical Humanities Can Shape Better Doctors*. Routledge: London.

Bleakley A. 2017. Six fallacies that hinder development of the medical humanities in medical education. *Medical Education*; 51:126–127.

Bleakley A., Bligh J., Browne J. 2011. *Medical Education for the Future: Identity, Power and Location*. Springer: London.

Blease C. 2016. In defence of utility: The medical humanities and medical education. *Medical Humanities*; 42:103–108.

Buchan J., Charlesworth A., Gershlick B., Seccombe I. 2019. *A Critical Moment: NHS Staffing Trends, Retention and Attrition*. The Health Foundation. https://www.health.org.uk/publications/reports/a-critical-moment.

Campo R. 2005. "The medical humanities" for lack of a better term. *JAMA*; 294(9): 1009–1011.

Cerecer D.A.Q., Cahill C., Coronado Y.S.G., Martinez J. 2019. "We the people": Epistemological moves through cultural praxis. *Cultural studies – Critical methodologies*; 19(3):214–221.

Commission on Social Determinants of Health (CSDH). 2008. Closing the gap in a generation: Health equity through action on the social determinants of health. *Final Report of the Commission on Social Determinants of Health*. World Health Organisation: Geneva.

de Almeida H. 1991. *Romantic Medicine and John Keats*. Oxford University Press: Oxford.

de Certeau M. 1984. *The Practice of Everyday Life*. University of California Press: California.

Desal K., Sanya B.N. 2016. Towards decolonial praxis: Reconfiguring the human and curriculum. *Gender and Education*; 28(6):710–724.

Durham University. 2018. Personification across disciplines. *Conference September 2018. Hearing the voice*. www.padonline.org.

Eco U. 2014. *From the Tree to the Labyrinth: Historical Studies on the Sign and Interpretation*. Harvard University Press: New York.

Engebretsen E., Fraas Henrichsen G., Ødemark J. 2020. Towards a translational medical humanities: Introducing the cultural crossings of care [published online ahead of print, 2020 Apr 27]. *Medical Humanities*, doi: 10.1136/medhum-2019-011751.

Engeström Y. 2019. *The Center for Research on Activity, Development and Learning, University of Helsinki, Finland*), Bleakley A. (Faculty of Medicine and

Dentistry, University of Plymouth, UK) AMEE. AMEE Annual Conference, Vienna, Austria, 24–28th August 2019. www.AMEE.org.

Fiske A.P. 1993. *Structures of Social Life: The Four Elementary Forms of Human Relations.*The Free Press: New York.

Fitzgerald D., Callard F. 2016. Entangling the medical humanities. Chapter 1 in *The Edinburgh Companion to the Critical Medical Humanities*. Whitehead A., Woods A., Atkinson S., et al. (eds). Edinburgh University Press: Edinburgh.

Foucault M. 1980. *Power/Knowledge – Selected Interviews and Other Writings 1972–1977.* Gordon C. (ed). Pantheon Books: New York.

Foucault M. 1973. *The Birth of the Clinic – An Archeology of Medical Perception.* Vintage Books: New York.

Frank A.W. 2017. An illness of one's own: Memoir as an art form and research as witness. *Cogent Arts and Humanities*; 4:1–7.

George R.E., Lowe W.A. 2019. Well-being and uncertainty in health care practice. *Clinical Teacher;* 16:298–305.

Gerada C. 2019. The making of a doctor: The matrix and self. *Group Analysis*; 52(3):350–361, doi: 10.1177/0533316418823117.

Gordon J. 2005. Medical humanities: To cure sometimes, to relieve often, to comfort always. *Medical Journal of Australia*; 182(1):5–8.

Greenhalgh T. et al. 2016. An open letter to The BMJ editors on qualitative research. *BMJ*; 352:i563. doi: ezproxy.library.qmul.ac.uk/10.1136/bmj.i563l.

Haidet P., Jarecke J., Adams N.E., Stuckey H.L., Green M.J., Shapiro D., Teal C.R., Wolpaw D.R. 2016. A guiding framework to maximise the power of the arts in medical education: A systematic review and metasynthesis. *Medical Education*; 50:320–331.

Hardacre J., Margetts A. 2020. Psychological PPE: Survival kit for creating a safer culture in the Covid-19 context. *BMJ Leader*. https://blogs.bmj.com/bmjleader/ 2020/04/15/psychological-ppe-survival-kit-for-creating-a-safer-culture-in-the-covid-19-context/.

Herman J. 2001. Medicine: The science and the art. *BMJ Medical Humanities*; 27:42–46.

Holland P.E., Garman N.B. 2010. Watching with two eyes: The place of the mythopoetic in curriculum inquiry. Chapter 2 in *Pedagogies of the Imagination*. Leonard T., Willis P. (eds). Springer Science + Business Media BV: Chicago.

Hutton P.H. (1988). *Technologies of Self*. Martin L.H., Gutman H., Hutton P.H. (eds). The University of Massachusetts Press: Amherst.

Jones E.K., Kumagai A.K., Kittendorf A.L. 2019. Through another lens: The humanities and social sciences in the making of physicians. *Medical Education*; 53:320–330.

Kahneman D. 2012. *Thinking, Fast and Slow*. Penguin: New York.

Kaptein A.A., Hughes B.M., Murray M., Smyth J.M. 2018. Start making sense: Art informing health psychology. *Health Psychology Open*. doi: 10.1177/ 2055102918760042.

Kristeva J., Moro MR., Odemark J., Engebretsen E. 2018. Cultural crossings of care: An appeal to the medical humanities. *BMJ Medical Humanities*; 44, 55–58. 10.1136/medhum-2017-011263.

Land R. 2019. #1 Plenary: Threshold concepts and troublesome knowledge: A transformational approach to learning (Emeritus Professor of Higher Education,

Durham University, UK). Presenter at AMEE. AMEE Annual Conference, Vienna, Austria, 24–28th August 2019. www.AMEE.org.

Lather P. (1991). *Getting Smart – Feminist Research and Pedagogy with/in the Postmodern*. Routledge, Chapman and Hall: New York.

Lechopier N., Moutot G., Lefève C., Teixeira M., Poma R., Grandazzi G., Rasmussen A. 2018. Health professionals prepared for the future. Why social sciences and humanities teaching in medical faculties matter. *MedEdPublish*. doi: 10.15694/mep.2018.0000195.1.

Leonard T., Willis P. (Eds). 2010. *Pedagogies of the Imagination: Mythopoetic Curriculum in Educational Practice*. Springer: Chicago.

MacNaughton J., Carel H. 2015. Breathing and breathlessness in clinic and culture: Using critical medical humanities to bridge an epistemic gap. Chapter 16 in *The Edinburgh Companion to the Critical Medical Humanities*. Whitehead A., Woods A., Atkinson S. et al. (eds). Edinburgh University Press: Edinburgh. https://www.ncbi.nlm.nih.gov/books/NBK379257/.

Marmot M., Allen J., Boyce T., Goldblatt P., Morrison J. 2020. *Health Equity in England: The Marmot Review 10 Years on*. Institute of Health Equity: London.

McFarlane J., Markovina I., Gibbs T. 2018 . Concluding commentary. The importance of the humanities in medical education: Where are we now? *MedEdPublish*; 7:83. doi: 10.15694/mep.2018.0000220.1.

Milne A. 2019. Uncertainty in the PreHospital Care environment. *PCP Academic Forum 29th October 2019*. Queen Mary University of London.

Moro M.R. 2018. A transcultural approach to psychiatry. *Cultural Crossings of Care*. Oslo University. Keynote Speaker.

Ney A. 2019. *Metaphysics: An Introduction*. Routledge: London.

Oslo University. 2018. *Cultural crossings of care – An appeal to the medical humanities*. Oslo, Norway.

Patel A. 2018. To be a good doctor, study the humanities. https://psmag.com/education/be-a-good-doctor-study-the-humanities.

Pearl R. 2014. *Medicine is an art, not a science: Medical myth or reality?* Forbes. https://www.forbes.com/sites/robertpearl/2014/06/12/medicine-is-an-art-not-a-science-medical-myth-or-reality/.

Peckham R. 2020. A health emergency is no time to sideline the medical humanities. https://www.timeshighereducation.com/opinion/health-emergency-no-time-sideline-medical-humanities.

Pickersgill M., Chan S., Haddow G., Laurie G., Sridhar D., Sturdy S., Cunningham-Burley S. 2018. The social sciences, humanities, and health. *Lancet*; *391*(10129): 1462–1463.

Puustinen R., Leiman M., Viljanen AM. 2003. Medicine and the humanities – Theoretical and methodological issues. *Medical Humanities*; 29:77–80.

Quine WVO. 1951. Two dogmas of empiricism. *Philosophical Review*; 60(1):20–43:39–40.

Saunders J. 2000. The practice of clinical medicine as an art and as a science. *Medical Humanities*; 26:18–22.

Scambler G. (Ed). 2008. *Sociology as Applied to Medicine*. Sixth Edition. Saunders Elsevier: London.

Schlozman S.C. 2017. Why psychiatric education needs the humanities. *Academy of Psychiatry*; 41:703–706.

Schwartz A.W., Abramson J.S., Wojnowich I., Accordino R., Ronan E.J., Rifkin M.R. 2009. Evaluating the impact of the humanities in medical education. *Mount Sinai Journal of Medicine*; 76:372–380.

Seth S. 2018. *Difference and Disease: Medicine, Race, and the Eighteenth-century British Empire*. Cambridge University Press: Cambridge.

Sinclair S. 1977. *Making Doctors: An Institutional Apprenticeship*. Bloomsbury Publishing: London.

Singleton J. 2015. *Cultural Melancholy: Readings of Race, Impossible Mourning, and African American Ritual*. University of Illinois Press: Illinois.

Slaby J. 2015. Critical neuroscience meets medical humanities. *Medical Humanities*; 41:16–22.

Stuckey H.L., Nobel J. 2010. The connection between art, healing, and public health: A review of current literature. *Framing Health Matters*; 100(2):254–263.

Taylor A., Lehmann S., Chisolm M. 2018. Integrating humanities curricula in medical education: A literature review. *MedEdPublish*; 6:28. doi: https://doi.org/10.15694/mep.2017.000090.2.

UK Foundational Programme. 2017. *UK Foundation Programme Career Destinations Report*. https://www.nhsemployers.org/your-workforce/plan/medical-workforce/foundation-programme-career-destination-report-2017.

Younie L. 2019. *Flourishing through creative enquiry*. https://www.creativeenquiry.qmul.ac.uk/.

Viney W., Callard F., Woods A. 2015. Critical medical humanities: Embracing entanglement, taking risks. *Critical Medical Humanities*; 41:2–7.

Wald H., Haramati A., Bachner Y., Urkin J. 2016. Promoting resiliency for inter-professional faculty and senior medical students: Outcomes of a workshop using mind-body medicine and interactive reflective writing. *Medical Teacher*; 38:525–528.

Wald H.S., McFarland J., Markovina I. 2018. Medical humanities in medical education and practice. *Medical Teacher*; 41(5):492–496. doi: 10.1080/0142159X.2018.1497151.

Walsh D., McCartney G., Collins C., Taulbut M., Batty G.D. 2016. *History, Politics and Vulnerability: Explaining Excess Mortality*. Glasgow Centre for Population Health: Glasgow.

Wear D. 2009. The medical humanities: Toward a renewed praxis. *Journal of Medical Humanities*; 30:209–220.

Whitehead A., Woods A., Atkinson S., et al. (Eds). 2016. *The Edinburgh Companion to the Critical Medical Humanities*. Edinburgh University Press: Edinburgh.

Wilkinson I. 2005. *Suffering: A Sociological Introduction*. Polity Press: Cambridge.

World Health Organization (WHO) 2019. Health evidence network synthesis report 67. *What Is the Evidence on the Role of the Arts in Improving Health and Well-being? A Scoping Review*. WHO: Geneva.

Wright Mills C. 2000. *The Sociological Imagination*. Oxford University Press: Oxford.

Wu H.Y.J. 2018. Six domains to develop critical medical humanities. *The Clinical Teacher*; 15:93–97.

5 The suffering self and burning woman

5.1 Introduction

We ended the last chapter with a quote from a medic that "I want to make it out of the next 18 months alive without crippling guilt about ethical judgement calls I had to make during a global pandemic."[1] His idea about himself was structured around survival and the emotional burden of moral and ethical dilemmas that threatened to cripple him; there is a real sense of the totality of that experience including individual, professional and social elements as well as the embodied sense of his self as potentially being crippled by these situations. His suffering was connected to the patients' suffering – the two were intertwined. There seems to be a fear akin to being lost in the woods.

Suffering is a particular form of being lost in the woods where a person may not be able to find their way out and keeps rushing around only to find they have become even more lost.

> [A]s long as I believed that life had meaning even if I could not express it, the reflection of life in poetry and in art. But when I began to search for the meaning of life, when I began to feel the necessity of living, I found this mirror either unnecessary, superfluous and ridiculous, or tormenting. I could no longer be comforted by what I saw in the mirror, namely my stupid and desperate position.

> If I had been like a man in a wood from which he knows there is no way out, I might have been able to live; but I was like a man in a wood who is lost, and terrified by this rushes around hoping to find his way out, knowing that with each step he is getting more lost, and yet unable to stop rushing about.

> (Tolstoy, 1987; p. 33)

Existentially, the search for a rational meaning can only intensify the feeling of being lost and what is necessary is a turn to the experiential. The lost feeling relates to a loss of intactness of the self. We begin this chapter on the suffering self by reviewing ideas about the self, where these came from and what they might mean in relation to suffering.

Descriptions of the experience of the suffering self are different from ideas about the self generally. The suffering self experiences a loss of intactness of self; as can be seen from the quote above, the hope is for a self that remains (alive) in spite of the onslaught on ethical dilemmas. This sentence shows that suffering is individually experienced as well as being socially constructed; the individual – "I want to make it out" – crosses over "without crippling guilt" with the social "ethical judgment calls I had to make during a global pandemic." This can produce a felt sense of a crossover in the body; the chiasma of social justice – the felt sense of reciprocity and reversibility, where we are both touched by and touching an ethical dilemma; where we both feel the sense of (in)justice in our bodies and respond to perceived injustice in a world where suffering is an understorey. The further descriptions of the experience of suffering include one of distress, loss of self, speechlessness, being on the wrong side of the fault line of life. The experience can often proceed alongside conscious awareness *without necessarily being aware of suffering* – continuing to function yet something feels awry. These embodied emotional experiences of suffering are not usually included in the ordinary constructions of the self which tends to be presented more like an abstracted (from context) ideal. That is, the ordinary self is seen as without suffering, and a state that the suffering self perhaps tries to return to.

Because ordinary selves are not usually seen as suffering, there is perhaps a rejection of the suffering self. The rejection makes an ethical response difficult since the abandonment of the suffering self can precipitate a reaction or projection. The felt sense of an individualised ethical dilemma reverberates on a perhaps invisible social level, on how we feel and how prepared we are to respond. On a relational level, health professionals may not know what to say or how to respond to patients and families, perhaps using touch and tenderness or rituals of healthcare practices as a communicative medium. They may not know answers, are immersed in uncertainty and feel compelled to respond in a positive way as to likely outcomes. Yet individually health professionals are often in situations of extreme suffering themselves. Perhaps their suffering takes the form of burnout, depersonalisation and emotional exhaustion as mentioned in previous chapters. Suffering of health professionals can be visible in behaviours such as professionalism concerns, excess substance and alcohol use and ultimately suicide.

The healthcare system tends to be run still on authoritarian relational lines where suffering is individualised and therefore seen as a personal responsibility. Wanting to survive without the emotional burden of role conflict with situational demands produces an anguish where the self is in conflict with idealised professional expectations. The individualisation and hence internalisation of suffering mean that emotions such as shame, guilt and thoughts about personal culpability are not addressed. That is, when a health professional is placed in a situation of having to respond to a suffering patient when they cannot be sure of the outcome as a professional, there is an anguished fusion of self as human and role as a professional, which can go underground if attention is not paid to this defining moment. There is a tension between suffering self and other, perhaps manifest in a lack of trust of being understood and related to cultural melancholy, a tension between not being able to value one's self enough to be able to do something – a languishing – and attempts at agency (Devisch et al, 2017). The languishing can be related to cultural melancholy; grief at an unconscionable loss which one will not allow one's self to see; there is displacement and disavowed mourning (Singleton, 2015).

From the above review of the suffering self, there are many different levels of understanding the suffering self. However, there is the idea of the self and then underneath that (as an understorey) is the experience of the self, but the two don't always match because of the epistemic break in what is perceived as real and knowable (ontology and epistemology or metaphysics). In the writing of this section, there is a dilemma in writing from the experienced suffering self or from the perspective of perhaps idealised versions of what a self is or could be because this general abstracted writing of the self does not reference suffering. Ultimately, these ideas about self then make suffering outside of self. As de Certeau (1984) claimed; "Writing repeats this lack in each of its graphs, the relics of a walk through language. It spells out an absence that is its precondition and its goal" (p. 195). As stated in Chapter One, we know that as we try to cross that space, we will be performing an absence if writing from a place that asserts suffering is elsewhere than us. Any organisation of knowledge that cannot account for suffering must seem as if it will fragment the discussion as it will exclude the experience of many people. Thus the self gets pulled out of itself into a social construction of the self. However, it does seem pertinent to consider what and how ideas around the self are organised at a general level whilst always bearing in mind that for many people – health professionals and patients – suffering is a part of the self and can often manifest in this anguish of an ethical dilemma. That is the moment when we know we suffer – when we resonate with those who suffer, in recognition.

For the purposes of this discussion, I will draw on three main levels of understanding the theorised self – the general universal felt sense of self ("I am"); the concept of the self from different academic disciplines including medical humanities, psychology and sociology; and the category of the self from a moral legal perspective (an individual person, a citizen, human rights). There is thus an experiential, embodied, felt sense of self (described by neuroscience, phenomenology and hermeneutics); a constructed self in relation with the social world (social psychology and critical theory); and a self that is instrumental as determined and judged by its role in society; which can also involve moral dilemmas formative in the development of self (these will be discussed in full in Chapter Six). Sources of self in the latter category of self occur through three primary social means – theistic, romantic expressivism and instrumentality (Taylor, 1989). There are overlaps within these; for example, the body is the citizen as evidenced by the Magna Carta Charter "*Habeus Corpus*" (late Middle English: Latin, literally "you shall have the body (in court)") (Jones, 2014). The citizen body is considered the site of operation of biopower (Danaher et al, 2000). The body is also considered in phenomenology, hermeneutics and neuroscience. Each of these levels are considered in Table 5.1 to show how they relate to one another. Each of these conceptions, levels and categories form part of the fabric of our lives and the quilt we make in this book. The self is constructed multiple times in different ways and from different perspectives depending on the theory and discipline from which this consideration is coming. I have placed the biomedical self in the instrumentality section of the table since it is most obviously associated with the scientific outlook. The point is that the self as multiple necessitates a multimodal form of knowing and learning.

Integrating a multimodal form of knowing and being is crucial and where the sense of moral self can arise. The integration required is between that of the dynamic relation between co-operation and defection (Wilson, 1998) as explored in Chapter Two. But rather than saying there is no such thing as a true self, we are required to understand more components of the self including the neuroscience, biology and epigenetic influences as well as social environmental, from a bottom-up synthesis (Wilson, 1998). We need both the social and the individual perspectives:

> "Psyche and culture are, in fact, 'coemergents'. There can be no culture, indeed, that is not experienced by a psychism and there can be no psychism that is perceptible without a cultural symbolism"
>
> (Cerea, 2018; p. 304).

Sources of modern identity come from each level, concept and category. For our purposes, moral judgments take a particularly prescient form in the relationship between doctor and patient. In the quote above, the physician expected to make moral-ethical judgments as part of the process of his self making it out alive. Moral judgments are made about the value of human life, dignity afforded on how we understand our role and beliefs about the kind of life worth living; these in turn are formative of both personal and professional identity.

Before going on to explore these categories of self, a caveat about discussions of the self. There is no one right idea of oneself, and differing levels of explanation relate to other levels. The self can be seen as a unifying agent, a code that makes sense of and organises our activities (Hollis, 1996). *How* the self is understood is itself a process that constructs ideas about the self in an iterative loop of reinforcement. For example, the construction of the self gives ideas about the mind. In fact, Mauss (1996) declared that the self equals consciousness and this is its primordial category.

Table 5.1 Levels, concepts and categories of the self

Item	Components	Theories
Experience of self (I am)	Experiential Embodied Felt Sense	Phenomenology Hermeneutics Neuroscience
Conceptual Constructed Self	Existing or produced by social Active agency or passive Intrapsychic or intersubjective Coherent or fragmented Produced in the moment or realised over time Disavowed unrecognised loss of self Split in self Id, ego, superego	Social psychology Critical theory Self-psychology – Kohut Psychoanalysis – Freud
Category of self (Person) Instrumental self Must give an account of moral sources that orient our lives Values of life goods fractured along these three strands (Taylor, 1989)	Theistic – relationship with God Instrumentality – citizen, economy Biomedical self Romantic expressivism – ethical relationship with self	Inwardness Radical reflexivity Articulated by Augustine Naturalism of disengaged reason Associated with scientific outlook Task of discovering and expressing what was hidden within Art as manifestation of self Moral evaluations mediated by imagination

This was not always so, as in the past a self was scarcely conceived of outside social roles (Hollis, 1996).

> From a simple masquerade to the mask, from a "role" (*personnage*) to a "person" (*personne*), to a name, to an individual; from the latter to a being possessing metaphysical and moral value; from a oral consciousness to a sacred being; from the latter to a fundamental form of thought and action – the course is accomplished.
>
> (Mauss, 1996; p. 22)

Work still evolves on this idea of a category of self; "far from existing as the primordial innate idea" (p. 20), the understanding of the self has revolved around debates on whether the self is an individual entity, a soul or substance, whether it is one and indivisible, or divisible, everlasting or finite, whether it is free, an absolute source of all action, and thereby responsibility or whether the self is socially determined – these ideas all make up the concepts of the self. These concepts themselves remain stable and will be drawn upon in the following discussions as they are inherent to ideas around risk and health promotion as noted in Chapter Two. The concepts are also implicit in moral and ethical dilemmas about healthcare.

In fact, I suggest that the concepts themselves are crucial mediators in transmitting a moral-ethical felt sense (into/out) of the body and thereby crucial in developing a sense of self, especially through the medium of a moral dilemma. All the levels of understanding of self – general universal sense of self ("I am"), the concept of the self from different academic disciplines including medical humanities, psychology and sociology, and the category of the self from a moral legal perspective (an individual person, a citizen, human rights) – are necessary and related to one another. Concepts of the self relate to the moral legal framework of category of the self, as applied to three main areas of social life – theistic, instrumentality (utility), and romantic expressivism (Taylor, 1989). The process of the self is similar to the process of perception and interpretation of knowledge that enables development of schemata as referred to in Chapter One:

> Sensations appear as interpretations of stimuli; perceptions as interpretations of sensations; judgments of perceptions as the interpretations of perceptions; particular and general propositions as interpretations of perceptual judgments; and scientific theories as interpretations of propositions.
>
> (Eco, 2014; p. 486)

Theories and schemata of self develop from sensations and perceptions of self. Through a shared language and understanding these also contribute to a universal sense of self over time and perhaps one that can be perceived as being lost through suffering. From Devisch et al (2017) we know that suffering has two axes of self-other and languishing-agency. Perhaps what is lost is the capacity to interpret and categorise experiences and perceptions since these seem to lie outside what is normal, of being the other side of the fault line of life. Therefore the interlocutor is lost; the speechlessness of suffering intervenes because of the devastation of events that lie outside what is considered normal. For both patients and health professionals, when faced with a moral dilemma, there may be a processing impairment which contributes to the feeling of loss of self. In addition, there is the displacement of an unconscionable loss on to the ego (Singleton, 2015).

These levels of analysis have implications for medical humanities and sociology at the curricular level – "what is the medical curriculum for?" – whether or not it is seen as technological and instrumental in itself or whether it supports broader social purposes of improvement of the societies we live in (Peddiwell, 2004; Wilson, 1998). That is, whether the self is seen as a tool of the state in its subjectivity or whether there is something beyond practices or technologies of the self (biopower) (Danaher et al, 2000; Foucault, 1973). Medical humanities has a particular role to play in understanding the theistic and romantic expressivism movements as sources of morality in developing the self by providing a different set of lenses to process events.

5.2 Medical humanities and sociology in service of the suffering self

We are not yet out the woods; there are many different approaches in sociology and medical humanities to cover what are contentious concepts related to the self, identity and the body and which evoke vociferous responses in defence of positions or concepts from each of the academic disciplines (Wilson, 1998). Yet these concepts are crucial to understanding suffering. That is to say, suffering can be seen as racialised and gendered, yet with debates about the constructed nature of race, gender and suffering, it is difficult to state anything without understanding the academic culture around these issues. Suffering seems to lend itself to existential questioning and finding some quite absolute truth which goes against many of the tenets of sociology.

Again, we are not out of the woods yet. In one of the conferences mentioned in Chapter Three, Moro (2018) suggests, "When you are lost, sit down." Figure 5.1 – Still in the woods – is the image for this chapter suggesting that while we sit and contemplate, the fires are raging, burning around us. I have used the words "burning woman" in the title to remind us of the gendered nature of suffering, too – how we see and respond to suffering. That in the crossover, it is often women who are caught in the crossfire, as Donna relayed in Chapter One, between abstracted policies and the practical implementation of these. The image also suggests the complementarity that Moro (2018) referred to, the use of two or more disciplines to explore but the difficulty in using these at the same time. That perhaps this is the greatest stumbling block to progress – the inability to think through and rationalise at the same time as keeping the wider sociological perspective. Chapter Two stated some basic assumptions which are explored further here:

1   People may not know cognitively the experience of suffering; it may be outside their awareness or consciousness because of the speechlessness that accompanies suffering.

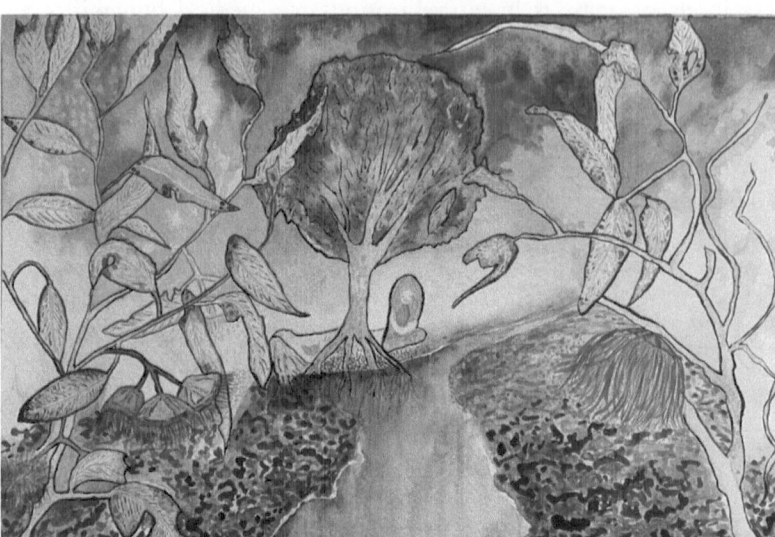

Figure 5.1 Still in the woods.

2　Both health professionals and patients are involved, intersubjectively, with/in suffering.

3　Any works on the self have to take into account the hole in the self. Therefore previous assumptions that prevail in mainstream about the self do not necessarily apply in the experience of suffering. Yet both suffering and not suffering belong to the self.

4　Critical race theory must be included in any exposition on suffering in order to counter knowledge and attitudes built upon colonialist projects of the self.

5　Given all the above assumptions, compassion is necessary to move beyond exclusionary practices and epistemic injustice. The epistemic gap is between suffering and mainstream practices.

Exploring the suffering self in more detail in order to find out what is really meant by this, what the implications are and by what it might mean to come undone when with a suffering stranger is in itself a way of coming undone. If we can expect to come undone (Orange, 2011) and know that no work is more important (Butt, 2002), then we must be prepared for the journey ahead. Ideas around self are complicated by sociological analyses of the self, arguing that there is no such thing as a true self – everything is constructed linguistically and culturally – there are only technologies of the self (Foucault, 1973; Hutton, 1988). The gendered self is performative and constructed (Butler, 1993) or an entanglement (Fitzgerald & Callard, 2016) or a knot in a sea of relations in pedagogy (Biesta, 2004). Yet people who suffer certainly experience this in/of their bodies and could be somewhat dismayed at this (transcended) post-structuralist position. It seems as if sociology and medical humanities have been involved in technologies that support biomedicine by writing the materiality of the body out of the equation of individuality.

Self and body are associated/synonymous in suffering. However, one of the reasons why post-modern and post-structuralists moved towards eschewing the idea of self or essence was precisely to address oppressive power relations and suffering as a result of gender, sexuality, disability, racial and socioeconomic culturally constructed fault lines, to suggest the idea that we are more fluid, connected and permeable than we believe ourselves to be. Yet these ideas about self also sit uncomfortably with the materiality of the body-self that lives, breathes, eats and suffers (Bynum, 1995a). Certainly, for the suffering person, the body is the medium and mediator of the experience and initiator of responses to suffering such as transcendence of the body, salvation and redemption, in a context of spiritual and existential crisis (Leder, 1990; Scarry, 1985; Sontag, 1991). Debates about the constructedness of the body and the body as the very condition of subjectivity (McLaren, 2002) are the discursive formations or epistemes currently available. These debates will be explored as they relate to suffering.

The gap identified in Chapter One – the epistemic break in knowledge due to the disconnect between life and death – will be explored since it is here that the curricular issues begin. To ask "what would a curriculum look like that took suffering into account?" means starting with basic concepts around life, death and suffering and how we respond. I start with ideas around life, death and suffering because suffering is incorporated in concepts of self; there is no split here or epistemic break. This means therefore that I will start with theistic sources of self as a category of self. For the section on theistic sources of self, I will draw on Caroline Bynum and her explorations of the medieval suffering self, body and social patterns (1995a, 1995b, 1991, 1987). I then turn to research on health professional education to explore instrumentalism as a category of self and how disengaged reason affects health professional self and practice particularly in relation to suffering. Disengaged reason is perhaps a reason why some people are not able to relate sincerely to suffering and may then act out in archetypal ways such as the hero, saviour or witchy woman (Wilson, 1998), i.e., as social formations (or roles) to link patterns of response to suffering to the mythopoetic curriculum. Then I will review the main psychological theories of the self (Damasio, Kohut, Jung, Freud) to establish the historical basis and some of the current psychological thinking on which ideas of the self originate, and notions of inside and outside. I do this exploration in a reversed order, from suffering self to what is considered usual self, so that I am addressing the epistemic break.

The epistemic break is then explored, on the back of the preceding points, at the basic level of concepts, ideas, schemata and patterns to continue the thread running through Sections 1.5, 2.3, 3.4, and 4.3.3. The theistic section outlines a paradigm shift necessary for thinking about suffering. This shift can be seen between medieval and current thinking, providing hints as to what we may need to move towards now. Medical humanities as a way of thinking differently about how we think about suffering – as a meta-cognitive strategy – can assist in the exploration of lacunae in medicine, health psychology and medical education at the epistemic and pedagogical level. Given that health professionals work with people from some of the most deprived locations and communities, there is an urgent requirement to address the inclusion of suffering at the curriculum level. This means moving beyond dichotomies prevalent in the medical humanities field in the service of suffering. Given that medicine's primary aim is to reduce suffering ("If the aim of medicine is to offer the hope of alleviating suffering, to invoke and influence human change, it needs more than science and technology": Francis, 2020; p. 25), then understanding the suffering self and body seems vital.

5.3 The theistic sources of the self

5.3.1 The (long) suffering body

Starting with the body is an acknowledgement of the concrete embodied experiential nature of suffering. Bynum (1995a) suggests that the reason why it is important to go back to the medieval past is to recollect that this is where the physical body was tied to identity, matter and desire, before and after death, and, most importantly, that this tying inherently included suffering. This means that the epistemic gap between life and death, as mentioned in Chapter One and upon which the framework is based in Chapter Two, can be addressed. This is important because as de Certeau (1984) argued, the break between life and death, where death is seen as a defeat by medicine, wraps it up in a shroud of silence, organises knowledge in relation to poverty and suffering as outside the field of medicine. The organisation of knowledge in the space between life and death means that existential issues such as suffering have been placed beyond the pale for discussion. Therefore it is difficult to reclaim the body unless we relate it to suffering and death (Becker, 1973). Rather than transforming illness into a scientific and linguistic category or object, the following explores how we can bring the human back into the discourse. How we do this will add another layer to the suffering framework.

Explicitly naming and acknowledging suffering, making this a starting point, changes our perception of the body, from post-structuralist tendencies to dissolve everything about the body into language, a movement which seems just as abstract as biomedicine in its effects, to acknowledging the body that lives and suffers as a material reality (Bynum, 1995a). The current post-structuralist concerns with sexuality and gender eclipse matters of suffering and death to their detriment. Explicitly acknowledging the body as a material reality seems important, as doing so brings cognition to the present debate and helps to avoid the trap of either representationalism or cognitive solipsism.

The lacunae currently about suffering and death in the medical curriculum are perpetuated by social science's and medical humanities' preoccupation with language or discourse, and dualist notions. Relying on discursive accounts of the body creates a body-as-trap where scholarly activity goes round in uncomfortable circles (Bynum, 1995a). Relying on a dualist notion of body-as-subject and body-as-object tends to arise from historical perceptions of body as despised, identified with chaotic nature and the female – passive, negative, irrational (Bynum, 1995a). There is no doubt these perceptions existed. However, they were not the only story as evidenced by Bynum (1987, 1991, 1995a, 1999b). She suggests that we want to be freed from a self that is reduced to an identity-position and a past that dwindles into a tradition of implausible generalisations (Bynum, 1995a).

However, therein lies the challenge since to move beyond restrictive binary positions means moving backwards to a trinary position or forward into multifold categories in how we know what we know as suggested in Chapter Four. This is a challenge because the plausibility and credibility of any modern-day scholar suggesting such an idea to a current medical education curriculum committee would probably be met with ridicule, to say the least. To suggest a trinary position of body, soul and spirit would undo all the distance that biomedicine has tried to create between itself and the psychosocial underbrush, which would not appear to be a palatable suggestion. Moreover, the admission that we are all human facing the same sea of existential uncertainty, albeit with different resources at our disposal, seems to be an a priori in even thinking about matters such as body, soul and spirit. Before rejecting these notions completely, though, it is worth understanding more about what was meant by this trinary idea of a person and what it meant to be human in the medieval ages. However, Bynum's (1991) point is that in the study of death, the human person was treated as a tight integral union of soul and body. A union dependent on redemption of suffering is a way of managing suffering and it is the redemption that informed relationships between medieval persons. This is an idea which comes up again later in Chapter Six when considering health promotion.

5.3.2 Resurrection and redemption

Resurrection and redemption occurred through the body and religious women were seen as providers of salvation in a twist of fate:

> Women understood the suffering that lay at the core of their lives to *be* both mystical ecstasy and active, innerworldly service of their fellow human beings.
>
> (Bynum, 1991; p. 74; emphasis original)

The two references to the inner life of the body linked to the social service of fellow human beings so that there was a relationship between the inner and outer, and in fact, the outer was seen as innerwordly. The return of body parts to reassemble wholeness, a tension between body as locus of pain and limitation and body as locus of personhood and therefore of salvation itself, was seen as predominant in societies where suffering and death were more visible (Bynum, 1991). The wholeness aimed for through the interaction between a united body, self and the social was an important aim for medieval life.

Bynum (1991) suggests that the notion of redemption and the doctrine of resurrection provides meaning from suffering and fragmentation. To assert wholeness in the face of decay and fragmentation was part of the human condition. This was an effort to assert that knowing, surviving and being must be embodied. Self was sensed as a psychosomatic unity (Bynum, 1995b). The body was seen as the site of manifestation of the soul's experience of God, and that the more perfect a body was, the more fully it experienced, including suffering (Bynum, 1995b). The body-soul-self was seen as inseparable, "a particularized, experiencing, glowing, and, at least partially, sensual person, moving ever deeper into delight" (Bynum, 1995b; p. 254). The cultivation of bodily experience was as a place for encounter with meaning, a locus of redemption, where the body was also an instrument of redemption (Bynum, 1995a).

Redemption was a yearning for stasis in an age of fear of biological change; a yearning for a particular body identity and material continuity (Bynum, 1995a). Identity referred to two related issues: spatiotemporal continuity (how I see myself) and identity position (how I think others see me). In this sense, soul was seen as carrying the structure of "me" that will arise at the end of time. Thus, identity was not like looking in a mirror image of infinite regress for a true self (Hutton, 1988). Identity was bound up in suffering and redemption; in the acts carried out in order to preserve stasis. The goal of human existence seemed to be chrystalline permanence:

> ... the self is a person whose desire rolls and tumbles from fingertips as well as genitals, whose body is not only instrument, expression, and locus of self, but in some sense self itself.
>
> (Bynum, 1995a; p. 33)

The hundreds of years in which a person was seen and experienced as a unity, a particular individual and a yearning towards communion and stasis also meant an inclusion of suffering and death in that conceptualisation which also provided existential meaning. Meaning was attributed and transferred through symbolism, metaphors and patterns of activities such as these including archetypes.

5.3.3 Symbolism, metaphors and archetypes

Bynum (1987) believed medieval religiosity, metaphors and symbols expressed the *experiencing* of the body more than *controlling* it. This emphasis on experiencing was necessary because medieval people could do little to decrease discomfort of any kind:

> They strove not eradicate the body but to merge their own humiliating and painful flesh with that flesh whose agony, espoused by choice, was salvation. Luxuriating in Christ's physicality they found there the lifting up – the redemption – of their own.
>
> (Bynum, 1987; p. 246)

Physicality meant suffering, which in turn meant glory. Food meant flesh; medieval religious woman went to God through suffering. Thus for the period 1200–1500 AD, humanity, understood as full physicality, was increasingly concerned with matter, corporality and so suffering as religious issues (Bynum, 1987).

Bynum (1987) makes the important point that medieval women had distinct emphases in piety associated with body and food. She was a symbol of humanity in the Middle Ages whose weaknesses – female flesh – restored the world. Bynum (1987) provides examples of women who attempted to become the suffering and feeding body on the cross, offered for the salvation for others. The realities of suffering and service, although universal for all humans, somehow pressed more heavily on religious women, perhaps because they could claim power through suffering. Perhaps this was the only power they could claim in many instances of poverty and lack of civil rights.

I cannot help but think of the similarities with women's stories in syndemic suffering (Mendenhall, 2019). What was striking was that in story after story across different continents and nations, women seemed to matter so little, except in their role as a caregiver. And yet this role prevented them from being able to look after their own health needs in the face of a chronic illness such as diabetes or HIV. Suffering was seen as suffering no matter the location. If women unconsciously suffer without this being acknowledged, then it is difficult to see how changes can be made. Each women was on the edge of her own life, an absent presence. Perhaps it is not just medieval religious women that suffer as a way of offering salvation for others, it is just that this is now carried out in silence and *in absentia*.

Seeing suffering as a way of providing salvation is a kind of turning point and provides an opening to the epistemic crisis. I include a number of quotes at length because I believe they are critical to understanding suffering and how suffering impacts on what and how we know. Symbolic reversals provide a liminality where boundaries are crossed and roles exchanged or rolelessness achieved. Symbols as dichotomies and therefore reversals seemed more prescient in men's spirituality than women's, where religious women's spirituality seemed deeper and more embodied:

> In union with the dying Christ, woman became a fully fleshly and feeding self – at one with the generative suffering of God. Woman's eating, fasting, and feeding others were synonymous acts, because in all three the woman, by suffering, fused with a cosmic suffering that really redeemed the world. And these three synonymous acts and symbols were not finally symbolic reversals but, rather, a transfiguring and becoming of what the female symbolized: the fleshly, the nurturing, the suffering, the human.

> Women's food images and food practices thus reflect a large pattern. For women's way of using symbols and of being religious was different from men's. It appears as a kind of sub-text within a larger text, dominated by dichotomous symbols and symbolic inversions, and it is always aware of male/female oppositions and of images of reversal. But women's sense of religious self seems more continuous with their sense of social and biological self; women's images are most profoundly deepenings, not inversions, of what "woman" is; women's symbols express contradiction and opposition less than synthesis and paradox.
> (Bynum, 1987; p. 289)

These are profound observations since they portray women at that time as having moved beyond dichotomies to fully embody suffering and take it in, digest it as food, as part of their humanity, which ultimately they saw as their salvation. It is fascinating to think of the current state of feminism and medical humanities as described in Chapter Four in relation to the perpetuation of dichotomies and preoccupation with these aspects of biomedicine.

For example, Bynum (1987) states how dichotomous symbols "tend to express *and support* the power of those identified with 'culture'" (p. 293). In the use of symbols and how they related to self, women tended to write about the soul or humanity. Women's sense of self was thus formed:

> It was from age-old notions that God, mind, and power are male, whereas soul, flesh, weakness are female that women drew inspiration for a spirituality in which their own suffering humanity had cosmic significance.
> (Bynum, 1987; p. 294)

Thus medieval religious women tended not to be rooted in dualism, a spirit entrapped by body – they were not a world-denying self-hating body-mind (Bynum, 1987). And rather than trying to emulate or imitate men, they struck out on their own. Instead they tended to plumb and realise all possibilities of the flesh, to become more human in order to save human being.

This was in alignment with philosophical beliefs that located the nature of things in their individuating matter and particularity:

> Symbols of self were in general taken from biological or social experience and expressed not so much reversal or renunciation of worldly advantage as the deepening of ordinary human experience that came when God impinged upon it.
>
> (Bynum, 1987; p. 295)

Women expanded suffering which was their continuation of self. All dualities were of less importance to women as they saw themselves as first and foremost as human beings – fully spirit and fully flesh. Religious women in the Middle Ages therefore took a different perspective on their own bodies as a symbol of humanity which had worth in the social world. The richness and depth of understanding of suffering in the medieval periods seems to have all but disappeared as we have lost all notion of what this means and do not speak about suffering. One has to think – where does all that suffering go? People are left with unbearable feelings and no context in which to situate them (Devisch et al, 2017). Whatever their practices, medieval religious women had a way of normalising and validating the experience of suffering and incorporating it into their lives to provide a sense of wholeness. It is no wonder nowadays therefore that people experience suffering do so as a loss of intactness in their self and a hole in what could be said. Therefore, the hole is of primary importance in and central to the following framework of analysis.

5.4 Epistemology – concepts, symbols, categories of self and framework

Perhaps more than anything else, Bynum (1987) shows the importance of congruency between the concept and the category of the self: The self "... appears as a kind of sub-text within a larger text, dominated by dichotomous symbols and symbolic inversions, and it is always aware of male/female oppositions and of images of reversal" (p. 289) and "[s]ymbols of self were in general taken from biological or social experience and expressed ... as the deepening of ordinary human experience" (p. 295). Therefore, the self as a concept, symbol and experience and a category were not always congruent with each other, which makes understanding and practices of the self both contested and challenging in experiences of suffering. There is the concept of the self and the category of the self used to explain the self to different effects and purposes, there is the abstract conceptualised categorised object and then there is the pragmatic practical experience underneath – subjectivity – which may not always match and which requires deconstruction.

The suffering framework (Figure 5.2) has three main areas of activity to address the epistemic gap between suffering and mainstream practices –

stitching across the social matrix, deconstruction through questions and containing as a metaphor for surviving suffering. This framework is used in the following sections in order to have conversations about the self in relation to suffering. The next section explores the stitching across health professional training and practice using a deconstructive approach to explore issues of the body, self and other. There is both deconstruction and stitching – an unpicking whilst looping back and stitching to other concepts reviewed in this chapter. The section works at trying to reconcile different perspectives of concept, category and experience of the suffering self.

Perhaps the difference in perspective between concept and category of self can be viewed through the lens of the chiasma. Suffering also involves an embodied crossover, a chiasma of the flesh between the social world and the individual. Between the felt sense of loss and social injustice, there is a world of suffering. Suffering is both of the world and in it as well as in and between the individual and the world – both reciprocity and reversibility. Therefore, both health professionals and patients are tied together in the crossover, much like the chiasma – the point of contact, the physical link,

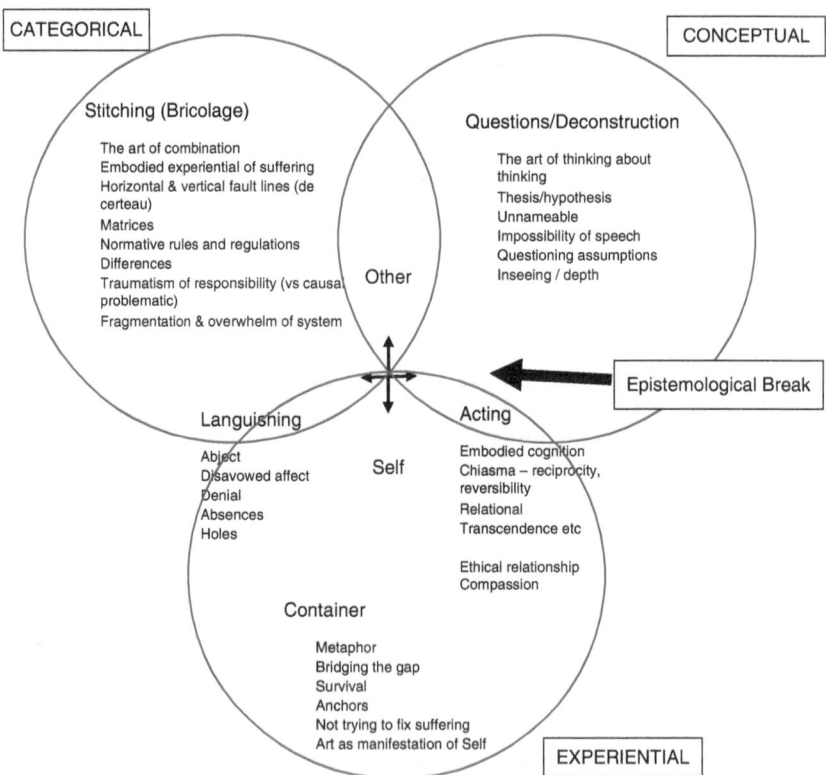

Figure 5.2 Suffering framework with conceptual, categorical and experiential imperatives.

between chromosomes of different genetic makeup. In spite of this, there are few conversations between patients and physicians about suffering (Epstein, 2017), and probably even less between health professionals. Perhaps this is because the pervasive distress, effect on identity and ability to be in the world precludes speech. Perhaps it is due to the epistemological break between concepts and categories of self, and the experience of self, especially in the case of suffering. Perhaps it is because doctors have learned not to see suffering or not "to use the word *suffering* for fear it casts patients as victims, denying them agency and personhood" (Epstein, 2017; p. 114; emphasis original). The lack of mention in the International Classification of Diseases Version 10 (ICD-10) creates a void around suffering, in both the literature and the clinic. Amongst other responses, Epstein (2017) suggests,

> My capacity to respond to the suffering of any patient depends on how well I can recognize that my imaginative projection of what the patient is experiencing is just that and no more.
>
> (p. 121)

Dreams, anxieties about patients, vulnerability, understanding the need for meaning and coherence – refocusing and reclaiming – as well as spiritual/ religious aspects of crusades against evil, transcendence, moral failure, testimony and witnessing, and redemption are all aspects of suffering between patients and health professionals and how we know what we know.

Yet as we have seen, health professionals can also be suffering from burnout and emotional exhaustion for a variety of reasons. Health professional knowing is haunted by epistemological vulnerability.

> Physicians remember their mistakes and are haunted by them. They hold them in silence for years, sometimes decades. Their stories reveal their psychological vulnerabilities – unrelenting perfectionism, unforgiving intolerance of error, unease in the face of ambiguity, a desperate need for certainty. While many physicians will acknowledge these vulnerabilities if asked, during everyday practice they usually lurk just outside awareness.
>
> (Epstein, 2017; p. 145)

Secondary trauma to clinicians – suffering as a result of patient suffering – has been acknowledged in some parts of the world and the UK, but compassionate care has yet to become mainstream (Dempsey, 2018).

As mentioned above, healthcare systems still tend to be run on authoritarian relational lines (Fiske, 1973; Foucault, 1973), where suffering is individualised, seen as a personal responsibility and divided into deserving and less deserving people according to value judgments on their lifestyles and behaviours. On the one hand, a focus on biomedical treatments and techniques helps to obtain the best possible patient outcomes and provides pathways for clinicians and patients through the sometimes harrowing work that has to be carried out; on the other hand, aspects of suffering can become pushed to the background. The relational aspects of epistemology influence categorisation and conceptualisation in a clinical context. The focus on clinical interventions and advice about diabetes has not comprehensively served populations well who suffer from poverty, violence, anxiety, depression and immigration (Mendenhall, 2019) – precarity, in other words.

Internalisation of suffering means that emotions such as shame, guilt, and thoughts about personal culpability on both sides are not addressed. How we know what we know is influenced by emotions and values. Issues around responsibility, choice and control are spoken about by health professionals with a glibness that belies complexity, which has occupied sociologists for many years (Foucault, 1973; Fox, 1999). This is a truly perplexing syndemic of suffering since healthcare professionals are heavily implicated in the perpetuation of health inequalities by not being able to find a way to adjust their training and work to meet the needs of people who are most disadvantaged or to even prevent the disadvantage and worse health outcomes in the first place. The limited epistemological coherence through concepts, categories and experiences of self in suffering means that there are real pragmatic effects of not being able to match up the different perspectives.

5.5 Instrumentality as sources of self: the body and self

In theistic sources of self, we explored how medieval women's religious practices expanded suffering as a way of developing their sense of self. They became more embodied as they suffered in the service of their social world, thereby incorporating the suffering to become flesh. Their religious role was their self and any moral dilemma they experienced became food for this self. This anguished fusion of their self and their role exposed their self (Hollis, 1996). This was a high price to pay for morality yet their suffering was a constitutive force of their self (Taylor, 1989). Their body was an instrument for the experience of suffering which they used to gain entry into experiences that deepened ordinary reality. In contrast, the instrumental sources of self were more concerned with economics, utility and the role of the self and were perhaps more disengaged (Taylor, 1989). That is, disengaged instrumentalism resorts to abstract representations of the body and self which leave the realm of bodily experience:

> Instead, the inhabitants will spend their time in the grand evocative biology of singular and composite feelings that will partially leave the realm of bodily experience for that of representation but will not roam too far.
>
> (Boyer, 2018; p. 110)

Boyer (2018) manages to write a sentence that encapsulates both the individual and social elements of embodied experience whilst proposing a formulary for a new feeling as a way of life, one that restructures how we encounter and endure feelings and somatic states in a more distributive sense across the population. She suggests that huddles of people have been self-and-other-allocated the role of feelings through the dual mechanism of projection and identification. Therefore, the social-cultural milieu cannot be separated out from the individual (which is a sociological position), yet there is also the fact of biological reality (biomedical position). What Boyer (2018) seems to be suggesting is that there is the possibility of both at the same time – that we leave the realm of bodily experience for representation but do not stray too far from this. This section will explore different subject positions on the body and self in the context of health professional training, thereby stitching together an actual example of how suffering becomes unwittingly sidelined in both health professionals and patients.

5.5.1 Theoretical background for health professional training and curricula phenomena

The research on which this part is based arose out of the desire to develop and implement a strategic plan of health promotion that reflected social justice principles and critical pedagogy. While the research drew on critical pedagogy, health professional rhetoric was concerned with empowerment and an assertive self, in order to address suffering. In practice, this rhetoric highlighted conflict and issues that were undoubtedly about the circulation of power. At the level of fundamental concepts, there was confusion about issues of self, choice and control and there was little understanding of a critical pedagogical approach to health. Exploring the link between learning and health specifically in order to address suffering relating to social injustice requires a post-structuralist approach with its emphasis on deconstructing notions of power. What is interesting to me now is that while motivation started off as wanting to address issues of suffering, I ended up writing about power, and that effectively erased issues with suffering even though the health professionals involved talked about this in relation to themselves and patients. Thus one of the effects of an analysis on power was to erase issues concerned with suffering caused by oppressive enactment of power.

The education of health professionals is based on a series of discourses of professionalism that privilege notions of control and choice (Riggs, 2004; Titchen & Higgs, 2001). These discourses are expressed through both explicit and implicit curricula which encourage the enactment of a particular construction of the "self" of both health professionals and clients or patients. This is the currency that people tend to trade in, in other words, and there is assumed to be a shared understanding of this between health professionals and patients (something like "we are all in this together"). The idealised self is one that is bound up with notions of control and choice, which may require struggle on an inner level with the self-regulation and self-policing (O'Grady, 2005) required to fit this norm. The struggles seemed to be relevant to suffering in that health professionals often did not know how to approach people who suffered the most from within their dominant discourse, and health professionals suffered, too. Yet there were still lacunae in this theorising: given that health professionals subscribe to and are complicit with dominant ideas yet also suffer with patients, there is no neat explanation of the self that can explain away the embodied experience of suffering.

The struggle for female health workers to link the abstract theorising with the actualities of their lives (Williams, 2002) seems to produce a paradoxical type of relationship with themselves and patients. On one hand, there is an expectation of conformity, compliance and obedience, which suggests more of a slippage of self while at the same time the expert-novice relationship characterising the health professionals' interaction with clients emphasises autonomy, control and empowerment of self. The mechanism of emphasising empowerment and choice in the uptake of healthy lifestyle behaviours, whilst at the same time expecting compliance and obedience, in contexts of deprivation and suffering seems an impossible dynamic to manage, one which places health professionals in an invidious position. The overselling of clinical interventions of diet and exercise in the management of diabetes to the detriment of understanding social factors such as poverty (Mendenhall, 2019) seems to be an unnameable suffering and one that works outside conscious awareness. However, with the curriculum focused on risk factors such as lifestyle behaviours, in order to achieve better health outcomes, there is little wonder that health professionals cannot see outside this.

Further, while health workers see themselves as having high levels of internal locus of control, this is in direct contrast to the helplessness and powerlessness they experienced and spoke about at work. The emphasis on evidence-based practice and scientific content was seen as reinforcing the dominant norm of the neo-liberal individual capable of self-regulation and self-policing. Given the practices of power that continue to disadvantage women in general and patients in particular in relation to their health and the institution, the lacunae in this sociological approach is the limited exploration or understanding of the embodied suffering and how this relates to the larger picture of structural practices.

Whilst it is possible to see how structural cultural meanings shape the illness experience and perspective of suffering, it is difficult to see how health professionals can unshape these experiences.

> The modern Western cultural orientation contributes to our experience of suffering precisely through this reciprocal relationship between the actual experience qua experience and how each of us relates to that experience as an observing self.
>
> (Kleinman, 1988; p. 27)

Suggesting that health professionals function as an observing self that can translate or decode the cultural and social narratives of the modernist project of health seems a big ask when they are as enculturated as much as anyone else and in fact tend to resist any sociological reflection. Health professionals become caught up in technologies of self (practices of the self) which implicate the body and observing self in a reciprocal relationship and is part of the stitching together of sociological theories about the self.

Sociological theories believe that the body could be seen as the main site of the enactment of the relationship between human agency (the individual) and structural constraint (the social) (Fox, 1999). Referring back to Fiske (1993), the authoritarian relationship between health professionals and patients can be seen as transferred to or governing that between an individual and her body. The body as a metaphor for managing structural virtual principles means that abstract ideas of health promotion are enacted on the body as dynamic and continually evolving outcome of resources and processes in a matrix of processes of social interaction (Sewell, 1992). Before teasing out this focus on the body as the interface of the relationship between the structural and the individual, different theoretical (or metaphorical) positions will be examined and summarised in order to inform this section. Fox (1999) presents the different theoretical positions – which body? – as follows:

1   The body as physical body – this was untenable for Foucault and poststructuralist others. The biological body, the "organism" or "body-with-organs" (Deleuze and Guattari, 1988; cited in Fox, 1999; p. 114) are discursively constructed. There was nothing seen beyond linguistics.

2   "Natural body" underpinning the "organism" – an essentialist position that acknowledges a natural body overlaid with cultural values having an existence that is determined phenomenologically through "experience," "faith" or "common sense."

3   "Natural" body beyond discourse and thus unknowable. Sociologists left with meaningless and pointless construct – "the sociology of?"

4   "Body-without-organs" (BwO) – a unified "body" that is the creation of power/knowledge, a social body throughout, a materially constructed, always already body (Fox, 1999; p. 114).

In Fox's (1999) view, the body is the metaphorical or metaphysical "surface" which connects the realms of the psychological and the social. Similarly, in relation to the self, "the anatomical body is not the carapace of the self" (p. 128): the carapace (or BwO), rather, is the territory that is constantly contested and fought over academically and clinically (Fox, 1999). Fox (1999) uses a metaphor to explain the social constructionist position.

The BwO is like a ball on a pool table stuck in some ruts or striations. It is not until the pool table is tipped and the ball moves out of one rut perhaps into another or perhaps into "smooth space" that any change can take place. The striations are known as territorialisations and are created by the construction process resulting from tension between the forces of the social and the BwO's will-to-power (Fox, 1999). This is like saying that people living in areas of high deprivation are likely to have worse health outcomes as they are stuck in these ruts or territorialisations where they are constructed through their subject position. Fox (1999) eschews any interior-exterior conception of subjectivity and embodiment, seeing this instead as an effect of the meaning of socialisation.

Similarly, Butler (1990) sees the boundaries between inner and outer as a set of fantasies, feared and desired:

> What constitutes through division the "inner" and "outer" worlds of the subject is a border and boundary tenuously maintained for the purpose of social regulations and control. The boundary between the inner and outer is confounded by those excremental passages in which the inner effectively becomes the outer.
>
> (Butler, 1990; p. 170)

The boundary of the body is maintained by the ejection of otherness and is an accomplishment of identity differentiation (Butler, 1990). The binary of inner-outer, where inner is privileged, is a social construction of the body in her view.

The mind-body binary has also been noted previously as a social construction. The mind-body has been variously represented as a mobius strip by Grosz (cited in Finlay & Langdridge, 2007; p. 178) where there is no clear distinction between inner and outer. Instead there is an inflection of the body into the mind and vice versa (Finlay & Langdridge, 2007). Merleau-Ponty's view was "that the body is the mind's body and the mind is the body's mind" (cited in Venn; p. 59):

> The idea, then, is of an intertwining of the world and the human, of interiority and exteriority, of the I and the Other; it evokes, analogically, the relation of a curve to its hollow. Such a relation is not representable as such; it can be apprehended only in the mode of the sublime .... the "throwness of being."
>
> (Venn, 2002; p. 59)

The intertwining of the mind and body and of the social and the individual has also been likened to relations of the exterior being "invaginated, folded, to form an inside to which it appears an outside must always make reference" (Rose, 1998; p. 188). Rose advocates abandoning "this 'fleshism' of the body once and for all" (p. 183). He would rather see social constructionism as the dominant concept similar to the BwO. However, Rose has a slightly different metaphor for embodiment even though he also draws on Deleuze to describe the relationship of the inner to the outer using the concept of the fold:

> The concept of the fold can give rise to a generalizable diagram for thinking of relations, connections, multiplicities, and surfaces – their formation of depths, singularities, stabilizations. This diagram of the fold describes a figure in which the inside, the subjective, is itself no more than a moment, or a series of moments, through which a "depth" has been constituted within human being. The depth and its singularity, then, is no more than that which has been drawn in to create a space or series of cavities, pleats, and fields, which only exist in relation to those very forces, lines, techniques, and inventions that sustain them.
>
> (Rose, 1998; p. 188)

These forces and tensions of the social and the individual are active in the formation of the folds or subjectivity. Similarly, in relation to agency: "agency is, no doubt, a 'force', but it is a force that arises not from any essential properties of 'the subject' but out of the ways in which humans have been-assembled-together" (Rose, 1998; p. 187–8). However, Fox (1999) would argue that the folds are not "in" the individual but are the fabric of the external (the pool table metaphor). The fabric of the external is constructed by social forces including pastoral power exerted by most state institutions.

Pastoral power was exerted by the state apparatus and public institutions such as health care services in a totalising and individualising manner such that the development of knowledge about "man" took place around two roles; one globalising and quantitative (totalising, e.g., epidemiology and statistics) concerning the population; the other, analytical, concerning the individual (Foucault, 1983). Pastoral power was thus formative in the territorialisations or striations of embodiment. The individualising techniques of power incited people to act on themselves to become subjects:-

> This form of power applies itself to immediate everyday life which categorizes the individual, marks him by his own individuality, attaches him to his own identity, imposes a law of truth on him which he must recognize and which others have to recognize in him. It is a form of power which makes individuals subjects. There are two meanings of the word subject: subject to someone else by control and dependence, and tied to his own identity by a conscience or self-knowledge. Both meanings suggest a form of power which subjugates and makes subject to.

> Generally, it can be said that there are three types of struggles: either against forms of domination (ethnic, social, and religious); against forms of exploitation which separate individuals from what they produce; or against that which ties the individual to himself and

submits him to others in this way (struggles against subjection, against forms of subjectivity and submission).

(Foucault, 1983; p. 212)

The subject is tied to him or herself through categorisation and imposition of a law of truth which other people then recognise and use. The role of recognition is explored further in Chapter Six. This may have relevance to the practice of health professionals as the subject is tied to him or herself and also divided within him- or herself and/or from others.

Historically, dividing practices included the isolation of lepers during the Middle Ages; the confinement of the poor, the insane, and vagabonds; the new classifications of disease and the associated practices of clinical medicine; the rise of modern psychiatry and its entry into hospitals, prisons, and clinics; and finally the medicalisation, stigmatisation and normalisation of sexual deviance in modern Europe, according to Foucault (Rabinow, 1984):

> In different fashions, using diverse procedures, and with a highly variable efficiency in each case, "the subject is objectified by a process of division either within himself or from others." In this process of social objectification and categorization, human beings are given both a social and a personal identity. Essentially "dividing practices" are modes of manipulation that combine the mediation of a science (or pseudo-science) and the practice of exclusion – usually in the spatial sense, but always in a social one.
>
> (Rabinow, 1984; p. 8)

Thus healthcare is a prime site for the manipulation of individuals through categorisation, the mediation of a science and the practice of exclusion in order to produce divided individuals both within and without.

The manipulation of individuals and the practice of exclusion may be part of the social construction of health professionals as they become tied to dominant identity norms, preferring to be privileged rather than not:

> Of particular significance is the link between self-policing practices and the maintenance of dominant identity norms. This type of contextual approach offers an important counterbalance to the individualistic impulse in much of western culture whereby, against clear evidence to the contrary, it often is assumed that who we are and how we live is solely a matter of personal decision of will.
>
> (O'Grady, 2005; p. 14)

This tying to one's identity through the maintenance of dominant identity norms along with self-policing may have relevance to the following participant comments. Different forces such as individualisation, totalisation, dominant identity norms, self-policing can all form differends (Fox, 1999).

Differends are described by the participants' responses. Differends are directly linked to the right to claim "knowledge" (Fox, 1999) and are thus very important in health care and the location of the body.

> The creation of a differend is an act of power which works at the margin or limit of a text. It frames that text (which may be a book or a social practice or a subjectivity), fabricating the distance between author and object, self and other, what is and what is not. Deconstruction identifies these framings, exploring the achievement of differends ..... Deconstruction reintroduces what has been left outside the frame.
>
> (Fox, 1999; p. 30)

Deconstruction as a knowledge claim or process then is constitutive of a different type of embodiment. There is a link between knowledge claims, deconstruction and embodiment. The participants' comments about health and their bodies construct their bodies and frame them. These constructions are then used to make knowledge claims. However, deconstruction is a knowledge claim based on deterritorialisation (Fox, 1999). All of these concepts are relevant to an instrumentalist source of self, that of disengaged reason. It is disengaged because of the differends. With these points in mind, I will now review the participants' comments.

5.5.2 Health professional training, curricula and instrumentality

Instrumentality, or disengaged reason, is explored here as a source of self to demonstrate how a techno-rationalist curriculum forms a self in practice and some of the consequences of that in relation to suffering. Health professionals are caught up in this practice, which can then impact patients and affect how prepared they are to respond to suffering. For example, Tom discussed "the obesity epidemic" frequently cited in the media and saw this as an opportunity for the media to judge people about their level of self-control and laziness:

> At the moment there's ... er ... almost a paranoia about, what they rave on as being the obesity epidemic and how we're all going to be scourged with serious diseases and we're all going to die, cause everyone's getting absolutely fat and I get a little frustrated with people who I think should know better, professionals in the area, health specialists and health experts. Cause we know the media are just, you know, they are just like sharks, feeding on a frenzy because it sells, it sells articles.
>
> (Tom)

Interestingly, Tom uses a metaphor of sharks having a feeding frenzy as a way of highlighting the behaviour of the media over bodies in the so-called obesity epidemic. Almost as if they were getting fat on the hysteria and stigma surrounding weight and health. Here, Tom is rejecting the media frenzy over a supposed obesity epidemic but still supporting the health education notion that people need to be empowered through education to control their own health. Tom believed in listening to the cues of your body and letting those determine your behaviour but still with the idea that people needed to be empowered to make the choice easy for them, in order for people to make a moral choice. The metaphors Tom drew on referred to the body in a particular way to describe the relationship between the social and the individual. That is, there was little conception of the potential suffering inherent in the discrimination and stigmatisation of the body.

The other way in which the body is the site of the enactment of the relationship between human agency and structural constraint is through the participation of the workers in their own oppression through the work they are required to do. The body is the vehicle for carrying out the tasks, there always being so much to do.

> So you come back and you got all your other more, more … you don't get time to read the patients' notes. You don't get time to do the extra things that can make a difference to that patient 'cos you're having to attend to the basic requirements of care. No sooner have they gone out the room and somebody's got some orders about something and the co-ordinator may give them to you, then you're starting to feed the patients because it's lunchtime then. Twelve o'clock. There's all the little older ladies and stuff and people that can't feed themselves so, if you're looking at power like in the nurses, you're so powerless. I felt so powerless I couldn't even listen in to what the doctors are saying and I, I felt I needed to know because I was the caregiver.
>
> (Louise)

The majority of participants described the workload as overwhelming, that work was about coping and just trying to get as much done as possible. The structural constraints included an enormous amount of administrative work, often generated by the increased use of technology. The differends in this case can be seen as paperwork including patient notes and administrative work, routines, basic requirements of care – care as something done "to" a patient (care as a vigil – Fox, 1999).

Paperwork can act as a differend because it frames the work that must be done and it writes the person as well as silencing other textualities like suffering (Fox, 1999). For example, Mary stated on a number of occasions the frustration she felt at the amount of paperwork she had to complete – admission records, medication charts and so on. These examples supply the control of the situation to doctors and yet they also limit what is considered within the frame of the patient.

> I described to somebody on the weekend, I said I work for the government and I do paperwork. *Laughs.*
>
> (Mary)

> Umm, so I get, I do get frustrated and I think, I mean the system does what it can because it is a government agency there are so many rules and protocols and safety and medical and legal issues that we just end up tangled in so much of that, that when it comes down to the common sense practical issue of what does this person need and it's like our hands are tied.
>
> (Mary)

Mary refers to her body as her hands being tied and therefore being unable to help patients where they might need it in relation to their suffering. There was also a form of suffering for Mary in that she seemed to lose a sense of herself and her purpose, becoming less agentic by paradoxically having to do so much paperwork.

Mary was clearly able to describe the effect that working in such a system had on her body:

> I would find myself being the fine point on which the whole thing balanced, because I would have to say look this patient needs a bed, ring all the different hospitals and be told no bed, no bed, no bed and have the emergency department staff saying we want this person out of here and not being able to find a place for them and that was the most stressful thing ... Er ... but in the end the reason I didn't continue is because I just found it, I was incapable of being the health system. You know I couldn't be that balancing point that it all hinged on and I got very stressed by that. (Mary)

> And I am so out of my body, I am so stuck in my head, I am so under time pressure, I am doing three things at once, I have got a pager going off, I have got a phone going off and then I get a call from a community clinic with somebody who needs to come in and that's the most pressure that I experience at work. (Mary)

> The thing that disembodies me is the time pressure. If I can take my time and just do one task and then another I can stay much more in touch with myself. I can do that. (Mary)

> So each day when I am driving to work, I am kind of consciously telling myself it's okay, just relax, just breathe, just keep, don't worry about your muscle tension, try to keep relaxed, it's not all up to you, it's only

the system, you can only do so much. I kind of had to say all those things to myself and just go in and try and just be myself and be calm. But through the day, invariably walking back to my car in the afternoon, I have to draw my bits of myself back from the atmosphere *laughs* cause they have run off during the day. By the time I get home I have usually got it back together again. *Laughs.*

(Mary)

Through time pressures, having too much to do, excessive paperwork, structural constraints and the emotional pressures of the work, Mary was able to describe how the only way she could survive the system was to become disembodied. That for her, human agency in terms of getting things done and meeting the requirements of the work meant she had to lose her relationship with her self and her body and participate in what she saw as an unhealthy environment. The way Mary was constructed within the environment was by being absent to herself and taking on the construction of the "system," being "that balancing point that it all hinged on." Mary became tied to that identity perhaps because it is these points that supplied the control of the situation to her – by *being* the balancing point.

The absence of the body was consistent in peoples' responses to questions about their relationship with their selves, with most people not understanding what was meant by this question. There was a fusion between their role and themselves. Most were able to talk about their relationship with self, when prompted, in terms of self-talk that was about coping with the system and not being defeated by it.

I think, I think that you just realize that if you, if you moan and groan too much its going to wear out onto other people and you are going nowhere and by, basically you can't change, often we have a defeatist attitude, you just can not change the system. So you have to make a decision. What is it actually better to be? Is it better to be moaning and miserable or is it actually better to be happy and positive?

(Louise)

I mean, and they can't, what's that saying, you can't change the way the wind blows, but you can alter the sails.

(Gill)

Generally, participants' relationship with self and body was minimal and seemed to exist mainly as strategies (self-talk and beliefs) to cope with work and the structural constraints. A few participants noted that they didn't look after themselves in the same way that they promoted a healthy lifestyle to the clients. The relationship with self was obviously not discussed during training or participation in the workforce as most participants were unable to articulate any relationship at all.

In terms of the body being the site of the relationship between human agency and structural constraint, it seems as though the structural constraints dominate the landscape, with most people leaving themselves and their bodies out of the discourse except in terms of coping and balancing commitments and responsibilities through a form of self-talk that enabled them to accept the status quo. The main theme in this section of the self and body was that there was a subjugation of the self and body in service to the health system or structural constraints with little discussion of suffering explicitly although suffering was implicit in what they described. Most people seemed to survive through a disembodiment and an acceptance of the status quo. Considering this to be so, then how do health professionals relate to suffering people, given that in order to comply with the system, they must become disembodied?

5.5.3 Instrumentality as relationship with suffering

Further exploration of the dynamic between healthcare professionals and patients shows the sort of fantasies and emotions when self and body reacted to a dilemma faced at work when a participant wanted to do something but felt constrained: "you want to say something that the system doesn't say" (Mary). When this sort of situation meets people who are suffering, there is a cognitive dissonance between what is required or advocated such as compassionate care (Dempsey, 2018).

> Well there's them and us really. *Laughs*. No it's true, those issues, the people with the problems are outside. They're the clients and I guess we noticed it because you are dealing a lot with people from lower socio-economic status type suburbs and different, this is the public system. You get people who can't afford private so you get poverty, they're your clients, but it wasn't explicitly discussed or there was no, sort of discussion about how do you think this patient perceives you, do you think there is a difference or, inequality in that area. That's just what you do... But I think, I know that people treat patients differently in private where the patients can afford to pay more. I think there is a lot more equality between consultant and client and there's a lot more respect I think probably. We had an attitude that well this is what you get if you come here cause this is public... And I mean that sounds really awful, but I am sure it is there in the atmosphere... It's unsaid... Public and private, yeah, yeah. Yeah, I mean its true, people without money don't have as much say in what happens to them. *Silence ~ five seconds*.
>
> (Mary)

The cognitive dissonance is a reflection of a system that perpetuates inequities and which health professionals are subsumed under. Using Gore's (1995a) categories of power, the comments made by Mary can be shown as examples of distribution – there's "them" and "us" with people with problems being on the outside; of classification – the ones with the problems are the clients who are also poor and without so much say in their care and therefore somehow deserving of less respect; exclusion – people with problems are not one of "us"; and of totalisation – people who are poor are the ones with problems. It is difficult to see how health professionals can respond to suffering adequately within such an instrumentalist approach to healthcare training and practice.

These comments are in addition to comments made earlier by the same participant about the punitive system of care in mental health:

> [A]lthough in medicine in psychiatry more than general there is a kind of punitive way of managing people who have got overwhelming distress. It's not very compassionate, it's not very understanding of where the distress comes from. It's much more like, we have rules and you can't behave like that here.
>
> (Mary)

The rules that delimit the sayable (Kendall & Wickham, 1999) are a manifestation of power at a time when people are most vulnerable. The rules apply to health professionals and patients although health professionals tend to be in a more privileged location than patients and perhaps have more access to resources. Idealistic visions of responding to suffering must be tempered by the context in which health professionals are working and are subsumed along with patients.

When discussing the difficulty presented by on the one hand wanting to be compassionate with people but on the other hand working within a system that was punitive, Mary made the following comments:

> There's a limit to it, but I am learning all the time and I am learning to watch myself and my own reactions and how I participate in that along with other nursing staff, you know, when the doors are closed and we joke about other peoples' misfortunes and there's this kind of rationale, it's okay to make jokes at the patients' expense because that's how we cope with the stress of working here. ... And that's part of the environment, and you know, we know it's not very nice, but that's what we do here and it's okay. And I go in and I really, the first few weeks I really shudder at that and I don't want to participate in it, and then within a few weeks I find I am in it and all of a sudden I am coming in rolling my eyeballs making a sarcastic comment about that person's parents and I don't want to be like that, but that's what the system encourages. ... Yeah, and not only an object but something that is just less, I don't know you are less respectful of them. You make them into the subject of humour. And yeah, part of me really doesn't like that. And yet part of me does that when I am here.
>
> (Mary)

"Gallows humour" has long been a strategy employed by health workers in order to survive a health system that encourages disembodiment whilst speaking the rhetoric of patient-centred compassionate care.

The pressure to conform to social norms within the work environment was also explained by Joan in terms of workers policing their own boundaries to maintain their clinical, rational, unemotional role within the health service.

> You know, umm a lot of people wanted to have that caring experience and had that compassion but from a business point of view or from a career point of view it didn't make sense. So then you've got a lot of these people going out into the workplace you have got nurses already policing their boundaries ... this is what we do, you do it our way, you socialize to our way or you don't socialize. You know and ... yeah and it's very you know it's very violent umm ... umm, so yeah that sense of umm and those boundaries give people power you know. ... You know, you know, there's I think there's also a direct relationship between knowing your boundaries but also if you can police them there's a sense of power about that you know.
>
> (Joan)

Protecting boundaries, territories and role delineation are all ways in which the gap between healthcare providers and patients is managed and can prevent a compassionate response to people who are suffering.

As an educator and nurse, Joan was involved with the training of students and was determined to ensure that students experienced what it was like to be on the receiving end of care and to keep powerlessness at the forefront of the training.

> No that's right because you have no concept of what it is to actually feel that powerlessness and umm that umm I mean it's perfect sort of experiential learning if you like, is that they, they know what it feels like.
>
> (Joan)

The mismatch in experience between worker and client seems to produce a power differential in the workers' favour if they are unable to empathise, understand and validate the patients' experiences. It wasn't until the workers had experienced healthcare as patients that they could be aware of power imbalances that thwarted a compassionate response to suffering.

There seems to automatically be a power imbalance when there is a lack of empathy since both worker and client are then made into particular types of subjects.

You know, like you have to be hard nosed and you don't crack and things like that and I thought about it this morning you know when we were talking about anxiety last week and health anxiety and umm I thought I don't think nurses have another way to cope or don't know any other way to cope with what they go through. So they literally have to shut down and turn off and you know and just do what they do and I mean otherwise it's a hard, it's a very difficult place to walk. I mean if you want to teach people about empathy can you go too far? Where I'm at a stage where I think I have gone too far.

(Joan)

This participant saw that in order to survive the type of work and situation she was in, she had to shut down or not work in that field, in other words, enforce rigid boundaries between herself and other people in order to survive. With little other recourse, in order to survive health, workers felt like they had to shut down and become disembodied.

Boundaries were reinforced in the face of suffering with success at work defined as having clear boundaries to their role (Louise, Betty and Katrin). In fact, Louise saw that cleaners and patient care assistants had more power than nurses because they had a very clearly defined role and were therefore able to say no.

Everything else but also if you are looking at these sort of power things umm in a way, people ... PCAs [patient care assistants] and cleaners have got more power than the nurses, ... They ... they know where they are. They know they are working within those boundaries. And they're more powerful bodies than the nurses are, ... Yes, yes. Whereas nurses feel they have to be all things to everyone. Because that's the expectation in their role, ... That's why they get so stressed, ... Feel so responsible. Yep. Because ultimately they're responsible for the patient. They're the one that goes to court if things go wrong ... And yet the ... the less qualified groups are really the more powerful groups. Yeah. They umm, they say no we won't do that. No. And that, which is ... They're doing the right thing. They're less stressed, that's for sure. *Laughs.* Yeah.

(Louise)

Both Louise and Katrin identified their profession as having to conform to expectations that they needed to be all things to everyone, with Louise relating this to the holistic approach to care of nurses. There seems to be a conception from doctors, to nurses, to occupational therapists that everyone else has got it easy and has far more power than the worker speaking at the time, when in reality all three were feeling the same effects of power. This could be seen as an effect of individualisation (Gore, 1995) within the health service where each type of worker is individualised and very little communication occurs across the different types of workers, especially about these sorts of issues.

For example, Cathy spoke about how she ended up internalising the issues due to an overwhelming caseload, when discussing how she was told by her line manager what she could and couldn't do. She complied with the direction and became a docile body that was productive in the workforce, though not without some cost to herself.

> Have this many sessions and that's it. So you, and that feels sad umm, personally and the clients and when I first started here and that was happening in the early years I very took that much to heart and umm, it really hurt me a lot, psychologically and then obviously physically you get sick and so on. But now I am much more, I'm having to accept it, you still ask questions.
>
> (Cathy)

Cathy describes the hurt both psychologically and physically as she absorbs the irrationality (Walkerdine, 1992) of the structure of the health services. The instrumentalist role of the individual, both client and worker, seems to be determined very much by the epistemic casting of the dominant medical model.

There is a culture of silence about any of the real issues impacting on people at work as exemplified by the relief and enjoyment people experienced by talking about these issues to someone else. There doesn't even seem to be the language available to people to articulate the issues that were covered in the interview. This means that any sense of agency is lost since the workers are always displaced outside of themselves in trying to be "good" health workers trying to live up to the norms and continually being involved in self-regulation and self-surveillance. It seems as though the best the workers can do is come to some sort of acceptance both of self and of the situation. Just as the clients they see may not have a choice in their behaviours, neither do the workers seem to have a choice about being critical either at work or in their training.

Cathy's view was that the lecturers tried to make them think for themselves "and to do that they basically didn't give us very much resources [*laughs*]."

> In terms of critical thinking, so, did they, did they umm, encourage us to think for ourselves. We had to! *Laughs.* We had to! Umm, we had to in the end. I mean, it was like we have got no two ways about it. Umm, probably too much so in my degree.

> Umm, they could have made us feel a little bit more secure about our profession and not, because once, when you're that critical about it, a lot of people, a lot of the students dropped out, because they were just so stressed about it. There's no umm there is no right answers in the discipline.
>
> (Cathy)

It seems as though the students were not supported in their endeavours to be critical about their work, with the emphasis instead being on self-reliance and greater self-regulation which actually worked to foreclose possibilities of agency. Again, it is very difficult to think beyond current circumstances and respond differently to suffering, unless there are explicit resources to do so.

One worker had an understanding of the complexities of working with other people who were seen as suffering, but this was not from her training. It seemed to come more from her experiences post graduation.

> But what came out of that was umm to me was, you can't you can't come from a middle class white privileged background and think, even begin to think, you know what those people want and need.
>
> (Donna)

> How do we, how do we start to umm learn, how do we start to just ask them, I can't even say work with them, because I mean, how do we, how do we start asking the questions of them that might enable us to work with them.
>
> (Donna)

This discourse is so different from the discourse around empowerment, which was done to and for the people. Instead the worker recognised that it was the workers that needed "enabling" to work with other people.

The silence about any other pedagogies means that what was known and taught about health and the body was limited, fragmented and always centred around the pathological causal problematic. The individual was seen as important as being the site of the problem but there was no engagement with the political or structural constraints – the body was just a vehicle for either pathology as a client or as a worker "to do." The body was not involved in the discourse as a possible consolidation of a sense of self (Niranjana, 2001) or as a container for experiential integration (Nathanson, 1992). There was no consideration of the contingencies associated with health and well-being and no consideration of what it means to be an individual or of the rhetoric around choice. In this way, the official curriculum seems to foreclose possibilities of agency to health dilemmas even though it speaks of the individual's responsibility, control, choice and empowerment. The patient would tend to be addressed by workers who could be suffering as a result of working in a system that precipitates fragmentation, chaos, crisis and displacement from one's self.

The evidence shows that participants are expected to learn and reflect in a disembodied manner, which seems to enable a focus on doing and being busy. Mary described the effect that being so busy had on her. "And I am so out of my body, I am so stuck in my head, I am so under time pressure, I'm doing three things at once." Furthermore, she describes the disembodiment being as a result of the time pressure she experienced and the effect at the end of the day was "invariably walking back to my car in the afternoon, I have to draw my bits of myself back from the atmosphere [*laughs*] cause they have run off during the day. By the time I get home I have usually got it back together again [*laughs*]." There is a difference between the ability to reflect and learn as part of professional practice, which participants described as a form of self-evaluation and embodied reflexivity.

Along with disembodiment and a reduction in affect, there also seemed to be no room for a self-reflexive cycle beyond heightened self-policing, which meant that workers could stay in their heads: be clinical, detached and objective by critically evaluating themselves. In the comments about the lack of critical pedagogy in their education, most workers showed evidence of a perception of critical evaluation being in terms of their practice in relation to what they "do" (Louise, Gill, Alice, Mary, Cathy, Emma, Polly). However, this type of "doing" or instrumentalism is in the context of a mechanistic approach to health service provision with a lack of reflection back of subjective experience. It is what is deemed necessary to complete workforce requirements.

Further evidence of the lack of reflection back of the subjective experience of being a health professional and instigating healthy practices was given by Ingrid when she said, "I haven't actually hit the right button with myself yet," in relation to herself and her own healthy lifestyle. The lack of reflection back seemed to allow incongruency between a worker's practice and the rhetoric of the health department. This incongruency was reflected in Fiona's comments as well. Louise, Betty, Cathy and Tom thought it was important to be a healthy role model. It seems almost as if the training encouraged disembodiment and a lack of congruency by its focus on doing and an absence of reflective practice of the subjective experience of the health workers, perhaps in order to manage their (unspoken) affective states. This type of practice forms severe constraints on the professional practice of health professionals.

Any references to the body as part of the professional practice were constrained. Polly stated that "you're sort of constantly thinking about what you are doing and trying to evaluate your own performance because you are still not sure what you are doing ... you are still trying to find your feet." Mary described herself as "being the fine point on which the whole thing balanced" and "in the end the reason I didn't continue is because I just found it I was incapable of being the health system. You know I couldn't be that balancing point that it all hinged on and I got very stressed by that." Some of Mary's strategies included "like I have to just draw myself in out of the situation and sort of try not to participate so much. Even though I am still physically present. Draw my energy back, hold my breath back and just say okay, this is what's happening I can't control it." The perception of the environment being out of control meant that the workers could not participate in the health system in the sense that they were non-relational, disembodied, disconnected and to a certain extent disengaged. The disengaged reasoning is a characteristic of instrumentalist sources of self.

Similarly Gill found that the feeling of being out of control almost led her into a major depression. "And then one day I woke up and I thought 'hey this isn't about me, it's not my fault that I can't see all those people' so I just stopped short of actually hitting rock bottom, which was an amazing thing." It was also amazing that Gill didn't talk about these feeling with anyone and she had to work through them on her own. The sense or feeling of being out of control was internalised and individualised, instead of seeing this as the feeling of what happens when the environment appears out of control due to overwhelming demand. There is little awareness of this or how to manage within the systemic constraints.

There must be a greater sophistication of knowledge production in health professional practice, to include a wider range of sources of knowledge like medical humanities, instead of arguing about what are essentially practices of the professional self, in order to raise awareness of the context. Since health professional practice and the health professional's self are constructed by social forces, inscripted, enfolded, then by finding out about individual experience (as in this research) we are ipso facto finding out about contextual experience as each participant can be seen as some reflection of their contextual experience. There seems to be an epistemic gap here which relates to how suffering is responded to, since there are not the words in training or practice to speak about this.

> A search for authenticity is crucial for professionals who need to be able to distinguish other people's 'false voices' from their own, since the ability to use experience to critique the voices of others is crucial to developing professional agency (Brookfield, 2005; p. 46). Patti Lather's notion of "embodied reflexivity" (1991; p. 48) provides an alternative pedagogic model that interrupts transmissive models of teaching in which individual's lived experiences are of little account.
>
> To value "embodied reflexivity" and "embodied learning," which is the "knowing that is discoverable in our experiences as embodied beings" (Gustafson, 1999; p. 250), is to value learning that resonates with lived experience.
>
> (Pearce, 2008; p. 45)

A curriculum for health professionals could benefit from the inclusion of a narrative for reflexivity that included acknowledgment of the health professionals' social being in relation to objective structures and suffering. In some cases, this may mean acknowledging the habitual absent body (Edvardsson & Street, 2007). Freire (1998) talks about a testimony of a progressive educator's practice, saying, "An educational practice in which there is no coherent relationship between what educators say and what they do is a disaster" (p. 55).

> I now focus on an analysis of the relationship between educator and learners, a relationship that involves questions of teaching, of learning, of the knowing-teaching-learning process, of authority, of freedom, of reading, of writing, of the virtues of the educator, and of the cultural identity of the learners and the respect that must be paid to it.
>
> (Freire, 1998; p. 55)

These thoughts apply equally well to health. There needs to be a coherent relationship between what health professionals say and what they do. If their curriculum could include some of the above points as part of the development of being a health professional, then the professions could go some way towards addressing the inequities in power and suffering currently present in the enactment of the curriculum. In this way, they could start addressing what it means to be in relationship with clients or patients and the relationship between what they say and do in their practice as health professionals.

Similarly, the relationship between subject and object needs exploring in the health professionals' practice. Health professional practice needs some notion of learning as described by Freire: "to study is to uncover; it is to gain a more exact comprehension of an object; it is to realize its relationships to other objects" (1998; p. 21). This requires some reflection back of the subjective experience which in itself requires some distance:

> "Immersed in the reality of their small world, they were unable to see it. By taking some distance, they emerged and were thus able to see it as they never had before"
>
> (Freire, 1998; p. 21)

This has resonances with the integrative capacity of the imagery of a clearing in a forest (Galvin & Todres, 2007). The role of the reflection back of the learning/health experience is precisely to place the subject's experience in context, which the subject who is in the middle of the subjectivity is unable to do on his or her own. Currently this ability to look back on one's self with the assistance of a reflective relationship is largely missing in health.

This type of learning is in addition to a reflexive spiral even if it is a form of an embodied reflexivity. Embodied reflexivity is said to include and acknowledge the ethical, political, cultural and social dimensions along with the idea that as we act we are also acted upon (Giddens, 1991). The context and social constructedness of self is emphasised here. I would like to emphasise, along with the aforementioned aspects, that for me the reflection back of my own subjective experience by another (that always keeps the context and constructedness in the forefront of their reflection back) has been vital for me in allowing my self in as part of this process of learning.

There is a difference for me between embodied reflexivity and reflection back of the subjective experience. Embodied reflexivity (Lather, 1991) is the reflective process that includes the body as part of those reflections and which is the essentially individual practice of reflective practice of action research and praxis. This is the practice that has been co-opted by the dominant neo-liberal epistemological discourses and turned into critical self-evaluation, i.e., more self-policing.

Reflection back of the subjective experience requires another person to reflect back, by which I mean mirror in an ethical manner (and this includes the contextual aspects of the experience) so that people can understand and make meaning out of their experience. Where people's experience has been grounded in silence and absence, embodied reflexivity is a privileged construct as there are not the words within to describe that experience. The two parts of reflection – embodied reflexivity and reflection back of subjective experience – go hand in hand.

The participant who most clearly identified the importance of connectedness, and feeling deeply connected, to know what it is like to be human was Joan. Her perception was that health is an experience of seeking life and that sharing that with other people was beneficial to her own health – the sparkly moment of palpable humanity. There is something deeply important about health, but this research indicates we are missing it currently in the health risk management approach. Health and suffering as self could be another way of perceiving health and that includes embodiment and a sense of being. But it seems as if these perceptions could only be held in a curriculum that emphasised relational pedagogy and a reflection back of the subjective experience of the health professional. Then personhood could be encompassed in the training, which means that health, suffering and learning are inextricably linked.

Fox (1999) suggests that health professionals can move out into "smooth space" after ongoing processes of deterritorialisation and reterritorialisation. By keeping an eye on the constructions of health work, health professionals can move out of ruts they may have been stuck in as far as their practice is concerned. Along with suggestions of questions that health professionals can ask themselves, he also has the following definition in relation to health:

> So a responsibility to otherness, in relation to issues of 'health' and 'illness', will suggest a radically different conception of the human potential, and this is what is meant by arche-health . Arche-health is a becoming, a deterritorializing of the BwO, a resistance to discourse, a generosity towards otherness, a nomadic subjectivity. It is not intended to suggest a natural, essential or in any way prior kind of health, upon which other healths are superimposed .... can never become the object of scientific investigation, without falling back into discourse on health/illness. It is not the outcome of deconstruction of these discourses, it is deconstruction: difference and becoming.
>
> (Fox, 1999; p. 11)

Fox (1999) posits that deconstruction is health and that lines of flight into smooth spaces become available from reflexivity, de-territorialisations and naming of differends. To me this is like saying the link between health and learning is deconstruction. However, again, this could be a big ask for health professionals grounded in a biomedical model and who rely on that model not only for achieving the best patient outcomes but also for their sense of professional and personal self. Some of the individual consequences of being socially trained in the biomedical model have been outlined here to highlight the relationship between the individual and social and the potential consequences on understanding and responding to suffering.

One key point is the disembodiment that occurs resulting in an absence of self at work – that in order to survive health, one has to make oneself absent. Leder speaks of this paradox:

> Yet this bodily presence is of a highly paradoxical nature. While in one sense the body is the most abiding and inescapable presence in our lives, it is also essentially characterized by absence. That is, one's own body is rarely the thematic object of experience.
>
> (Leder, 1990; p. 1)

While a post-structural analysis has identified the absences and gaps in the field of healthcare workers, this may be because a post-structural account is designed to highlight these sorts of issues. Post-structural analysis has done little to embody the self and in fact perpetuates ideas of non-embodiment. This means that in terms of suffering, there is little wonder that health professionals find it difficult to know how to respond to suffering and yet feel impelled to do so. Whilst post-structuralism was useful in analysing structures of power which could then be used more productively and less oppressively, in theory, there are some difficulties with integration of these ideas in the healthcare field. Probably most health professionals would feel comfortable with the idea of a "natural body" underpinning the "organism" – an essentialist position that acknowledges a natural body overlaid with cultural values having an existence that is determined phenomenologically through "experience," "faith" or "common sense" (Fox, 1999). But I can't see many taking on the idea of a body without organs.

Health professionals want to respond to suffering and often choose activist roles in order to do so. Critical pedagogy as a means of challenging conceptions of the self in a relationship that fails to recognise the effects of social structures and forces is crucial (Usher et al, 1997). Yet the effects of social structures and forces make the construction of self a continual social practice that takes place within the healing relationship or meeting place (Foucault, 1973) of the health professional and client or patient. The continual practice of the self through awareness of relations of power is also important.

However, what can no longer be missed is an understanding of suffering and how this impacts on individuals and the healthcare relationship.

Foucault (1973) argued that development of practices of freedom needed to operate at the level of developing techniques designed to incite individuals to relate to themselves and others, according to a different set of designated norms for governing conduct. Thus Foucault (1973) is concerned with working at the limits of existing regimes of practice to invent alternative modes of relating to ourselves in an ethic of care for the self. This means working at the limits or edges of the dominant construction of self as the neo-liberal self in health, one in pursuit of freedom from oppressive forces – the motivation provided by much of neo-liberals' rhetoric (Harvey, 2005).

5.5 Working at the limits or edges of the dominant construction of self

The biomedical individual has been constructed by psychology and the medical and social sciences as one who is able to control their behaviours in an attempt to achieve freedom from outside control (Ogden, 2001). This self has become increasingly constructed as autonomous, detached and self-reflexive (Ogden, 2001) whilst also coming increasingly under the control of institutional surveillance (Petersen & Lupton, 2000). Health is framed in terms of compliance and evidence-based practice (Freshwater & Rolfe, 2004) of the health professionals' self.

Further definitions or constructions of the self include the following:

- The self as an experiential integration (Nathanson, 1992)
- The self is one that makes meaning, i.e., has agency of meaning (Lather, 2007)
- The self is a knot in a web of relations – no relation means no self (Bingham & Sidorkin, 2004)
- The self is consolidated largely through the body (Niranjana, 2001)

However, these definitions are not mainstream and their use is restricted to post-positivist social sciences. Feminist ethicists argue that subjectivity and morality are inseparable and that what is needed is a radically different notion of the subject to that offered by "the strictly individualistic, rational, moral subject of modernist thinking" (Usher, 2000; p. 22) and to that offered by the patriarchal biomedical model. Post-structuralists take exception that most writing about the self tends to fall into binary or dichotomous variables – self-not-self or self-other; object-subject; inside-outside; male-female; conscious-unconscious; with the exception of Freud, curiously enough.

Freud proposed a system of interpretation of the self as comprising id (largely unconscious drives associated with the body), ego (the negotiator between drives and perfectionism or idealism) and superego (reflective of higher authority – religious, familial, social). At the time, Freud's scientific model of the self influenced thinking and popular culture so much that we now take for granted terms like the unconscious. The same could be said for the word self – common usage indicates that most people believe they have self and act as if they do. Therefore it comes as a shock to experience suffering and a sense of loss of self.

Understanding the self is thus important because otherwise how do we know what, and how, has been lost? This is tricky because, as Singleton (2015) points out in cultural melancholy, the loss is disavowed, unmourned and barred from recognition; "a loss that claims yet cannot be claimed" (p. 4). The barring of conscious recognition of loss and the displacement of the loss unconsciously onto the ego mean that any description is constantly coming up against the boundary of experience. One could be forgiven for thinking that perhaps post-structuralist thinkers were suffering from a loss of self that they could not recognise because they eschewed the importance of experience in their theorising. But as Ney (2019) states about our knowledge or beliefs, "the total field is so undetermined by its boundary conditions, experience, that there is much latitude of choice as to what statements to re-evaluate in the light of any single contrary experience" (p. 129). Suffering is a boundary experience of the self, an invitation to liminality where experiencing is more important than controlling suffering (Bynum, 1987).

Starting with experience, Damasio (2010) suggests that consciousness of our contextualised experience is a process, that it is a connection between the social and individual that is sensed and is a starting point for understanding what a self is. The self includes the felt experience of consciousness, the content of the mind and the holder of that experience and content. He analyses self from two perspectives: (1) self as an observer appreciating a dynamic processual object (self-as-object) and (2) self as knower, the process that gives a focus to experiences and eventually allows reflection on those experiences (self-as-knower). The division is produced by the perspective and not by any inherent split between the two. The latter is based on the former, through distinctions between "me" and "not me." The self-as-object or material me perceives, generates emotions and feelings, or somatic markers, that enable these distinctions, which give rise to feelings of knowing, or self-as-knower. His definition of the material me is "a dynamic collection of integrated neural processes, centred on the representation of the living body, that finds expression in a dynamic collection of integrated mental process" (p. 9) or the mind, or core self. These neural patterns are simultaneously mental images which can become known if a rich enough self-process subject is generated. What he calls an imaginarium of the mind-self-body-brain (problem). If no self is generated, images are still there but no-one knows of their existence.

However, as the scope of the self expands, gradually an autobiographical self forms whose terms are of biographical social nature:

The conscious minds of humans, armed with such complex selves and supported by even greater capabilities of memory, reasoning, and language, engender the instruments of culture and open the way into new means of homeostasis at the level of societies and culture. In an extraordinary leap, homeostasis acquires an extension into the sociocultural space.

(Damasio, 2010; p. 26)

Damasio (2010) makes an extraordinary leap in the text to include a model of self that seemingly starts off as a biomedical model but then expands its scope to extend into the sociocultural space as both a constructer and constructed process in search of survival and well-being.

Damasio (2010) effortlessly relates the social and individual through a biomedical concept of homeostasis:

The investigation of sociocultural homeostasis can be informed by psychology and neuroscience, but the native space of its phenomena is cultural.

Both basic homeostasis (which is unconsciously guided) and sociocultural homeostasis (which is created and guided by reflective conscious minds) operate as curators of biological value.

(p. 27)

Basic and sociocultural homeostasis promote the same goal of survival of living organisms even though they are in different ecological niches; to the extent that some deliberately seek well-being; although this may come at a cost to others. For example, neo-liberal well-being requires the exploitation of vulnerable workers. Sociocultural homeostasis is seen as a fragile work in progress. Perhaps this has never been more apparent than during a global pandemic.

Even though Damasio (2010) does not mention suffering explicitly, by invoking the term survival, he begins to imagine how complexity works between the materiality of individuals and sociocultural practices. Indeed, he goes on to justify the exploration of conscious minds through the brain science by linking art, spirituality and social justice:

Understanding ... allows us to judge perhaps more wisely than before the quality of knowledge and advice those conscious minds provide. Is the knowledge reliable? Is the advice sound? Do we gain from understanding the mechanisms behind the minds that give us counsel?

(Damasio, 2010; p. 28)

Placing the construction of conscious minds in the history of biology and culture opens the way to reconciling traditional humanities and modern science, so that when neuroscience explores human experience into the strange worlds of brain physiology and genetics, human dignity is not only retained but reaffirmed.

(Damasio, 2010; p. 29)

The connection between the science of the mind, the self, and sociocultural context as co-constructing each other places consciousness as a key faculty and process in understanding suffering. Sharpe (2016) concurs, stating "rather than seeking a resolution to blackness's ongoing and irresolvable abjection, one might approach Black being in the wake as a form of *consciousness*" (Sharpe, 2016; p. 14; emphasis original).

To live in suffering and formulate consciousness from there means to produce something out of the nothing of black social, material and psychic death: "to think and be and act from there" (Sharpe, 2016; p. 22). And that producing something is possible: "even as we experienced, recognized, and lived subjection, we did not *simply* or *only* live *in* subjection and *as* the subjected" (Sharpe, 2016; p. 4; emphasis original). Surviving, continued vulnerability to inexplicable and overwhelming force constituted self both as a something and as a nothing known to themselves and each other (Sharpe, 2016). Yet Sharpe's (2016) writing does not seem divided against itself. It seems to resonate with Bynum's (1987) idea that sufferers are non-dualists in themselves perhaps *because* they experience or perceive themselves as on the wrong side of the fault line of life.

Both Sharpe (2016) and Damasio (2010) link sociocultural context with the materiality of the body, self and conscious mind. This is significant because traditionally sociocultural (or post-structural) analyses tend to focus on linguistic and practice formations or norms that exert power over the body whilst failing to take into account the materiality and phenomenology of the body (Ortega, 2014). The failure to take these into account is seen as a characteristic abjection by social constructionism that cannot include such things as flesh, blood, vomit, etc., since they escape symbolisation and threaten ideal body images: "These are all parts of myself which must be expelled so that I can inscribe myself in the symbolic order" (Ortega, 2014; p. 9). The abjection of the flesh in an attempt to reach symbolism reinforces a duality in thinking about the social and the individual which is not necessary as Sharpe (2016), Bynum (1987) and Damasio (2010) demonstrated. It is important to be clear about this because so many analyses get stuck in this body-as-trap (Bynum, 1995a).

Reinforcing binaries or dualities does not serve people who suffer the most. Whilst acknowledging the effect of power in issues of social justice is vital, as well as taking political action to change these effects, when thinking about the body, mind and self, dualities that separate these out are not useful to an individual. In a critique of Foucault, Ortega (2014) argues that dualism prevents an understanding of the effects of normalising power and the resistance inherent in that:

Foucault's aversion to psychology and psychoanalysis has led him completely to neglect the individual psyche and to reduce interiority to that which power and its coercive mechanisms produce inside bodies.

This is important because the lack of understanding produces a void in relation to suffering. Consciousness of the void created by both neo-liberalism and post-structuralism enables us to see that the human minds behind these practices can be as fallible as each other.

For example, Sharpe (2016) shows how power works to both act and erase at the same time, perhaps producing the unconscionable loss of self that Singleton (2015) discusses. Therefore, understanding embodiment and the self as inseparable is crucial:

> [W]hile even as that terror visited on our bodies the realities of that terror are erased. Put another way, living in the wake means living in and with terror in that much of what passes for public discourse *about* terror we, Black people, become the *carriers* of terror, terror's embodiment, and not the primary objects of terror's multiple enactments; the ground of terror's possibility globally.
>
> (Sharpe, 2016; p. 15)

We are required to link embodiment, the self and context in prolonged cultural suffering in order to understand and mitigate against how a sociocultural void is created around these experiences and in addition how discourses about human rights can often perpetuate the status quo by propping up the neo-liberal regime (Butt, 2002). Realising this seems to be more important than critiquing the use of biomedical neuroscience to discuss and explore the self as long as context is accounted for as much as possible, which it seems to be by Damasio (2010) and Sharpe (2016).

The idea of a sociocultural void around the experience of suffering is important to explore since this could be a manifestation of the social construction of suffering. As Wilkinson (2005) wrote, sociology does not have a theory of suffering as the words are frustratingly elusive. Yet the sociocultural void persists because suffering is not discussed, normalised nor validated as a legitimate experience of life and self. The epistemic break in how we know what we know about the self in relation to suffering and death means that a void is socially constructed about and in the self; we do not have the words for this. Perhaps the silence about the suffering self is because of *avoidance* or fear of finding something terrible in suffering.

Therefore, not only does the experience of suffering mean a perception of a loss of intactness of self and unbearable feelings of distress, there is also the void linguistically and socioculturally which can only reinforce the experience. The hole in what can be said and done changes the figure-ground relationship between the self and the social to a becoming-around-a-hole that is co-constructed, paradoxically in order to survive. The tension between agency and languishing is united under the umbrella of performativity whilst looking for a reference point (or person) such as the normatively valued hero – white male heterosexual autonomous neo-liberal person. This seems to be a cultural phenomenon. In addition, there is always the tension between self-other, with both being determined along cultural historical lines. What this may mean is that the hole is skipped over; there is a papering over the epistemic gap.

What may it mean to hang out with this individualised sociocultural hole in terms of the self? When contemplating this, I drew on Ney's (2019) thoughts about the boundary of experience in relation to undetermined thoughts and belief. That is, coming up against the boundary experience of suffering changes thoughts and beliefs – the ability to feel understood and trust that understanding by other people (Devisch et al, 2017) – so that in effect what disappears is the cultural norm of the neo-liberal self; this is experienced as a hole. Staying with the hole in thoughts and beliefs is like an experience of running your finger around the rim of a glass to produce a note that resonates in a sustained way. The so-called empty self of suffering produces a note, a something in the face of the nothing, that ripples out in sound waves from the container and is perceived by and perhaps resonates with other receptacles (people). Suffering registers on many different levels. For me, a powerful evocation of this was the spectacle of Italian people singing from their balconies in their time of lockdown, over empty streets, the ripples of sound meeting and harmonising with other's suffering.

Rather than covering over the hole of suffering, people were *connecting through* their suffering. What does this mean in terms of the self? It means that in spite of a sociocultural hole in suffering, the empty streets and a lack of engaged consumer activity, there was something arising out of collective selves. And in order to transmit and receive this something, there did have to be embodied materialised selves albeit acting in unison. Poststructuralists may argue that this example is simply a demonstration of practices of the self – subjectivity, authority and discourses. It may well be; I have no argument about that. However, it would not have been possible at all without a physical body.

To me, the post-structural debate about the lack of self or natural body beyond discursively constructed practices falls down on the fact that whilst basing itself on the notion of a body as a site of competing discourses, at the same time it refutes the existence of a physical material body. In the intersection of the individual and the social, whilst undoubtedly there are cultural influences and oppressive practices, there has to be a body in place as a manifestation of the self. Taking this material phenomenological body as a baseline to explore suffering is a must. Establishing such a normative baseline is in opposition to attributing all suffering to sociocultural constructed experiences without exploring how the individual body processes that. The extended consciousness Damasio (2010) talks about reached out into the collective in an attempt at social homeostasis, with this observation based on the assumption that the social homeostasis was possible because of the biological homeostasis of the core self or core consciousness, and there was also an awareness that elusively perceived and conducted all this.

Damasio (1999) invites us to consider the existence of a core self by an experiment. He suggests viewing the page you are reading, then turn to view the wall off to your right, then the room around us and noticing that while part of our consciousness was involved with changes in perception in our visual field, there was another part that was stable and able to register the changes in the body (Damasio, 1999; p. 21–22). Part of how we know what we know is through registering change in the body – there is some level of consciousness that was aware of movement, by not moving. That in order to perceive change there must be a reference point, part of us that is still, and this is related to core consciousness.

This may be nonverbal and elusive to understand yet comforting to know that all the while there is a part of us aware at this somatosensory level of perception: interoception. Interoception (the sense of self-generated from inner experience or internal reality of proprioception, vestibular apparatus, nociception, chemoreception and osmoreception) leads to perceptions such as hunger, thirst, suffocation, nausea or vomiting. "These are all parts of myself which must be expelled so that I can inscribe myself in the symbolic order" (Ortega, 2014; p. 9). At first, I wrote this with a typo – symbiotic – but this also makes sense since the abjection characteristic of social constructionism, that cannot include such things as flesh, blood, vomit, etc. – is a reflection of a symbiosis with the dominant order of transcendence of the body in order to achieve symbolisation and ideal body images.

Social constructionism could be seen in this light of yet another masculinisation of the embodied experience that takes away the value and legitimation of expanding our embodied suffering (Bynum, 1987). Perhaps the social constructionist and post-structural refusal of the physical body is another example of living life abstractly, jettisoning the stuff of "me" as expressed in the body and "I" as a person that continues to exist, to be "I" through time (Bynum, 1995a). Whilst the anti-essentialist position is understandable as a reaction to Cartesian and Enlightenment dichotomies (Bynum, 1995a), which is where the debate between the social and individual was cemented, there is also a need to reclaim the body, me and I. My suggestion is that while there may be a hole in what we can say or do in the face of suffering, there is a core part of us that survives and that can "sing" on the edges of that experience. The resonance of this song is picked up on by attuned others and joined with.

Perhaps the reason why a sociological theory of suffering is difficult to articulate is because of the lack of resonance with the notion that there is an inner reality. Sociological analyses, as previously mentioned, tend to eschew any idea of essence or absolute truth because there is the assumption that selves are co-constructed socially and are primarily performative (Butler, 1993). Feminist analyses have "dethroned the notion of a self-centred, rational, unitary subject" (Venn, 2002; p. 53). It may have been necessary to dethrone the autonomous neo-liberal subject but ideas around "[a]n I by itself does not exist" (Ricoeur, 1992; p. 18 cited by Venn, 2002; p. 57) can be perceived as equally disempowering when "I by itself" is all there is in times of solitude and survival.

There is no reason why an "I" cannot exist alongside an "I-we" of extended consciousness in social science theory. And that to throw out the "I" in favour of an "I-we" that is heteronomous is again making abject an artefact of culture and a faculty of human being. In fact, there seems to be little difference between the quotes previously from Damasio (2010) and the following by Venn (2002):

> A who or 'self' 'happens' at the relay point or points where the history of a culture, sedimented in its stock of knowledge, its narrations, its 'texts', joins with the history or biography of a particular individual. In this way every self is sutured in history. But this suturing, or folding, requires the participation of others: as interlocutors, imagined or not, as models or ideal egos, as those in the gaze, of whom recognition is bestowed or refused, as elements of the lifeworld that validate particular selves.
>
> (p. 58)

He goes on to say that the subject is always in process, the same as Damasio (2010) stating that the self is a process as much as consciousness itself. Odd that there should be such resonance between texts of different epistemological positions that almost sound like a unity. This unity is what Wilson (1998) has been proposing. The difference is that Venn (2002) stays at the register of the communal becoming whereas Damasio (2010) provides accounts of biological and social registers of the self. The consciousness of the social sciences is to deny the individual materiality of the body to the extent that agency as a concept becomes lost.

The difficulty arises because social sciences have privileged language as the co-constructor of both the social and individual world. Therefore, it has been difficult to imagine, and downright refuted, that anything exists extra-discursively. However, as Damasio (1999) argues,

> If language operates for the self and for consciousness in the same way that it operates for everything else, that is, by symbolizing in words and sentences what exists first in a nonverbal form, then there must be a nonverbal self and a nonverbal knowing for which the words 'I' or 'me' or the phrase 'I know' are the appropriate translations, in any language.
>
> (Damasio, 1999; p. 107–108)

The exact phrase "I know" suggests "the presence of a nonverbal image of knowing centred on a self that precedes and motivates that verbal phrase" (Damasio, 1999; p. 108). *And* that self – extended autobiographical consciousness – will also be co-constructed by others, circumstances and social practices. Consciousness is always consciousness of something, not of nothing.

However, there is a difference in acknowledging that co-construction of selves and then denying there is no such thing as an individual "I." As a process, an "I" exists – the body that lives, breathes and suffers (Bynum, 1995a).

> As you look at this page and see these words, whether you wish for it or not, automatically and relentlessly, you sense that *you* are doing the reading. I am not doing it, nor is anyone else. You are.

> *Consciousness* is the umbrella term for the mental phenomena that permit the strange confection of you as observer or knower of things observed, of you as potential agent on the scene. Consciousness is a part of your mental process rather than external to it.
>
> (Damasio, 1999; p. 127; emphasis original)

No doubt that consciousness is influenced and constructed by a myriad of practices and people. Yet it would be disingenuous to suggest that an individual perspective, ownership of thought and agency are not part of the self process, the very feeling of you that is required to know of your own existence and of the existence of others (Damasio, 1999).

The relevance of this to the suffering self is that while there may be speechlessness and distress at the individual level of experience, there is still an individual experience at the nonverbal register of being which can be legitimated and known, perhaps not through acts of speech so much as a level of resonance and attunement, perhaps through somatosensory conveying and touch. That a theory of suffering can start with the concept of an individual, albeit one who experiences a loss of intactness of self, because there is this level of understanding of core consciousness. Moreover, even though there is a perceived loss of intactness of self, it is reassuring to know that there is still a boundary, a body, an organism and life:

> The specification for survival that I am describing here include a boundary; an internal structure; a dispositional arrangement for the regulation of internal states that subsumes a mandate to maintain life; a narrow range of variability of internal states so that those states are relatively stable.
>
> (Damasio, 1999; p. 136)

Consciousness of the pre-categorical, pre-cognitive, pre-conceptual stage is possible and provides the way out of the woods referred to in Chapter Four and further developed in this chapter. Chapter Four suggested we needed to think differently about the self in order to change the status quo, to develop curricula committed to disrupting forgone conclusions about social relations and the relationship between the individual and social.

We briefly left the realm of the representational and have not strayed too far in order to explore the relationship between the individual and social. Deconstructing post-structural representations of the self and the body meant seeing below the surface of linguistics to consciousness, returning to a biomedical model to understand the relationship between the self and the body as well as that between the individual and social. Having travelled across this epistemic gap, various subjects have arisen for suggestions for a curriculum. I have no illusions that these could be incorporated into a medical curriculum, for example. I am not sure that that is their place at the undergraduate level even though when I was that age, that is what I thought I was going to university for. Working at the limits or edges of the dominant construction of self means continually cultivating consciousness of both the individual and social aspects of suffering. We have not covered much about affects in this section and will be doing so in the next chapter as we explore more about curriculum issues and how this works in a transcendence, of absence of self and body, in a biomedical model of suffering. In so doing, we will explore further the romantic expressivism sources of self, as well as how these relate to suffering and knowing. This is important because as we have seen, there are competing ways of thinking about the self and how this impacts on practice as well as suffering, how we survive and find a way out of the woods as well as dealing with the kind of ethical concerns highlighted by the quote at the beginning of the chapter.

Box 5.1   Reflection

A symbolic reversal occurs in healthcare whereby through means of the body and different technologies patients are displaced from their own knowing and become reliant on health professionals in this strange new world they find themselves inhabiting. Patients require pathways out of the woods, out of their own existential experiential suffering. They need to know footsteps, pathways, bridges and so on through this strange liminal land, where health professionals feel so at home that they refer to their NHS "family." Patients can feel like they are guests in someone else's house, trespassing on routines and rituals. The embodied crossover is this feeling of being in someone else's home that does not quite make sense and you are not entirely sure of your welcome.

The paradox seems to be though that due to time pressures, systems of overwhelm, punitive ways of managing this, and the intense quality and quantity of tasks, there may be nobody home. Perhaps the ethical dilemmas that bother our sleep are our ways of waking up to what was real in the day, a way of knowing, a way of breaking through the hamster wheel of rhetoric that enchants us, when something doesn't go according to plan. Perhaps ruptures are a good way to interrupt the frictionless smooth space of uninhabited bodies. The mythopoetic curriculum speaks of the violence of consciousness emerging (Holland & Garman, 2010).

Concepts, symbols, imaginaries, narratives form a web of the social matrix; it is the social matrix. This forms a veil over what we can know and see; a veil which can cover our insight. But there are lacunae we can fall through. Falling into the abyss is not necessarily a bad thing if we are to understand more about suffering and ourselves. Ethical dilemmas may well expose the self that was covered over by the matrix of social roles and expectations. Finding the right tools to find your way out is part of the process of emergence.

Questions for reflection

1   How do you digest events and information from the day?
2   What emotional voids do you see as being formed and encouraged in healthcare and how do they contribute to suffering? How do voids relate to the culture of consumerism?
3   In what sense does the above passage resonate with you or not? How?
4   In what sense does gender play in salvation and redemption narratives of suffering through different roles in healthcare?
5   How do people who are traditionally and materially marginalised and disadvantaged fall through the social matrix or safety nets of redemption and salvation in healthcare?

Further Resources

Knapp. C. 2004. *Appetites: Why Women Want*. Counterpoint LLC: New York.

References

Barad K. 2007. *Meeting the Universe Halfway: Quantum Physics and the Entanglement of Matter and Meaning*. Duke University Press Books: New York.

Becker E. 1973. *The Denial of Death*. The Free Press: London.

Biesta G. 2004. *"Mind the Gap!" Communication and the Educational Relation in No Education Without Relation*. Bingham C., Sidorkin AM. (eds). Peter Lang Publishing: New York.

Bingham C., Sidorkin AM. (eds). 2004 *No Education Without Relation*. Peter Lang Publishing: New York.

Boyer A. 2018. *A Handbook of Disappointed Fate*. Ugly Duckling Presse: Brooklyn.

Brookfield S.D. 2005. *The Power of Critical Theory - Liberating Adult Learning and Teaching*. Jossey-Bass: San Francisco.

Butler J. 1993. *Bodies that Matter: On the Discursive Limits of "sex"*. Routledge: New York.

Butler J. 1990. *Gender Trouble: Feminism and the Subversion of Identity*. Routledge: New York.

Butt L. 2002. The suffering stranger: Medical anthropology and international morality. *Medical Anthropology*; 21(1):1–24; discussion 25-33. doi: 10.1080/01459740210619.

Bynum C.W. 1995a. Why all the fuss about the body? A medievalist's perspective. *Critical Inquiry*; 22(1):1–33.

Bynum C.W. 1995b. *The Resurrection of the Body in Western Christianity*, 200 – 1336. Columbia University Press: New York.

Bynum C.W. 1991. *Fragmentation and Redemption: Essays on Gender and the Human Body in Medieval Religion*. Zone books: New York.

Bynum C.W. 1987. *Holy Feast and Holy Fast: The Religious Significance of Food to Medieval Women*. University of California Press: Berkely.

Cerea A. 2018. Culture and psychism: The ethnopsychoanalysis of Georges Devereux. *History of Psychiatry*; 29(3): 297–314.

Damasio A. 2010. Self comes to mind: Constructing the conscious brain. Pantheon/Random House: New York.

Damasio A. 1999. *The Feeling of What Happens: Body, Emotion and the Making of Consciousness*. Vintage: London.

Danaher G., Schirato T., Webb J. 2000. *Understanding Foucault*. Allen and Unwin: Australia.

De Certeau M. 1984. *The Practice of Everyday Life*. University of California Press: California.

Deleuze G., Guattari F. 2009. *What Is Philosophy?* Verso: London.

Dempsey C. 2018. *The Antidote to Suffering: How Compassionate Connected Care Can Improve Safety, Quality and Experience*. McGraw-Hill: New York.

Devisch I., Vanheule S., Deveugele M. Nola I., Civaner M., Pype P. 2017. Victims of disaster: Can ethical debriefings be of help to care for their suffering? *Medical Health Care and Philosophy*; 20:257–267.

Eco U. 2014. *From the Tree to the Labyrinth: Historical Studies on the Sign and Interpretation*. Harvard University Press: New York.

Edvardsson D., Street A. 2007. Sense or no-sense: The nurse as embodied ethnographer. *International Journal of Nursing Practice*; 13: 24–32.

Epstein R. 2017. *Attending: Medicine, Mindfulness and Humanity*. Scribner: New York.

Felitti V.J. 2019. Origins of the ACE study. *American Journal of Preventive Medicine*. doi:10.1016/j.amepre.2019.02.011

Felitti V.J., Anda R.F., Nordenberg D., Williamson D.F., Spitz A.M., Edwards V., ... Marks JS. 1998. *Relationship of childhood abuse and household dysfunction to many of the leading causes of death in adults: The Adverse Childhood Experiences (ACE) Study. American Journal of Preventive Medicine*; 14(4): 245–258.

Finlay L., Langdridge D. 2007. Embodiment. Chapter 7 in *Social Psychology Matters*. Hollway W., Lucey H., Phoenix A. (eds). Open University Press: Maidenhead.

Fiske A.P. 1993. *Structures of Social Life: The Four Elementary Forms of Human Relations*. The Free Press: New York.

Fitzgerald D., Callard F. 2016. Entangling the medical humanities. Chapter 1 in *The Edinburgh Companion to the Critical Medical Humanities*. Whitehead A., Woods A., Atkinson S., et al., (eds). Edinburgh: Edinburgh University Press.

Foucault, M. 1983. *The Subject and Power – Afterword in Michel Foucault – Beyond Structuralism and Hermeneutics.* Second Edition. Dreyfus H.L., Rabinow P. (eds). Chicago Press: Chicago., pp. 208–226.

Foucault M. 1973. *The Birth of the Clinic – An Archeology of Medical Perception.* Vintage Books: New York.

Fox, N.J. 1999. *Beyond Health – Postmodernism and Embodiment.* Free Association Books: London.

Francis G. 2020. The art of medicine Medicine: Art or science? Perspectives. *The Lancet*; 395:24–25.

Freire P. 1998. *Teachers as Cultural Workers – Letter to Those Who Dare to Teach.* Westview Press: Colorado.

Freshwater D., Rolfe G. 2004. *Deconstructing Evidence-based Practice.* Routledge: Oxford.

Galvin K., Todres L. 2007. The creativity of 'Unspecialization': A contemplative direction for integrative scholarly practice. *Phenomenology and Practice*; 1(1): 31–46.

Giddens A. 1991. *Modernity and Self Identity. Self and Society in the Late Modern Age.* Stanford University Press: Stanford, CA.

Gore J.M. 1995. *On the Continuity of Power Relations in Pedagogy. International Studies in Sociology of Education*; 5(2):165–188.

Harvey D. 2005. *A Brief History of Neoliberalism.* Oxford University Press: Oxford.

Holland P.E, Garman N.B. 2010. Watching with two eyes: The place of the Mythopoetic in Curriculum Inquiry. Chapter Two in *Pedagogies of the Imagination.* Leonard T., Willis P. (eds). Springer Science .Business Media BV: Chicago.

Hollis M. 1996. Of masks and men. Chapter 10 in *The Category of Person: Anthropology, Philosophy, History.* Carrithers M., Collins S., Lukes S. (eds). Cambridge University Press: Cambridge, pp. 216–233.

Hutton P.H. 1988. *Ch2 in Technologies of Self.* Martin LH., Gutman H., Hutton PH. (eds). The University of Massachusetts Press: Amherst.

Jones D. 2014. *Magna Carter: The Making and Legacy of the Great Charter.* Head of Zeus: London.

Kendall G., Wickham G. 1999. *Using Foucault's Methods.* Sage Publications: London.

Kleinman A. 1988. *The Illness Narratives: Suffering, Healing, and the Human Condition.* Basic Books: New York.

Lather P. 2007. *Getting Lost: Feminist Efforts Toward a Double(d) Science.* State University of New York Press: Albany.

Lather P. 1991. *Getting Smart – Feminist Research and Pedagogy with/in the Postmodern.* Routledge, Chapman and Hall: New York.

Leder D. 1990. *The Absent Body.* The University of Chicago Press: London.

Mahendran A. 2019. *Moments of Rupture: The Importance of Affect in Medical Education and Surgical Training.* Routledge: London.

Mauss M. 1996. A category of the human mind: The notion of person; the notion of self. Chapter 1 in *The Category of Person: Anthropology, Philosophy, History.* Carrithers M., Collins S., Lukes S. (eds). Cambridge University Press: Cambridge, pp. 1–25.

McLaren M.A. 2002. *Feminism, Foucault, and Embodied Subjectivity*. State University of New York Press: Albany.

Mendenhall E. 2019. *Rethinking Diabetes: Entanglement with Trauma, poverty and HIV*. Cornell University Press: London.

Moro M.R. 2018. A Transcultural Approach to Psychiatry. Cultural Crossings of Care. Oslo University. Keynote Speaker.

Nathanson D.L. 1992. *Shame and Pride – Affect, Sex and the Birth of the Self*. W.W. Norton and Company: New York

Ney A. 2019. *Metaphysics: An Introduction*. Routledge: London.

Niranjana S. 2001. *Gender and Space – Feminity, Sexualization and the Female Body*. Sage Publications: New Delhi.

Ogden J. 2001. *Health and the Construction of the Individual: A Social Study of Social Science*. Routledge: London.

O'Grady H. 2005. *Woman's Relationship with Herself – Gender, Foucault and Therapy*. Routledge: London.

Orange D.M. 2011. *The Suffering Stranger: Hermeneutics for Everyday Clinical Practice*. Routledge: New York.

Ortega F. 2014. *Corporeality, Medical Technologies and Contemporary Culture*. Taylor & Francis: London.

Pearce J. 2008. Narratives for reflexivity: Understanding the professional self. *Creative Approaches to Research;* 1(2):45–54.

Petersen A., Lupton D. 2000. *The New Public Health – Health and Self in the Age of Risk*. Sage Publications: London.

Peddiwell J.A. 2004. *The Saber – Tooth Curriculum. The Classic Edition*. The MacGraw-Hill Companies: New York.

Rabinow P. (Ed.). 1984. *The Foucault Reader*. Pantheon Books: New York

Ricoeur P. 1992. *Oneself as Another*. University of Chicago: Chicago. Translated by K. Blamey.

Riggs D.W. 2004. Challenging the monoculturalism of psychology: Towards a more socially accountable pedagogy and practice. *Australian Psychologist;* 39(2):118–126.

Rose N. 1998. *Inventing Our Selves: Psychology, Power, and Personhood*. Cambridge University Press: Cambridge.

Scarry E. 1985. *The Body in Pain: The Making and Unmaking of the World*. Oxford University Press: Oxford.

Sewell W.H. 1992. A theory of structure: duality, agency and transformation. *American Journal of Sociology*. 98(1):1–29.

Sharpe C. 2016. *In the Wake: On Blackness and Being*. Duke University Press: Durham.

Singleton J. 2015. *Cultural Melancholy: Readings of Race, Impossible Mourning, and African American Ritual*. University of Illinois Press: Illinois.

Sontag S. 1991. *Illness as Metaphor & AIDS and Its Metaphors*. Penguin Modern Classics: London.

Venn C. 2002. Refiguring subjectivity after modernity. Chapter 4 in *Challenging Subjects: Critical Psychology for a New Millenium*. Walkerdine V. (ed). Palgrave: Hampshire.

Taylor C. 1989. *Sources of the Self: The Making of Modern Identity*. Cambridge University Press: Cambridge.

Titchen A., Higgs J. 2001. A dynamic framework for the enhancement of health professional practice in an uncertain world: the practice-knowledge interface. Chapter 28 in Practice Knowledge and Expertise in the Health Professions. Butterworth Heinmann: Oxford.

Tolstoy L. 1987. *A Confession and Other Religious Writings*. Penguin Classics: London.

Usher P. 2000. Feminist approaches to a situated ethics. Chapter 3 in Simons H., Usher R. 2000. *Situated Ethics in Educational Research*. Routledge-Falmer: London, pp. 22–38.

Usher R., Bryant I., Johnston R. 1997. *Adult Education and the Postmodern Challenge – Learning Beyond the Limits*. Routledge: London.

Walkerdine V. 1992. Progressive Pedagogy and Political Struggle. Chapter 2 in *Feminisms and Critical Pedagogy*. Luke C., Gore J.M. (eds). Routledge: New York.

Walsh D., McCartney G., Collins C., Taulbut M., Batty G.D. 2016. History, politics and vulnerability: Explaining excess mortality. Glasgow Centre for Population Health.

Williams L. 2002. *In Search of Profession – A Sociology of Allied Health in Second Opinion – An Introduction to Health Sociology*. Germov J. (ed). Oxford University Press: Oxford.

Wilkinson I. 2005. *Suffering: A Sociological Introduction*. Polity Press: Cambridge.

Wilson E.O. 1998. *Consilience: The Unity of Knowledge*. Abacus: London.

6 Pilgrimages – how can medical humanities think differently about suffering?

6.1 Introduction

Without affirming the reality of suffering as a valid part of life and our experience, it can seem as if we are living a fiction. bell hooks describes the feeling of relief and release when the reality of her experience is affirmed; that is, it was the act of living the fiction that produced the anguish.

> And at that moment of her acknowledging the truth of what I had experienced was such a relief! The moment she affirmed the reality of what had taken place, I was *released*, because somehow what we all know in our wounded childhood experiences ...: it's the act of *living the fiction* that produces the torturous angst and the anguish ... the feeling that you're mind-fucked.... I love it when that moment of truth – breaking through denial and reentering one's true reality – becomes the hopeful moment, the promise: when we can know ourselves and not live this life of running in flight from reality.
>
> (bell hooks, 1994; p. 267)

Likewise, the aim of this chapter is to affirm the reality of suffering as part of the usual lived experience of health professionals and patients in order not to perpetuate the anguish of denial. Medical humanities has a role in bringing to the table discussions about suffering and thereby to develop in conjunction with sociology a theory of suffering in healthcare organisations that will promote appropriate responses to both health workers and patients. Previously, in the exploration on instrumentalist sources of self, health workers demonstrated a shut down, disembodiment and a fusion between self and role in response to overwhelming work environments and not knowing how to deal with suffering. There were few discussions about suffering although it was perceived to be all around them. There was also a sense of wanting a return, a recognition and reflection back of the circumstances which an instrumentalist approach to healthcare was not able to provide.

So how can medical humanities help us to think differently about suffering? Core to the answer to this question are issues to do with what we consider to be a concept of self, a category of a person and the other to that self. The intersubjective space – what happens in between health professionals and patient – is important to consider as are the modes of communication. There are issues concerned with the body as noted in the previous chapter: what happens when suffering is not responded to, or responded to in a way that denies suffering as a core human experience. The development of a so-called false sense of self gets constructed in a void of response from mainstream society. We need to think differently and for that we need different tools to traverse the void, the lacunae in our lives, in order to not prolong suffering unnecessarily or at least move from unbearable to bearable suffering. Suffering is not talked about enough by health professionals; there is an avoidance as evidenced by all the mainstream approaches to health and well-being, essentially creating a silence around suffering by aiming to make the suffering self something other than it is.

In order to start thinking differently about how we think about suffering, there are a number of assumptions that must be made explicit. One new radical assumption suggested at the end of the last chapter is that the suffering self IS the self; it is not an aberration of human nature. Suffering is who we are just as much as joy, anxiety, equanimity. How could it be otherwise given the amount of suffering in the world, over the entirety of the human existence?

> While I certainly did not wish to suffer, suffering was also the embodied reality, the truth, of my situation. Some part of my integrity was to suffer; not to have suffered would have been to fail to experience myself fully in the situation I was in.
>
> (Frank, 2001; p. 359)

Another assumption is that we have forgotten how to be with suffering. That the fear of encountering our suffering is the fear of opening a Pandora's box and not being able to shut the lid on it again. Part of the anguish for health professionals when encountering suffering is the feeling of not knowing what to say or do, and this not knowing can be experienced as overwhelming, leading to an abrupt end to conversations or a regression to roles and scripts as the only way of knowing what to say. As health professionals encounter suffering continually at work, there must be a way to negotiate a passage through suffering without shutting it down or disconnecting. These latter strategies only serve to intensify the experience of suffering as there is a refusal that obstructs any further progress.

In addition, the avoidance and denial of suffering caused by mainstream policies, institutional curricula that do not even mention suffering alongside cultural ideals of what it is to be a human being and a health professional, produce a form of ghosting and living in a kind of fiction, which in itself forms an anguish beyond the realms of bearable suffering. This is the sort of thing that Frank (2001) is talking about when he does not want to be made into an object and when he advocates for a recognition of suffering in research:

I feared professionals who were unable to encounter suffering as the hole – the unspeakable and perhaps the incomprehensible – in what they could say and do. I feared them seeking to explain me as an object of suffering, rather than remaining silent in the face of what they could not speak.

(Frank, 2001; p. 359)

What is at stake in these questions is whether qualitative research can enhance a recognition of suffering in society or whether — research becomes, however unconsciously, an organizing practice through which medicine and society can avoid recognizing suffering.

(Frank, 2001; p. 356)

Avoidance or treating people who are suffering as objects is a form of symbolic violence. No wonder in these instances the sufferer withdraws from a lack of being able to trust mainstream society and a languishing in place of an agency (Devisch et al., 2017).

Agency can be built on a false predication of what a concept of self is. The way we think differently about suffering has to address the epistemic break at the level of embodied symbolic cognition in order to be able to even begin to hope that there could be a change. By adhering to old notions of self, censored suffering increases and crystallises:

And because, to be a good medical treatment citizen, I have to pretend I share the premises of the system, my censored suffering "crystallizes into a gigantic fund of anxiety," just as Baudrillard (1998) aptly described it. That compounding of suffering is what I dreaded.

(Frank, 2001; p. 361)

As demonstrated in chapter four, health professionals are committed to a particular view of the self, a particular fiction that enables them to continue to do the work they do. And yet this view of self may ultimately be detrimental for their own health and well-being when what they experience does not fit that system of analysis.

It is that system of analysis that is so damaging to the person who suffers, be they a health professional or patient. How we conceptualise, categorise and schematise people within the biomedical model is necessary to carry out the difficult work that people have to do and it is also a source of alienation and suffering:

But I suffered at the prospect of what I could call going back into it. I suffered at having to submit my suffering to medical workers for whom I was another instance of a category requiring that this and that be done. In treatment, I knew I would become a task that workers would have to address as one of a series of tasks that were part of a working day. I would be something else to get done. Being treated that way is

> tolerable when I do my banking or get my driver's license renewed;
> I expect to be treated that way. But to be treated that way when I am
> suffering turns my suffering into one of the things that do not fit.
>
> (Frank, 2001; p. 361)

Why is this way of being treated so prevalent? How does this fit into the overall scheme of suffering? Barad (2007) states that it is not possible to elucidate intentionality and that we cannot know all our thoughts afore-thought. Therefore, assuming that health professionals are not being in-tentionally mean or cruel, what else could be operating? Suffering itself and its avoidance is in operation. By focusing on a technical rational curri-culum, a to do list, where each step is focused on to minute detail, is a way of making it across the abyss of suffering. Staying at a fairly shallow level of analysis is a survival technique for healthcare workers. But this also puts the professional at peril since to go through that one-way looking glass is also to submit to a training that makes the probability of mental ill-health more likely (Sinclair, 1997).

What this means is that students and clinicians come up against situa-tions and patients where they do not have the words themselves to navigate their way through particularly in relation to interpersonal issues of suf-fering. For example, a medical student was telling me recently of an ex-perience with a patient where she had come away thinking, "What right do I have to say he will be OK? What if he isn't? He may die," after she had responded with reassurance in order to attend to his distress. She felt mortified that she had breached a level of trust by wanting to reassure him with what she felt was perhaps a premature gesture *but didn't know what else to do.* She questioned by what authority she had the right to say these things and by what right the patient believed her. "Who am I to be in this room?" She seemed to feel as if there was some sort of fiction going on at some level and yet didn't know how to articulate this initially let alone even manage it. But the student had hit on a very important aspect of clinical practice. The conflict that can occur between the clinical sense of profes-sional self and the personal sense of self that picks up on distress and doesn't know what to do. Coming back to bell hooks: "it's the act of *living the fiction* that produces the torturous angst and the anguish" (1994; p. 267). This is where the epistemic break can occur.

Part of the break that can be so damaging to health professionals is the awareness of confronting an ethical dilemma and not having the tools to process this (beyond the four pillars of non-maleficence, beneficence, justice and autonomy) as a process of self formation. That this living the fiction is a particular form of damage that occurs in medical school and beyond. At the moment of an anguished fusion of self and role during such a dilemma, the self is exposed. What this means, to return to the example in the preface, is that as a health professional with a legitimated role to carry out with a pa-tient, I experienced suffering alongside the patient, in knowing how to be a human as well as a professional, in order to attend to her suffering, with the latter constraining the former. That in part of that exchange, the self as knower was present in both of us and, at some level, beyond individual roles, can see through those roles to the humanity of the situation. This knowing through suffering must be acknowledged and honoured and is a vital connection that mediates any disengaged instrumentalist knowledge. This is the substrate that provides traction for the technical rationalist approach.

Therefore, this chapter explores the ethical dilemma of humanity versus professional self, in the idea of romantic expressivist source of self, through the art of connecting up what tends to be erased in circumstances described above. That is, in the heat of the clinical encounter when health professionals feel like they don't know how to respond, what to say or do, how much to share, or that they feel like they are being false somehow by sticking to professional guidelines, there can be a fusion between self and role that can be erased because people tend not to talk about this. The moral anguish exposes the self but then becomes erased and then the hidden anxiety and suffering around this goes underground or perceived as other. Cognitive dissonance produces identity dissonance. This notion is explored here through the epistemological constructs of self, pilgrimage as an act of embodied cognition drawing on literature as well as the film *Rabbit Proof Fence* and finally through pedagogies of encounter that encourage the exploration of affect in teaching and learning (Mahendran, 2020). The chapter then goes on to discuss some of the common forms of epistemic breaks constituting health professional and patient suffering such as PTSD, depersonalisation and burnout. Finally, the chapter picks up the thread of wandering lines again to explore different ways of thinking about these, drawing on concepts from medical humanities such as Rilke's inseeing, art as an idiom and expression of self, mythopoetic curriculum, Nietzsche's call to danger, Soldjer's call for a pedagogy of acrobatics and Bauchelard's poetics of space in acts of restoration of the suffering self. In terms of the suffering self, the ethical encounter (Butler, 2005) is of most importance, so that will be the focus on in this chapter.

6.2 Mapping the landscape of learning (epistemological constructs of self) by including the Black Anthropocene

This section explores the different sources of self in relation to the romantic expressivism ideas in the context of the Black Anthropocene. That is, whilst acknowledging the importance of the romantic expressivism as a source of self in healthcare practice in order to be able to deal with the moments of anguish of knowing what to say in the face of suffering, there is always a context in which this expressivism takes place, that of the Black Anthropocene (Yusoff, 2018). This will hopefully deal with the contested ideas about the essence of inwardness in relation to the other. The contested ideas of self are relevant here because some theorists locate the self as an expression of inwardness, of art as an expression of self, whilst others see the expressivism as occurring in an intersubjective space which necessarily includes the idea of the other, whilst others see the psyche itself as occurring intersubjectively and that there is no such thing as an individual self or psyche (Winnicott, 1954). These are difficult matters to contemplate, yet they are vital in addressing suffering as occurring in part between healthcare professionals and patients as well as an embodied experience. Understanding this means that a link is formed between the individual and social through an appreciation of the moral nature of suffering.

6.2.1 *The romantic expressivist source of self*

There are sources and ideas of the self as discussed in Chapter Four; theistic, instrumental and romantic expressivism as proposed by Taylor (1989). This section focus on ideas about the self from a romantic expressivism perspective, with reference to the arts, as experience of the self. The ideas about the self and the experience of the self do not always match because of the epistemic break in what is seen as real and knowable. This is particularly the case when thinking of a decontextualised self. That is, a self can be seen as a monolithic idea that is abstracted from context, according to white colonialist thinking, which has important consequences for those seen as outside the colonialist project of self. Those outside the colonialist project of self are seen as others and they constitute the boundaries of experience of what is seen and knowable, as eloquently described by Sharpe (2016). If we know that blackness constitutes the outside and that the very notion of justice produces and requires black exclusion and death as normative (Sharpe, 2016), then we have a moral ethical duty to consider this in ideas about the expressivism of self and how this is perpetuated by the epistemic break.

The epistemic break feeds the instrumentalist sources of self that are seen as belonging to a fragmented and disconnected social world (Taylor, 1989). The understanding of the different sources and concepts of self is important because the ideas connect to moral sources and notions of inwardness. The process by which a self is formed is seen to be through the continual "search for moral sources *outside* the subject through the language which resonates *within* him or her" – an order linked to a personal vision (Taylor, 1989; p. 510). Therefore, the personal vision looks for resonance in the outside worlds by means of God (theistic), rational (instrumental) or nature (romantic expressivism). Nature is seen as a source of self and moral good in the world.

Thus for the example above, where a medical student described her moral anguish about not knowing what to say in the clinical situation, she is inherently looking for a source of understanding, a source of self beyond the technical-rationalist instrumental curriculum. When she asks, "Who am I to be in this room?" she is directly appealing for a source of self that is linked to a personal vision of moral worth that is also connected to the social world – to be in this room. Part of her dilemma, the moral anguish, is through experiencing an epistemic break between her concept of self provided through her role and between that as a human, what she is experiencing. The disconnect is apparent in what she sees in her response to the patient – what she is able to provide based on her professional knowledge – and what she knows as a human with her understanding of the unknowability, or uncertainty, in the situation.

The disconnect is between the reflection back to herself through the patient's view and requirements of her to perform, and what she knows in herself. In her mind, her language does not seem to resonate with a personal vision of herself because this personal vision, perhaps of knowing certainty of patients' outcomes, perhaps provided through professional expectations, is not true for her. Thus a moral conflict arises of a self that falls through the lines of professional conduct. She shows courage in being able to see and acknowledge this break in epistemology and by being able to discuss this rather than dismiss it as unimportant and moving on. And in fact, by engaging with this matter, she is developing a self that arises out of her ethical stance (Butler, 2005). The important point is to see these sorts of occurrences as an epistemology of sorts, or an epiphany, that involve recovering contact with a moral source. These sorts of epistemological movements have not always been available as when the self was completely identified with the social role one occupied.

For example, Hollis (1996) draws on the example of Antigone who buries her brother despite her uncle's edicts not to. She ends up being entombed by her uncle's orders in a cave and dies there. What Hollis (1996) perceives is the moral anguish she suffered in her role as a citizen (and niece of the ruler) and that as a sister of a beloved brother. During this moral struggle, her self was exposed through being trapped in conflicting demands and roles. The fusion of the identity and role in the Greek tragedy offers a "category" of self that secures a precarious space between social factors and innerworld, with neither extreme seen as the ultimate reality (Hollis, 1996). That is, Antigone is doomed *because* of her category of a self as sister and niece citizen with no other recourse to make a decision. Her social self is her self which is what dooms her. The precarious space is secured by our epistemological process of conceptualizing, categorizing, symbolizing, imagining, abstracting, synthesizing and differentiating. These processes of the self act as anchors in our perception and interpretation of the world:

> Concept of what a person is forces at most a distinction between core and penumbra and a well-chosen core can be ambiguously policed forever by pointing out the hermeneutic options involved in mapping terms in one language onto those of another.
>
> (Hollis, 1996; p. 232)

These hermeneutic options and self-policing are in contrast to Antigone, who Hollis (1996) believes chooses the path which dooms her, not as an individual consciously processing options (a modern self distinct from both roles who must choose), but as a person who *is* her mask as a citizen and a sister. The question is whether health professional training continues to produce model Antigones who are not able to navigate successfully between professional and personal selves and thereby who continue to objectivise patients' suffering, as they are not able to attend to their own suffering, let alone anyone else's. For health professionals to know they are more than their mask, just as patients are more than their illness, is to go beyond shallow interpretations by having an epistemological process to follow.

Having an epistemological process to follow seems to be along the lines of de Certeau's (1984) efficacious meanderings along wandering lines in order for health professionals to retrieve from institutions what perhaps has gone underground, like Antigone into her cave. Institutions thrive on roles and responsibilities, boundaries, tasks, hierarchies and an occupation of space. De Certeau (1984) in a poetics of making do suggests that we can retrieve ourselves from within these spaces, but there are no specific suggestions on what might be at stake. The efficacious meanderings by silent discoverers means finding what works in the moment by a particular form of consciousness and may be how medical humanities can contribute to thinking differently about thinking about suffering. In contrast, Taylor (1989) suggests that moments of awareness that break through our usual consciousness are opportunities for transformation, and this could be where medical humanities has a role to play in developing resources for addressing suffering.

Taylor (1989) suggests that these moments of awareness are connected to an inwardness, a transfiguration matched with inner depths, in romantic expressivism. They are key to great moral or spiritual significance, "to a certain depth, or fullness, or seriousness, or intensity of life, or to a certain wholeness" (Taylor, 1989; p. 422). The form of the art, or awareness in this instance, designates the moral drive and cannot be separated out from issues of social justice. The social world triggers an inwardness – the two are relational. To his mind, the self is in a social world that itself manifests an acting out of polarities between axes of good and evil, in a spiral form of moral evolution (Taylor, 1989). That is, social movements are constantly moving between one polarity or the other, creating a spiral, in which the self occupies a precarious space. The inwardness, or inner self, is a response to and a resource against these social forces.

The inwardness is also connected to the natural world as a source of self and goodness, a deep source waiting to be tapped into, a source which is an inner impulse of nature. Taylor (1989) sees the return to the goodness of nature as a way of making something out of the nothing of instrumentalist sources (the place of logos) of self, a way of connecting, reconciliation and redemption. Art is thus a way of escaping degradation and fragmentation through creative imagination and a much richer conception of nature which has an inner dimension. However, there are disagreements with the ideas of romantic expressivism as a source of self, and many poststructuralists take issue with the idea of an inner essence as somehow reifying or reinforcing oppressive categories of a person.

These ideas may have been presented as if they represent an un-complicated reality and a straightforward translation between the in-dividual and the social. However, whilst this understanding is not the case, there are lacunae in the way that romantic expressivism is presented without due consideration of the structural forces at play and how they influence any relationship with the inwardness as demonstrated by Singleton (2015). Taylor (1989) is keen to point out conflict and incon-sistencies between ideas. In fact, he seems to suggest that the artist occupies a marginalised, more liminal space, in relation to society:

> What is revealed lies beyond and against what we normally understand as morality. The artist is an exceptional being, open to rare vision; the poet is a person of exceptional sensibility. ... But this also opens the artist to exceptional suffering. ... [F]orces him or her to forgo the ordinary satisfactions of life, to forgo successful action and fulfilled relationships.
>
> (Taylor, 1989; p. 423)

He cites D.H. Lawrence as describing the call of the artist into "the cru-cifixion into isolate individuality" (p. 423). While on the one hand Taylor (1989) is referring to a going beyond social norms through exceptional suffering, on the other hand he is reinforcing the idea of the autonomous individual albeit within a state of precarity and increased vulnerability.

Fareld (2012) takes Taylor to task for this point, for failing to fully ex-plicate ideas on vulnerability and suffering. She suggests that a return to oneself, in the inwardness, is less an act of appropriation but more as an experience of losing a part of the self in order to attain a self-relation:

> Returning to self is thus a double movement where self-consciousness is attained at the price of 'abdicating' from the position as self-sufficient and sovereign. Rather than being affirmed by others, the act of recognition is about negating oneself, as only through a self-negation does one enter the realm of intersubjectivity (which is the only access point to oneself). Hence, the self appears to itself only at the cost of renouncing the claims to sovereign self-determination.
>
> (Fareld, 2012; p. 129–130)

The recognition of the self, in her view, is about recognising the vulner-ability, suffering and fallibility of being human. Denial of this recognition of vulnerability and suffering in self and other, in service of autonomy, is denial of one's self. Recognition entails a dispossession then of the sovereign autonomous self and an affirmation of the suffering self.

Fareld's (2012) focus on the intersubjective space as the place where the self manifests, or is exposed, is a particular interpretation of Taylor (1989).

This interpretation sees the face as always being turned to others and as being put outside ourselves as well as being vulnerable to others. In an echo of Winnicott (1954), who believed that the mind-psyche was localised by the individual and placed either inside the head or outside the head (because the head could not be seen by oneself and so was not believed to exist as part of oneself) but was rooted in a need for a perfect environment, Fareld (2012) highlights the primacy of the intersubjective space:

> This means that the dialectical relation between myself and the other, which makes me exposed, is not to be understood as a movement where something inner is externalized and shattered in my encounter with the other, but rather as manifesting that this unity which is 'I' is always already lost to me, as a precondition for my self-relation
>
> (Fareld, 2012; p. 131).

Thus to be an "I" means to not be fully apparent or accessible to oneself. Fareld (2012) quotes Nancy: "Self is what *does not find itself*" as it remains exposed (Nancy [1997] 2002; p. 56). The precarity of this position makes any fixed identity position impossible to maintain; dialectic is the movement that persistently undermines fixed categories and binary structures, thereby making a return impossible, and why such an attempt at return apparently has to be repeated again and again, paradoxically making us into ourselves. The apparent/seeming failure of the restoring self-unifying movement is a pre-condition for the development of self.

What this means, in the example given above, is that the medical student experiences a loss of self and vulnerability in responding to suffering, but the loss of self is more in the way of loss of sovereignty and autonomy of self, that is, the normative ideal of self. In a double loop of reflexivity, Fareld (2012) identifies that the self which does not find itself (the normative autonomous idealised self) in the intersubjective space, is what constitutes the self. Self-making involves working again at the limits of experience and particularly in the context of suffering. The precarity of this self, in the liminal space at the edge of experience and in the intersubjective space, between the social and the individual, feels insecure and untethered, yet it is the connection between the individual and the other, between them and their environment, beyond normative ideals of what it is to be a self. The discomfort apparent in this perception of the self goes against perhaps more solid instrumentalist ideas of the self. Perhaps this is why people sense a retreat or return into the self is required as a way of escaping the discomfort and precarity.

Taylor (1989) seems to argue that in encounters with and sensitivity to suffering, a person has inwardness, connection with nature and a source of self to turn to, an inexhaustible deep source of self waiting to be tapped, which is an inner impulse of nature. This implies a source of stability amongst intersubjective repetitions of return where the self does not find itself and is displaced. Moreover, if we consider the self-as-knower (Damasio, 2010) (Section 5.5) the experience of subjectivity, liminality, precarity and vulnerability is the feeling of what happens in a relation, and this all happens to a dynamic collection of mental processes, the imaginarium of the mind-self-body-brain. Damasio (2010) suggests that if no self is generated, images are still there but no-one knows of their existence. Clearly, in an imaginarium, there is still a self that is aware of the existence of the self that exists or is lost in the return to self, but the two are not mutually exclusive as Fareld (2012) seems to suggest. Confusing, yes, but not exclusive.

The struggle between self and other is perhaps exemplified by Rilke who was acutely sensitive to the world inner space and the yearning for internalizing (Corbett, 2016). Rilke's relationship with Rodin, a sculptor, produced creativity and exploration of questions of the self and life. For example, in reference to a statue of Apollo, what some may see as a sleeping stone, Rilke related to it as a mirror on which to project his inner life and out of the absences of a broken anonymous statue, crafted an experience of the world as a poem: "for here there is no place that does not see you. You must change your life" (Rilke cited by Corbett, 2016; p. 211). The empathic union of poet and statue, of object and beholder, author and reader created a consciousness of art, a communicative medium. The consciousness or awareness was likened to a window; the eyes, a frame of vision or a measurement of expectation (Corbett, 2016).

The idea of windows is related to the in-between space of the world, between nature and the individual, or between the social and the individual. Rilke coined the term *Weltinnenraum* or "worldinnerspace":

> to describe the space where the barriers between the internal and external collapsed onto a single plane. It is a realm where the self is like a bird flying soundlessly between the sky and the soul, he said. Rilke accepts the concept as both a contradiction and a reality in a poem titled "Worldinnerspace": "... O, wanting to grow, / I look out, and the tree grows *in* me," he writes.
>
> This in-between realm was the only place Rilke understood as home, the space where all things came to settle at last. For him, the house was a container and he was the air slipping out its windows; the cat running away at night. He was a ghost and a myth.
>
> (Corbett, 2016; pp. 260–261).

Having mastered the art of inseeing which meant the penetration of the interior world of objects and animals with his mind, he could also use this strategy in reverse to defend himself by stretching his contours, to fully outline himself and thereby imagine strengthening his body's borders. Rilke demonstrates the consciousness of inner and outer awareness as well as the interplay between and what that experience was like. The relationship between drawing an observer out into the world, whilst the observer also draws the work or object back into his or her body was one of mutual co-creation as well as empathy and potential loss of self.

The relationship between art and empathy has been explored and is one of the premises upon which medical humanities interventions are based. Empathy was believed to be of four types and a way of freeing an individual from the solitude of the mind:

1   General apperceptive empathy – when one sees movement in everyday objects;
2   Empirical empathy – when one sees human qualities in the non-human;
3   Mood empathy – when one attributes emotional states to colours and music; and
4   Sensible appearance empathy – when gestures or movements convey internal feelings (Corbett, 2016; p. 100).

The two-way gaze tethers lives together and fulfils the beholders involvement. The *einfühlung* "feeling into" was both a bodily and emotional form of resonance, of tuning in to forms, and an act of lived recognition. The act of recognition is about negating oneself, a drawing into and out of, attribution of perception, reassembling of perceptual fragments in a vast empty space, somewhere between the lines, as a person who might experience them but only through a self-negation in order to enter the realm of intersubjectivity. This movement itself was art functioning as an articulation of the self. There was structure out of an impulse, a piece of ground on which one could stand and not lose one's self, through a window or portal that also implied precarity and vulnerability.

From a sociological perspective, the movement between empathy and abstraction in art, and the point on the spectrum between these two poles where society was located, was a reflection of the psychological health of the society that produced it (Corbett, 2016). Worringer (1997) proposed that the objectified sense of delight in self experienced through representational forms of art was a manifestation of identifying with the object as a source of beauty and goodness and an innate sense of confidence in the world as it is. This identifying with was in fact a form of empathy through which persons could source self *as long as* the identification was within mainstream practices of self. Anything outside that was treated as other. In contrast, during times of social turmoil, the urge to abstraction in art, the decontextualisation of the object, was a reflection and expression of man's insecurities. Therefore, the notion of medical objectification of the human, as an abstraction from their context was in some sense a sign of confidence in the representation, interpretation and classification of the human as an episteme, as a way of knowing. However, this dialectical relationship with both object and abstract, as a form of mobius strip, was foundational on notions of recognition and return between redemption, spirit and soul.

Worringer (1997) relates various insecure states of man to the value of art for inner psychic exaltation.

> Since for us the whole of art's capacity for bestowing happiness is comprised in the possibility it provides us of creating an ideal theatre for our inner experience, in which the vital forces of our organic vitality, transferred onto the work of art by means of empathy, are able to live themselves out uninhibitedly. (p. 132)

The abstraction was to produce an absolute, a world beyond appearance, "in which it may rest from the agony of the relative" (p. 133). Redemption was gained through silencing deceptions of appearance, gaining possession of things through identification with them when animated and transfigured, through transcendental feelings, that produced a "glorification of that relation of interdependence between man and outer world, the consciousness of which had given rise precisely to the transcendental humour of the soul" (p. 133). Thus, even though an abstraction may appear as cold and humourless, it is in fact a desire for redemption through identification with the object. Moreover, this reversal is a reflection of insecurity, where the imagination required soothing. The abstract forms were seen to be the highest form in which humans can rest from the confusion of the world (Worringer, 1997). The soothing required for the confusion was a return to the abstract orderly mathematical forms in the turmoil of chaotic lives (Worringer, 1997). This was in contrast to the representational form of art which had dimension and depth, as reflections of a blissful reality where beauty was identified with beauty of self (Corbett, 2016). Therefore art was a reflection of the dynamics of society in which it is situated.

From the above, it can be seen that romantic expressivism as a source of self is tied up with notions of recognition, inseeing, feeling into, empathy, worldinnerspace, the space between the social and the individual, precarity, vulnerability, suffering, identification with as well as abstraction, reassembling perceptual fragments in a vast empty space, liminality and discomfort through a perception of self-negation. There is one last piece of the puzzle to stitch into place for this section. Acknowledgment must be made of the will to power over the self as the constant overcoming of self in order to control "inherent differential energetics of the existence that works hard on itself" (Sloterdijk, 2013; p. 65). This pedagogy of acrobatics comprised a tension between immanence and transcendence with works on the self and constant vigilance of the source of the self which combines theistic and instrumentalist sources of self, embedded in a romantic expressivism.

In a pedagogy of acrobatics, the elementary facts of life were being covered up "by trivial moralities, humane chumminess and wellness programmes" (Sloterdijk, 2013). Both Nietzsche and Kafka were working towards the same cause of identifying that the rope for acrobatics was the path of humanisation, of socialisation, fraught with danger and caught between two poles of immanence and transcendence. Acrobats were "practised in the art of crossing the abyss of the 'sensual world' [*Sinnenwelt*] with the balancing pole of asceticism" (p. 64). The metaphor of the rope in acrobatism only works if it is under tension, has anchors and modalities of power transfer, and therefore attention must be paid to these. The tension was supplied by a pull from above, from the metaphysical intentions and constant vigilance in order not to fall. In *Thus Spoke Zarathustra*, Nietzsche writes, "You have made danger your calling: there is nothing in that to despise." These ideas work in well with precarity and walking over the abyss that seem to arise from not knowing what to say or how to respond to suffering. In order to explore these ideas of sources of self, and precarity within that, a film is now drawn upon to show how self and other are related through categories of self enacted through colonialism.

6.2.2 *Rabbit Proof Fence*

The film *Rabbit Proof Fence* (Noyce, 2002) is used as a background for exploration of instrumentalist categories of person and how these relate to romantic expressivism sources of the self as described above – precarity, inseeing, worldinnerspace, pedagogy of acrobatics, vulnerability and suffering. This is being done in order to demonstrate the impact on Indigenous peoples' health and how health professionals have struggled to speak to their suffering as shown in the last chapter. These issues are important because they directly effect the relationship between health professional and patient and are perhaps most stark when there is a focus on health promotion in the face of enormous suffering, to the detriment of understanding the history and impact of colonialism. The disconnect here in health professional practice is longstanding and reminiscent of the roles played by religious and governmental authorities in the original early days of colonialism. In the search for recognition, roles may be re-enacted with subsequent moral anguish about knowing what to say and how to be unless awareness is brought to these interactions. Medical humanities has a role to play in promoting understanding and resistance to colonialist practices by learning to think differently about these types of suffering which are based on displacement and acrobatic existentialism. Medical humanities seems to be the ideal place to think beyond healthy lifestyle behaviours, or humane chumminess, to understand more about why people do or don't do the things they do, why some people continue to answer the call to danger and how we are all hungry ghosts at the threshold of experiences of our lives. That perhaps these ethical ruptures are glitches in the mainstream matrix, a rent in the veil, in order for us to be more aware. By not attending to suffering we become abstracted from our own lives and those around us; we become hungry ghosts living on the edge of our experiences.

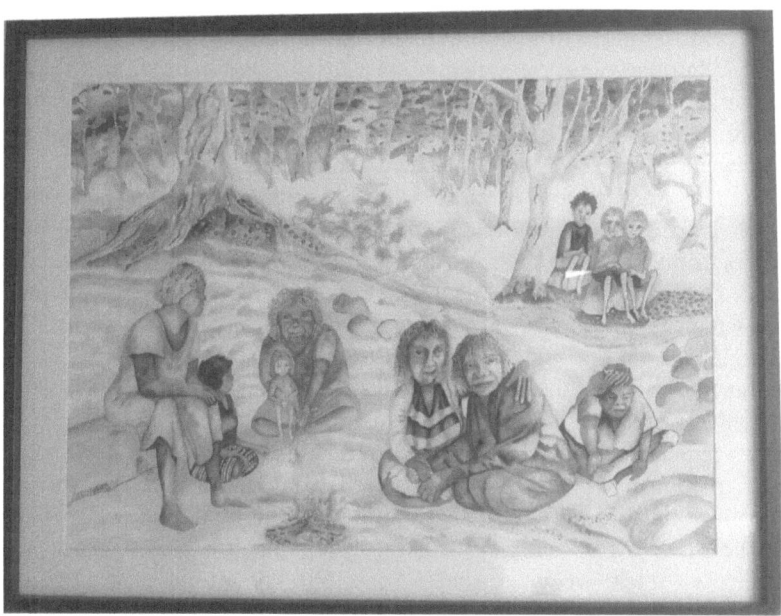

Figure 6.1 Clearing in the woods.

Rabbit Proof Fence, along with my experiences in Australia, was the inspiration for the painting providing the structure for this chapter (Figure 6.1). The painting shows a group of indigenous women sitting around a fire, in a dry creek bed, in a clearing in the bush. The sands form lines around them dappled by the sunlight filtering through the trees. *Rabbit Proof Fence* is a film about a young girl, Molly, and her family and how they survive the imposition of white policy of removal of children and incarceration in British institutions during white colonialist rule in Western Australia in the 1930s (Pendreigh, 2003). This is a true story of Molly, Daisy and their cousin Gracie's violent removal from their mothers at the Jigalong camp in the northern Western Australia, to placement in an institution in Moore River Native Settlement as it was then known, and their subsequent walk back following the Rabbit Proof Fence, a journey of approximately 1500 miles which took nine weeks, over some of the harshest terrain in the world. It is a story of immense suffering which still reverberates in current Australian life (Commonwealth of Australia, 1997).

The events were founded on British categories of a person; categories were by colour which was determined by the chief Protector of Aborigines Mr Neville. According to his system of categorisation, children and adults were sent to various domestic occupations according to their colour, which he believed determined their intelligence. The lighter colour persons were deemed to be, the more intelligence they were assumed to have, since they were seen as more like white people than different from them. This campaign of terror was designed to assimilate Aboriginal people into white culture, losing their families, culture, language, pride, land and heritage in the process, with a view to complete assimilation and elimination in the long run: "Are we going to have a population of one million blacks in the Commonwealth, or are we going to merge them into our white community and eventually forget there ever were any Aborigines in Australia" spoke Neville in 1937 (Martin, 2014). He also spoke of saving Aboriginals from themselves as he was their chief protector and undertook all decisions about their lives from the purchase of new shoes, giving approval or not for marriage, to what they could wear, live and eat. This policy continued until 1970, even after Aboriginal people were finally given the vote in 1967. Thousands of children were abducted from their families becoming what is known as the Stolen Generation (Commonwealth of Australia, 1997).

Molly's tenacity and determination to return home takes her across vast distances of inhospitable land where she relies on her instincts and knowledge of that landscape to survive. She sees into the land – inseeing – and people she meets along the way, trusting her ability to discern, track and cover her own tracks of where they'd been. She knew how to walk in the river so their footsteps could not be tracked, to lay decoys, how to use the weather to her advantage. She follows the Rabbit Proof Fence, which connects her to her mother, who meanwhile keeps a vigil at her end, tapping the wire to send messages to her daughter, calling her home. Molly is exhausted, starving and often stumbles as she carries Daisy across the salt pan. The lowest point is when they both collapse on a vast dried out salt lake, a lacunae, unable to go any further. To all appearances, they have lost and are about to die. The cry of an eagle brings her to – her mother had told her to keep an eye on the eagle as it would always look after her. The girls slowly rise and Molly sees the longed for hills – "home." Meanwhile her mother senses she is near and wards off the approach of a police officer on the lookout for the children. The family are reunited and disappear to live in the desert. However, the story does not end there, sadly. There are repeat institutionalisations as Molly and then her children are not able to escape the authorities. Molly walks the length of the Rabbit Proof Fence again with her young daughter Annabelle. She loses both her daughters to the authorities.

> For individuals, their removal as children and the abuse they experienced at the hands of the authorities or their delegates have permanently scarred their lives. The harm continues in later generations, affecting their children and grandchildren.
>
> (Commonwealth of Australia, 1997; p. 4)

The categories of person were used to separate and displace families and then abuse them. This is a familiar governmental approach to children from poor and deprived families in the UK, too:

Many were subjected to crimes; torture, rape and slavery.... From their evidence, a number of common themes emerge. They and their families were lied to, many parents were told that their children had been adopted by loving families, some children were told their parents were dead. Some have learnt after years of searching for their records that their parents tried to get them back. One foster mother campaigned to have her foster daughter returned to her from Australia.

(Laville, 2017)

Home Children was a child migration scheme founded in 1869 and under which more than 100,000 children were sent to the colonies from the UK. The Forgotten Children (Hill, 2008) were the subject of a recent film *Oranges and Sunshine* (Loach, 2011) which portrays the attempts to reunite families across a cultural, emotional and geographical divide.

However, the reuniting of families was not always possible – the return was not possible. And in this way, the survivors may have been doomed to repetitious acts in order to recognise themselves in the absence of any family or connectedness. Through the displacement and loss, people were forced to rely on their instincts to survive. This took them to places beyond the social order, beyond themselves as categories to a more precarious existence. The abstraction of people and children from their contexts was a sign of the unhealthiness of society at the time, so it is no wonder that these people took on the behaviours of the way society treated them and became marginalised in their own existence.

In addition, the forced African migration of slavery (Sharpe, 2016) and ongoing settler colonialism have been ending worlds for as long as they have been in existence (Yusoff, 2018). Millions of people have been killed or displaced through the Holocaust, wars, genocide, poverty or "ethnic cleansing." Currently the official figures for those who have been displaced through violence and persecution in 2016 stands at nearly 66 million people globally (United Nations Hugh Commissioner for Refugees (UNHCR), 2017). The threads of extraction, assimilation and displacement are key here for understanding how those affected continue to have the worst health, living conditions and history of exclusion in the world.

Yusoff (2018) uses the term Black Anthropocene to refer to the process of white categorisation of the person by colour, followed by extraction "racialization belongs to a material categorization of the division of matter (corporeal and mineralogical) into active and inert" (p. 2). She takes specific task to the measurement and categorisation of the mapping of binaries of human and inhuman matter and the terrible atrocities that result.

[T]o understand Blackness as a historically constituted and intentionally enacted deformation in the formation of subjectivity, a deformation that presses an inhuman categorization and the inhuman earth into intimacy. ... as a node of extraction of properties and personhood.

[A]t the same time, this forced intimacy with the inhuman was repurposed for survival and formed into a praxis for remaking other selves that were built in the harshest of conditions. The proximity of black and brown bodies to harm in this intimacy with the inhuman is what I am calling *Black Anthropocene*.... Literally stretching black and brown bodies across the seismic fault lines of the earth, Black Anthropocene subtend White Geology as a material stratum.

(Yusoff, 2018; p. xii)

These fault lines exist in the form of syndemic suffering (Mendenhall, 2019) and are closely related to cultural melancholy (Singleton, 2015). The hole in formation that will not be recognised culturally and personally as not only an extraction from the earth and communities but also in the personhood of black lives.

The fault lines of syndemic suffering and cultural melancholy are "given without the possibility of resettling, insists that you must stay with and in the displacement" (Yusoff, 2018; p. xi) and that refuse redemption. Voiding subjects and a relation to the earth that was embodied and organised created a void of extractive dispossessions in service to the refiguring of humanness. The idea that categories of person or human contribute so much to ill-health through dispossession is distressing when there seems to be little recourse to change and when these essentialised categorical differences run so deep:

The geologic claims on and in black and brown flesh establish stratigraphic traces that are both bone deep and intergenerational, marking bodies with nuclear radioisotopes and skin with codes of disposability in the proximity to power and toxicity.

What is at stake and what is on the front line are defined through the colour line.

(Yusoff, 2018; p. 51)

The categorisation of human versus inhuman is of note for medical humanities because of the "unseen fragment," as subject and relation, that both erases and perpetuates the fault lines: "*humanness* is no longer a *noun*." Being human is "a praxis and cannot be taken for granted as a self-explanatory category or reason" (Yusoff, 2018; p. 52). Therefore any praxis by medical humanities must be aware of how we are educated into being around the colonialist project through concepts of colour, measurement, as well as categorisation into roles and inhumanity. Such notions are inherently tied in with ideas of salvation and redemption, which in themselves can be seen as both a cause of and response to suffering.

This suffering, of which categorisation of race is foundational, marks a "black hole" of humanity (Weheliye, 2002):

Humanity continues to persist in its current forms of inhumanity precisely because it is a humanity that is racially constituted and where racial difference is produced as an oppositional form on the outside when it is really, as Silva argues through spatialized and subjective modes, internal to the formation of such humanity.

(Yusoff, 2018; p. 55)

The black hole in humanity, internal to its formation as the colonial man, creates a void internally reflective of the external one. Whereby one's role in society is synonymous with one's colour, personhood and self become fused in yet another moral anguish that goes unrecognised in white epistemology.

The key themes of categorisation, dispossession, extraction, assimilation, displacement and creation of a void seem to be properties of how society treats groups of people, who then also have the worst health. If these themes are then tied in with the VIDDA (violence, immigration, diabetes, depression and abuse) model, there seems to be a correlation between the social and individual figures of suffering. As Sharpe (2016) reminds us, black deaths are the constitutive aspect of democracy, the idea of justice and human rights produces the conditions of black death and exclusion as normative. The social activities that reinforce this exclusion and death are strategies of containment, regulation, punishment, capture, captivity and cavity.

6.3 Indigenous health in Australia

At present, exclusionary practices are operating within health that define non-Indigenous Australians as having health while, generally speaking, Indigenous people do not. This is a setting of a boundary and the inculcation of a norm (Butler, 1993). Indigenous Australians have been positioned as "other" to the non-Indigenous Australians in health whilst also being excluded from the mainstream health services by practices such as limited visiting, predominantly complex English language signage, overt hostility and prejudice as well as discrimination. Indigenous health is an example of how the imposition of colonizers' ideologies continues to disadvantage Indigenous people at the same time as it accrues advantage to non-Indigenous people (Moreton-Robinson, 2003, cited in Riggs, 2006).

Indigenous health has been the subject of many papers that seek to identify why Indigenous people continue to show the worst indicators of health of all Australians (Australian Institute of Health and Welfare [AIHW], 2019). White colonisation in Australia has resulted in such a shameful picture of Indigenous health. Health professionals have minimal contact and information sharing with Indigenous people during their training. The role of privilege in perpetuating health inequities needs to be examined in the context of ongoing practices of ownership and belonging on the part of white people and exclusion from white society on the part of Indigenous people.

The curricula of most health professional university courses pay minimal attention to issues surrounding different genders, races and ethnic groups. There is a silence on the impact of white colonisation of the health of Indigenous people. One could think that because Indigenous people are most sick more often they would form a greater proportion of the work of health professionals. And therefore that more of the curriculum would be devoted to the way that white colonisation/behaviour has impacted on Indigenous peoples' health. However, to the best of my knowledge, Indigenous health tends to be but one option to choose from amongst many topics. Understanding the nuances of relations between race, ethnicity, culture and white exclusion is vital to understanding disparities in health.

The exclusion of Indigenous people from Australian society is said to be the root of the shameful current state of health of Indigenous people (Eades, 2000). The exclusionary practices experienced by Indigenous people form the process of materialisation (Butler, 1993) that give shape and boundaries to the body of the Indigenous person and meaning to them about what it means to be human. The life course perspective, a theory referred to in relation to Indigenous health, agrees with the process of materialisation and sees the physiological status as a marker of the past social position of Indigenous people (Eades, 2000). Thus diseases that are endemic today in Indigenous people include obesity, hypertension, diabetes, renal failure, coronary heart disease, cancer and arthritis (Jackson and Ward, 1999) and could be seen as largely auto-immune diseases, i.e. as the body attacking itself. The prevalence of auto-immune diseases could also be seen as the biological stress response being activated too often and for too long (Eades, 2000). Epigenetics is believed to also play a role through the environment changing genes in response to trauma (Yamada & Chong, 2017; Rozek et al., 2014).

The stress response and the view of the body attacking itself make sense in a life where exclusionary practices have been the norm. Indigenous people who have survived being a part of the Stolen Generations show clinical pictures that are "consistent with a contemporary understanding of the harmful impact of chronic trauma on the developing self" (Petchkovsky, San Roque, Napaljarri and Butler, 2004). The degree of distress experienced by these people was suspected to be "merely the tip of a monstrous iceberg" (Petchkovsky et al., 2004). The monstrous iceberg encompasses trauma, re-experiencing (recollections, dreams, flashbacks, cues/triggers with emotional or physiological responses), overwhelming threat, hyperarousal and dissociation, intrusive recollections, recurrent nightmares, avoidance or numbing, loss of memory, diminished interest in life activities, estrangement from others, affect restriction, foreshortened future, hypervigilance, insomnia, concentration difficulties and irritability, lifelong duration often with exacerbations to major depression proportions, not feeling at home in either culture, somatisation (chronic headaches, irritable bowel syndromes, chronic body aches and pains), alexithymia (a characterological style which struggles to identify emotions and allow an inner life of fantasy and imagination)

(Taylor, 2000 cited in Petchkovsky et al., 2004), self-harm, chronic shame, suicide, social withdrawal, chronic fatigue or tiredness, feelings of pessimism, despair or hopelessness and feelings of inadequacy (Petchkovsky et al., 2004). Such experiences made up the fabric of these people's lives.

The process of materialisation for Indigenous people who were part of the Stolen Generations ends up making them abject in relation to the white culture:

> [W]hat is *abject*, on the contrary, the jettisoned object, is radically excluded and draws me toward the place where meaning collapses. A certain "ego" that merged with its master, a superego, has flatly driven it away. It lies outside, beyond the set, and does not seem to agree to the latter's rules of the game. And yet, from its place of banishment, the abject does not cease challenging its master.

> Not me. Not that. But not nothing, either. A "something" that I do not recognize as a thing. A weight of meaninglessness, about which there is nothing insignificant, and which crushes me. On the edge of non-existence and hallucination, of a reality that, if I acknowledge it, annihilates me. There, abject and abjection are my safeguards. The primers of my culture.
>
> (Kristeva, 1982; p. 2)

Indigenous people play a role in white culture through the process of materialisation of abjection. They and the symptoms they can exhibit have been radically excluded from white society and continue to be so. There must be a collapse of meaning for people who experience such extreme symptoms as listed above, which means there can be no agency of meaning (Lather, 1991). By being merged with a non-Indigenous culture where the position of being Indigenous carries with it a passivity and a victim role, there must still be a subtext that Indigenous people are somehow wrong and must change either through behavioural or social determinants of health policy. It is no wonder then that Indigenous Australians display the worst health indicators in the nation, which is a cause for national shame (Eades, 2000).

The fear is that by health professionals remaining ignorant of the distress of these events, history is repeating itself as Indigenous people are confronted with health professionals who exhort them to exercise ("It's not a big exercise campaign") or give up smoking or who just can't understand why they can't lose weight. Dis-remembering is the denial, rationalisation and trivialisation of cultural forces and, it may be said, feelings, which work to systematically edit the reality of inflicted harm (Petchkovsky et al., 2004; p. 11). Overriding of distress in order to get a job done seems to be the implicit rationalisation in the health professional curriculum that is silent about cultural events such as this.

The silence on the reality of inflicted harm is part of the in-between, of the space or gap, between the educator and the educated. Another part of the space in between educator and educated could be what Petchkovsky et al call the "attacks on linking" with culture, family, and emotional connection of Indigenous people:

> Emotion is hated, emotional connections are actively attacked. A style of function that is 'logical, almost mathematical, but never emotionally reasonable' prevails. Consequently, 'the links surviving are perverse, cruel and sterile.'
>
> (Petchkovsky et al., 2004; p. 12)

What is in-between the educator and educated includes the materialisation of the bodies and the negative effects of chronic trauma along with possible attacks on linking and emotions. It could be that any encounter with a white middle class health professional who espouses advice and information based on the idea of an individual who is a rational autonomous human being, without contacting or connecting to their feelings or subjective experience, will only re-enact the trauma experienced by Indigenous people, as it has been said that "it is the systematic attacks on all this linking [with extended feelings, family, land, animals, dreaming tracks and culture] that constitute the core trauma of the Stolen Generations story" (Petchkovsky et al., 2004; p. 13). This represents the core trauma of a person not being allowed or able to exist within their primary relationship. These points of complexity also lend weight to the idea that even in extreme cases of materialisation where social practices of health and education have been formative, a person's subjective experience needs contacting, acknowledging and containing within the understanding that the person's (patient's or client's or health professional's) context is all important.

The failure of mainstream health services for Indigenous people has been widely documented (Brideson, 2004; Brideson & Kanowski, 2004; Elliott-Farrelly, 2004; Ellis, 2000; Hunter, 2004, 1993; Jackson & Ward, 1999; Martin, 2004; Riggs, 2004; Saggers & Gray, 1991; Vicary & Westerman, 2004; Westerman, 2004; Riggs, 2006). Some believe that reconciliation is the answer (Eades, 2000; Jackson & Ward, 1999) but it seems to be an ever-retreating horizon (Loff & Anderson, 2000). It seems that we do need a more socially accountable practice (Riggs, 2006) of health care, one that focuses on the way that racialised understandings of subjectivity are dominant in most countries and one that acknowledges the "whiteness of psychological epistemologies" (Riggs, 2004) as well as other epistemologies. The whole idea of an autonomous individual progressing upwards towards a state of good health is closely connected to colonial narratives of civilizing primitive cultures (Riggs, 2004). By disowning parts of Indigenous health, such as suffering, the white health epistemology seems to reject other standpoints. It seems as if there can never be any real change in the location of epistemological standpoints until all that is disowned is taken back and owned by the white people. The number of references over a long period of time are included here to demonstrate how little has changed over the decades in spite of activists' efforts.

The example of Indigenous health is included here to highlight how Western ideologies and epistemologies of health have contributed to the exclusion and banishment of Indigenous health and peoples from mainstream training curricula and health services. These phenomena are highlighted by Indigenous health and the same could be true for marginalised populations in the UK and US. Part of the banishment could be seen as a result of the imposition of the neo-liberal autonomous instrumental individual along with the binary notions surrounding health with its focus on (perfect) health and the consequent banishment or abjection of all perceived imperfection and suffering. In such extreme conditions of materialisation and abjection, even though the context can clearly be shown to be responsible for the materialisation that occurs, the personal subjective experience also needs including in the health encounter. The complexity of the health encounter and health professional practice cannot be overstated. These ideas will now be developed further in the next section.

6.4 How will a return be enacted?

Categories of self underlie many of the disconnects between health professional and patients, especially those who have been categorised outside mainstream ideas of what constitutes a person and self. Instrumentalist categories of self underpin the disconnect between learning objectives and curriculum and the people who are involved. These are difficult notions to explain to health professionals, clinicians and medical curriculum personnel. Different approaches are required and those seem to come from the medical humanities within medical education. Fundamentally, questions of what we do, who we are and what we exist in require careful analysis because clearly the current status of health professional education, practice and health promotion is implicated in the increasing inequalities between those who are suffering from long term chronic illness, earlier onset, lower quality of life, lower life expectancy, poverty and deprivation and those who have longer healthier life expectancies. Along with the gap in inequalities, there is a gap in knowledge about how these occur and have been perpetuated over the years in spite of the efforts to bring political awareness to the detrimental effects of austerity (CSDH, 2008; Marmot et al., 2020).

Marmot et al. (2020) identify the impact of adverse childhood experiences (ACEs) mediated by poverty, deprived areas, less opportunities for development and neglect. However, the literature on ACEs is at risk of decontextualizing and thereby individualising these phenomena because social, institutional, economic and political causes of ill-health and trauma, as exemplified by the situation of Indigenous Australians above, have proven so difficult to address. The Black Anthropocene highlights the fundamental effect of consumerism on perpetuating extraction, displacement and hence trauma on populations globally (Yusoff, 2018). We are all implicated in the perpetuation of neo-liberal consumerism with some people affected more than others, some who have less resources to fall back on and are more at risk in the first place. The risk of violence and trauma from inequalities has proven to be a stable indicator in communities that suffer the most (United Nations Development Programme (UNDP), 2019). Amongst many factors, what mediates these forms of suffering in people are poorly adjusted institutions whose staff do not know or have not been trained in evidence based approaches, that take the context into account, to manage violence and trauma, for example.

Trends in expenditure on various commodities show a massive contrast between cigarettes, alcohol, narcotic drugs and military spending compared with basic sanitation, health and education (United Nations Development Programme (UNDP), 1997). For example, in 1997, global expenditure on cosmetics was US$8 billion, ice cream US$11 billion, alcoholic drinks in Europe stood at US$105 billion, narcotic drugs US$400 billion, military spending US$780 billion compared with additional expenditure to achieve basic education for all US$6 billion, water and sanitation for all US$9 billion, and basic health and nutrition US$13 billion (United Nations Development Programme (UNDP), 1997). The disparity between what is spent on essentially self-medication is shocking compared to the little believed necessary to reach basic health and education as a human right.

There is the ethical issue of choice and a need not so much for more consumption or for less but for a different pattern of consumption for sustainable human development. The environmental, developmental, technological and moral arguments present a critique of consumption patterns that are inimical to human development (United Nations Development Programme (UNDP), 1997), yet there seems to be little cultural support to change these patterns given the election of governments in the biggest consumerist countries that continue down the same old path. This is in spite of the increasing evidence of relations between inequalities, homicides and violent conflict. There are more homicides in countries with higher income inequality across all categories of human development (United Nations Development Programme (UNDP), 2019). For high and very high human development countries the association is strong: Income inequality explains almost a third of the overall variation in homicide rates, even after years of schooling, GDP per capita, democratisation and ethnic fractionalisation are accounted for (United Nations Development Programme (UNDP), 2019; p. 90). Violence and trauma cannot be separated out from consumerism.

Trauma is the leading cause of death for people aged under 44 in the UK (Trauma Audit and Research Network (TARN), 2020; Public Health England (PHE), 2018). The World Health Organisation states that, globally, some 470,000 people are victims of homicide every year (World Health Organisation, 2017). Hundreds of millions more men, women, and children suffer non-fatal forms of interpersonal violence, including child maltreatment, youth violence, intimate partner violence, sexual violence, and elder abuse, with many suffering multiple forms. Such violence contributes to lifelong ill-health – particularly for women and children – and early death. Not acknowledging the possible cause of ill-health as trauma, as in a trauma informed approach, could be seen as a form of inequity.

London itself is a city rife with inequalities and marginalisation of disadvantaged groups of people (Cunningham & Savage, 2017). The four London Trauma networks have seen a rise in gunshot injuries since 2016 (Norton et al., 2018). Between 2500 and 3000 people with penetrating injuries are treated by London Trauma teams each year: of those, 250–300 are firearm injuries and the rest from knives (TARN, 2020). Doctors at the frontline of care in Accident and Emergency departments described the level of brutality and violence of knife injuries as shocking. The level of violence related to gang membership has been escalating with 116 murders in London in 2017. Several A&E consultants are calling for a preventive approach to violence. Whilst the London Trauma system is saving more and more lives, they would rather not have to in the case of violence.

Women have been subjected to violent attacks with one woman dying every 2.6 days from domestic violence in England. In contrast to knife injuries, women can present at primary care seeking help from doctors, who they identify as their most trusted health professional. Long term survivors of domestic abuse often have chronic health problems such as gynaecological disorders, chronic pain, neurological symptoms, GI disorders and self-reported heart disease. The difficulty in separating from violent partners has been noted as a desperate attempt to or fantasy of repair their own childhood distress (Metz et al., 2019).

Thus, violence often disrupts the lives of individuals for decades. Beyond death, physical injury and disability, violence can lead to stress that impairs the development of the nervous and immune systems. Consequently, people exposed to violence are at increased risk of a wide range of immediate and lifelong behavioural, physical and mental health problems, including being a victim and/or perpetrator of further violence. Violence can also undermine the social and economic development of whole communities and societies.

Violence is said to be one of the most devastating national and global challenges we face. Violence behaves like other contagious diseases in that there are characteristic signs and symptoms causing morbidity and mortality, and it is transmissible, causing more of itself. Furthermore, violence also demonstrates population and individual characteristics of contagious epidemics such as clustering, geo-temporal spreading and person-to-person transmission. Incubation periods are variable with some manifestations of violence not becoming apparent until years after being subjected to child abuse, for example, or perhaps there is immediate violence through retaliation in gang warfare.

People at heightened risk for violence have acquired this through exposure to violence in the first place. Victimisation or visual exposure is then mediated by the brain, which processes violence into scripts, copied behaviours and unconscious social expectations. Processing then leads to several situational adaptive responses including aggression, impulsivity, depression, stress, exaggerated startle response and changes in neurochemistry. Violence begets aggression which then increases the likelihood of more violence. Past exposure to violence is thought to be the strongest predictor of violent behaviour.

Not all persons exposed to violence go on to be perpetrators. Other factors influence uptake such as proximity, dose and age, like other contagious factors. Poverty, limited education and family structure also act as modulators. Specific strategies are required to interrupt the transmission in the community. Treating violence as an epidemic health problem, mediated by brain and social processes, is seen as a scientifically grounded understanding of violence and holds the potential for health professionals to contribute to the recognition, prevention and treatment of the perpetuation of violence (Slutkin et al., 2018). Health professionals are currently underutilised and under-resourced in multisectoral approaches to violence reduction.

Healthcare workers are at the front line of having to deal with the aftermath of government policies that only encourage consumerism amidst policies of austerity, inequality and associated violence. There are some new initiatives that aim to prevent violence and the re-traumatisation of people who attend healthcare through an awareness of the impacts and effects of trauma such as the trauma informed care (TIC) approach and public health approach to knife crime prevention. One approach by the Centre for Disease Control in the US and trauma networks in the UK is a trauma informed approach to healthcare through the awareness and prevention of ACEs. The trauma informed care approach started with the observation that intractable public health problems such as obesity seemed to represent a way of coping with the symptoms of trauma (Felitti, 2019). Furthermore, ACEs are also implicated in the perpetration and perpetuation of violence (Scottish Violence Reduction Unit, 2020).

A public health approach to knife crime involved frontline clinicians realising that a person presenting in an emergency department provided an opportunity for a teachable moment (Purtle et al., 2015) or reachable moment, a period of self-reflection precipitated by a real sense of mortality and vulnerability (Brohi et al., 2019), although this is usually referred to reaching people and communities who are isolated from mainstream services (Purtle et al., 2015). However, relatively few approaches have been rigorously evaluated for their effectiveness and evaluation has not been a high priority. Not enough programmes are aimed at primary prevention in the community or societal levels, compared with secondary or tertiary prevention. Programmes operating at the community or societal levels are under-emphasised compared with those aimed at individual or relationship factors which could be because the major government sectors involved – health, education, housing, social care, police and justice – have been underfunded for years (Butler et al., 2019). There is a pressing need to develop or adapt, test and evaluate many more prevention programmes in developing countries (WHO, 2002). It seems as if these programmes are too little too late as by the time a person reaches an emergency department it is likely that they will be involved in repeated acts of violence (Scottish Government, 2019).

Using a life course perspective, researchers found that people who struggled to cope were more likely to have suffered cumulative trauma over their life-times. Using an ACEs scoring system the researchers found that respondents were 52% more likely to have suffered abuse, neglect and dysfunctional households (Allen & Donkin, 2015; Felitti et al., 1998; Hinch, 2014). There was a graded (dose-response relationship) between ACEs and ischemic heart disease, cancer, chronic lung disease, skeletal fractures, and liver disease. Later studies have found links to cancer, HIV, obesity, headaches, depression, IV drug use, smoking and alcohol use, chronic pain, premature mortality, "per-sonality" disorders, PTSD, Complex Post Traumatic Stress Disorder, early sexual activity, violence (victim and perpetrator), poor diet, and lifetime in-carceration (Allen & Donkin, 2015). In Wales, 47% of 3885 respondents of a survey of reported at least one ACE, whilst 14% reported experience four or more ACEs (Hughes et al., 2017).

There is a problem with these approaches in that there is a merging of the individual effects and social impact in understanding. Typically, the three "e"s of individual trauma were an event, series of events or set of circumstances that is experienced by an individual as physically or emotionally harmful or life threatening and that has lasting adverse effects on the individual's func-tioning and mental, physical, social, emotional, or spiritual well-being (Substance Abuse & Mental Health Services Administration [SAMHSA], 2014). Yet these definitions do not take into account the social and economic circumstances that predispose people to vulnerability to violence such as economic inequity as mentioned above. For example, county lines (Coomber & Moyle, 2017) and government policy contribute to a complex picture of knife crime in some of the most deprived communities such as Newham and Lambeth in London: government cuts to policing, government policy of austerity and its effects in local areas, housing and cuts to youth services were all cited as reasons by respondents for the rise in knife crime and violence (Roberts, 2019). She found that young people felt a sense of hopelessness and despair, that gang membership was perceived as the only way out of their situation as it gave them a sense of belonging in an environment where they have felt isolated (Roberts, 2019). Trauma takes place in an environment of suffering of isolation, alienation, marginalisation, violence, intergenerational uprooting and displacement as often different ethnicities cluster together.

6.4.1 The symbiotic relations between capitalism, race and trauma

The harrowing accounts provided by black writers of the effects of capitalism – where blackness constitutes the very outside of capitalism's experience – are characterised by evidence of extraction and assimilation through colonialist projects (Yusoff, 2018) and human development projects (United Nations Development Programme (UNDP), 2019). The consumption of various goods such as alcohol, tobacco and drugs seems to indicate that there is a universal approach to self-management based on altering one's physiological state. Perhaps we are all hungry ghosts looking for sources of self in our consumption and retail therapy. I say this because of the phenomenal amount spent on these substances seems to indicate that culturally we are compelled to enact the repetitious ritual of taking something in to assuage our living and perhaps attempt a livable life. A repetitious ritual such as *La Coatlicue* is a means by which awareness is kept at bay and prevents one's attention being captured or consumed by anything or anyone else (Anzaldúa, 1999). The hamster wheel of medical practice coincides with the statistics of violence and crime in deprived areas to keep health professionals busy and unaware of the bigger global picture. Perhaps there is a fear of looking to see the bigger picture. Fear holds one frozen in stone, with the consuming internal whirlwind, dealing with contradictions, dualities, reversals and suffering. There is a crossing over, a chiasma:

> Why does she have to go and try to make "sense" of something, she has to "crossover," kicking a hole out of the old boundaries of the self and skipping under or over, dragging the old skin along, stumbling over it.
> (Anzaldúa, 1999; p. 71)

Processing and becoming aware of the hole is not simple or easy; there is a silencing of the wild tongue in relation to suffering (Anzaldúa, 1999). Perhaps it is more culturally acceptable to consume, to try to fill the hole of empty ghosts (Maté, 2018), in keeping with the colonialist project where white men were perceived as ghosts by indigenous cultures (Clarke, 2007), rather than confront suffering in the world.

Suffering in the form of PTSD, DPD, and burnout will now be described generally in relation to the population as a whole and then specifically as they relate to health professionals. The intention with these descriptions is to look beyond individualisation, to see what can be learned culturally or socially in order to further understand suffering and how health professionals can respond. Whilst PTSD, DPD and burnout may be considered specific medical diagnoses or domains, they are so in a culture dominated by consumerism and neo-liberal ideology. Therefore there may be threads of resonance running through that may help to understand suffering. I am also including this section as part of my metaphor of lacunae: going back to the bone is a necessary step since often in the experience of trauma, the self is believed to retreat to the bone structure, a place where the self feels safe from impingement from the outside world. Perhaps this is best explained by Anzaldúa:

> In looking at this book that I'm also finished writing, I see a mosaic pattern (Aztec-like) emerging, a weaving pattern, thin here, thick here.

I see a preoccupation with the deep structure, with the gesso under painting that is red earth, black earth. I can see the deep structure, the scaffolding. If I can get the bone structure right, then putting flesh on it proceeds without too many hitches.

(Anzaldúa, 1999; p. 88)

This suggestion is a different form of source of self to those suggested by Taylor (1989). Going back to the bone is a way of finding a return in amongst sociocultural constructions of self, a re-memorializing and a recognition of the self that hides from the self during times of severe trauma and the prolonged aftermath of that. In this context, a return requires a different source of self whilst probably still drawing on other forms previously described too.

6.4.1.1 Post traumatic stress disorder (PTSD)

PTSD is a Diagnostic and Statistical Manual of Mental Disorders Version 5 categorisation of 20 symptoms across 4 clusters (intrusions, avoidance, negative alterations to cognition and mood [NACM], and alterations to arousal and reactivity [AAR]) (Price et al., 2019) experienced by an individual. The diagnosis developed out of classification of generalised anxiety disorders and stressor related disorders. PTSD is characterised by hyperarousal, intrusive memories or flashbacks, and other symptoms after experiencing a specific event that is conceived as a trigger. About 20–25% of people experiencing traumatic events eventually develop PTSD; therefore 75–80% of people do not (Price et al., 2019). There are different types of PTSD and recovery depending on how many traumatic events have been experienced and whether or not or how much any have been resolved, how well-resourced persons are, what support they have, whether there are any other family issues such as abuse or neglect, and how much help they have been able to access. Various theories have been developed to underpin interventions such as the polyvagal theory (Porges, 2011), psychophysiology and psychoeducation (Rothschild, 2000; Scaer, 2014), neurobiological approaches to structural dissociation and working with fragmented selves (Fisher, 2017), memory and information processing (van der Kolke et al., 2007), somatic experiencing (Levine, 1997, 2010), ego state therapy (Emmerson, 2007; Forgash & Copeley, 2008) and a range of other evidence based techniques (Courtois & Ford, 2009). Active outsiders can help in the aftermath of disasters by knowing about somatic experiencing and psychoeducation (Ross, 2003, 2007). Psychoeducation focuses on how to manage overwhelming physiological states and affects (fight, flight or freeze) which can lead to dissociation and fragmenting (Fisher, 2017; Rothschild, 2000; Scaer, 2014).

The social impact of PTSD is mainly in terms of whether it is recognised and validated as a set of symptoms and, if so, how they are viewed by the general public (Herman, 2001). Stolorow suggests we are now in an era, an "Age of Trauma":

Because the tranquilizing illusions of our everyday world seem in our time to be severely threatened from all sides – by global diminution of natural resources, by global warming, by global nuclear proliferation, by global terrorism, and by global economic collapse.

(Stolorow, 2010)

He believes that the essence of emotional trauma lies in the shattering of absolutisms of everyday life – the system of illusory beliefs that allow us to function in the world, which in turn is experienced as stable, predictable and safe. However, a significant proportion of the global population have not experienced such a world and continue to live without either tranquilizing illusions or absolutisms.

Stolorow (2010) suggests that we need a collective relational home, an empathic civilisation, where we meet as "siblings in the same darkness," deeply connected with one another through holding and caring for devastating emotional pain, as a shared ethical principle. This, in contrast to resurrective grandiosity, or various forms of dissociative numbing that either try to bring back illusory beliefs or avoidance of them all together, is enabled by looking at our existential structure to take into account our shared vulnerability and form identities from there.

As with definitions of suffering, the experience of psychological trauma includes a sense of alienation, estrangement, aloneness and isolation. The experiential chasm that separates a traumatised person from other human beings is characterised by unbearable affect, particularly when attunement from the relational surround to assist in tolerance, containment, modulation and integration of that unbearable affect is absent (Stolorow, 1999). There is a difference between an attunement that cannot be supplied by others and an attunement that cannot be felt by the traumatised person because of their aloneness in their suffering (Devisch et al., 2019). There is also a difference in horizons of experience between people, where the traumatised person is certain that one horizon cannot accommodate the other. This essential incommensurability in horizons works by the network described by Ney (2019) where we are all living on the edge of our experiential realm. These boundaries of experience contain belief systems, or absolutisms, that allow people to exist on a continuum of functioning.

When absolutisms are shattered through trauma and no safety or continuity can be assured, the person is exposed in "the unbearable embeddedness of being" (Stolorow & Atwood, 1992; p. 22):

As a result, the traumatized person cannot help but perceive aspects of existence that lie well outside the absolutized horizons of normal everydayness. It is in this sense that the worlds of traumatized persons are fundamentally incommensurable with those of others, the deep chasm in which an anguished sense of estrangement and solitude takes form.

(Stolorow, 1999; p. 467)

At the same time as people experience alienation and isolation, they also yearn for someone who is able to understand these experiences in a deepening of the concept of twinship (Kohut, 1984). There is a sense here of what Frank (2001) was describing when he wanted health professionals to understand and not treat him as an object in his suffering. There is also a sense of the fiction of the autonomous rational person as shattered in circumstances beyond his or her control. This idea is taken up in the next section on depersonalisation.

6.4.1.2 Depersonalisation

Depersonalisation is a term used to describe the feeling or experience of being a stranger to one's self or of there being a stranger inside (Abugel, 2010). There is a loss of mood, of affect: "Imagine thinking with all feeling removed. You become a thing that sees words passing through your head, moment by moment, like subtitles in a movie" (Abugel, 2010; p. 25). Feeling "unreal" can happen to anyone from time to time but it is also associated with severe stress and acts as a defence mechanism to distance an individual from overwhelming circumstances (Simeon & Abugel, 2006).

> For depersonalised people, the world within, or the world around, may seem strange and unreal for prolonged periods of time. They feel detached from the sense of self they once took for granted and struggle, often for many years, in fruitless searches for answers that are hard to come by.
> (Simeon & Abugel, 2006; p. 3)

Pierre Janet proposed a sense of incompleteness of self, of being out of sync with one's normal self, a disconnection between primary and secondary psychic activity that disrupts, leading to an echo, usually used to create the illusion of a continuous flow of activity.

Various other notable figures all attested to the phenomenon of depersonalisation – Freud, William James, Mayer Gross; referring to the veil, sick soul, or the reality of the unseen, with a feeling of imminent insanity threatening, lying at the heart of the condition. Freud hinted at conflict, guilt, as perhaps being a trigger for depersonalisation or derealisation (the strangeness of and alienation from reality) (Simeon & Abugel, 2006). That is, depersonalisation is an ego's or self's defence against a variety of perceived negative feelings, conflicts or experiences. A poorly integrated ego or sense of self means that negative self-representations are kept outside conscious awareness through practices such as habitual behaviours, routines, repetitive compulsive rituals and such like. This dissociative experience therefore interferes with identity formation, perhaps explaining why adolescents are more vulnerable to depersonalisation (Simeon & Abugel, 2006). Identity and awareness are instead focused on the sense of being or feeling like an automaton, machine or puppet (divided within) which must be observed compulsively. The split is seen as between the observing self and the experiencing self; "the danger is experienced pertinent to the participant self, and can thus be distanced from the observing self" (Simeon & Abugel, 2006; p. 60). The dreamlike quality of depersonalisation relates to feelings of unreality and the split of the sense of self into an observing self and a participating self.

The dreamlike quality of depersonalisation can also lead to an altered sense of time including an inability to evoke the past readily or clearly, to distinguish the present from the past or future, and a sense of time stopping and deepening, losing sense of time passing either quickly or slowly. The change in perception of time may have something to do with the hyper-awareness of one's self. At the same time as the drive to intensify alertness, there is also a dampening of potentially disorganised emotion because escape or avoidance seems impossible. All this is mediated by fear of the self or of existence itself (Simeon & Abugel, 2006). There is also a disturbance in the perception of space so that a person may feel vertigo when navigating the way around (Lopez et al., 2018). Disturbances of self and body representation were found with 12% of the patients have experienced distorted own-body representations (their hands or feet felt larger or smaller), 37% reported abnormal sense of agency, 35% reported disownership for the body and 22% reported disembodiment (Lopez et al., 2018). Emotional numbing or loss of affect, changes in body experience, visual derealisation, loss of agency and changes in subjective experiences are core features of depersonalisation and naturally cause distress to the individual, leading to withdrawal and isolation (Simeon & Abugel, 2006).

Cultural and social influences on ideas of the self lend credence to the idea that depersonalisation is a feature of modern life (Abugel, 2010; Simeon & Abugel, 2006). The idea that depersonalisation is a feature of modern life is evidence not only through the use of illicit recreational drugs but also by centralised bureaucracies that dehumanise individuals through excessive routinisation and humiliation of the workforce, which in turn fosters disengaged instrumentalism and detachment of the self. Valuing material achievements, rewards, financial success and overidentification with corporatisation through marketing and branding have been encouraged through social media and the promotion of celebrity lifestyles, which few will ever reach. Although conducted a long time ago, perhaps in a foretelling of what was to come, the Whitehall studies showed that there was a gradient of ill-health and mortality inversely proportional to the position one occupied in civil service (Marmot & Steptoe, 2008). Whilst limited in its scope in terms of inclusion of diversity, the studies demonstrated the relationship between social position and health. Perhaps, rather than just control or power, the level of depersonalisation and hence disengagement was a source of higher morbidity and mortality.

Watching atrocities unfold on the news or social media can lead to emotional numbing, disengagement and a sense of unreality as each new horror becomes yet another source of fodder for the masses. "Real life 'seemed like a movie' to the national consciousness" when people viewed the Twin Towers collapsing on live television on 9/11 (Simeon & Abugel, 2006; p. 64). When people experience these world events of horror, unless there is attunement with those around them, as opposed to distorted messages, mixed messages, double-binds or non-messages, there can be a distortion of the sense of self and hence vulnerability to depersonalisation.

Theoretical constructions about depersonalisations affect how it is seen by clinicians with some arguing that the condition reflects an alteration of consciousness rather than a structural dissociation of the self (usually perceived as a splitting between the observing and experiencing ego) (Simeon & Abugel, 2006). Van der Hart and colleagues suggest in a simple structural dissociation model that two aspects of the personality comprise an "apparently normal part of the personality" (ANP) and an "emotional part of the personality" (EP) with the latter a more sequestered part focused on past trauma (van der Hart et al., 2006; p. 5). Simeon & Abugel (2006) suggest, in an apparent reversal, that in depersonalisation the ANP **is** the depersonalised self, whereas EP would be the prior feeling state because it feels (p. 67). This is important because what the latter are suggesting is that the personality remains accessible via affect. Moreover, the nature of depersonalisation is that it takes over the whole of the personality so that the person thinks that is the whole of who they are. The reason for understanding this is that forewarned is forearmed since both patients and health professionals suffer from depersonalisation from the dehumanising effects of healthcare systems. These effects and nature of healthcare systems are something to look out for in the attending to suffering.

Further detail that may help to understanding suffering more comes from research conducted on depersonalisation and dissociation. Holmes et al. (2005) suggest that the key poles are detachment (of body, sense of self, or external world) and compartmentalisation (a deficit in the ability to deliberately control processes or actions that would normally be amenable to such control). This is important because there is accumulating evidence from descriptive, cognitive and brain-imaging studies that information-processing pathways are quite distinct between detached and compartmentalised states. In detached states, there is a distinction between attention and encoding which presents difficulties in forming new emotional memories, whilst in compartmentalisation memories are stored but not easily retrieved. Therefore one of the key differences is the formation, storage and retrieval of emotional memories or affect. This could contribute to the feeling of suffering – of being on the wrong side of the fault line – if the person is also suffering from depersonalisation and detachment. There is overlap between PTSD in that depersonalisation could be seen as a chronic form of PTSD:

> There is considerable overlap between the concept of detachment and many of the phenomena associated with trauma and PTSD that have attracted the dissociative label. (p. 6)

"Full-blown" flashback experiences, in which the individual reports becoming totally immersed in the traumatic memory to the point of believing that the event is happening again and losing touch with their current surroundings, are relatively rare. They could even be conceived as an extreme form of detachment in their own right, in the sense that they involve an altered state of consciousness characterised by a sense of separation from reality.

(Holmes et al., 2005: p. 6)

Not understanding the relationship between the different states means that health professionals can be working in the dark in relation to patients as well as themselves. Understanding the role of affect and attention, encoding and information-processing pathways is also crucial. Perhaps the role of imagination is crucial here as shown by the number of painters and writers who have written about depersonalisation in one way or another.

The cultural heritage of depersonalisation includes artwork such as Edvard Munch's painting *The Scream*, depicting a detachment from all things outside one's self, as mentioned in the preface. These experiences, including a heightened awareness of the infinite and the eternal, have been described in the literature including the Bible, by Shakespeare, Dostoevsky and Henri Amiel's private diary, *The Journal InTime* (Simeon & Abugel, 2006). In the latter, a theme predominates:

The world and everything in it, including his personal identity, felt unreal, unfounded, and without substance. True reality, he concluded, beyond the veil of the day-to-day world, consisted of the eternal, the infinite, God. The more the self disappeared, the closer one came to the truth and to God, he rationalized.

(Simeon & Abugel, 2006; p. 129)

Amiel uses words like "a molecular whirlwind" to describe individual life, where a "glass screen" was interposed between himself and the life around him, leaving him only the role of the looker-on. There are echoes of Taylor's (1989) sources of self here – between theistic and instrumentalist sources of self – but Amiel demonstrated more complexity in his understanding in himself and the world. He believed he never had the "quantum of illusion" to risk the irreparable; his insight prevented him from joining life as well as preventing a descent into madness (Simeon & Abugel, 2006).

Amiel coined the term "depersonalised" and added many words to an otherwise unspeakable experience. Words are included at length here in order to address the speechlessness of suffering, in case they may be of use.

Amiel exhibits the things that psycho-pathologically primordial about depersonalisation – the existential essence of the experience. Depersonalisation is one of the very few, if not the only state, which discloses the basic, elementary fabric of being, the feeling of this fabric, the experience of this fabric. The tragedy is that depersonalisation discloses itself in a 'negative form', as absence, such as inner pain after an amputation, which still tells us about something we once had, but lost. With depersonalisation the individual does not know exactly what he had, but still experiences something that is 'lost'. That is why depersonalisation can be so painfully hopeless, groundless. That is why there are no words to express because literally, there *are* no words in language to express it. (Bezubbova cited by Simeon & Abugel, 2006; p. 134; emphasis original)

Amiel provides words for the frustration and sorrow resulting from living with one foot in this world and one foot in another (Simeon & Abugel, 2006). These experiences have been described in the literature as *le coup de vide* (the blow of the void) (Simeon & Abugel, 2006).

Sartre (1965) in *Nausea* described the experience of depersonalisation by using the voice of depersonalisation. His and others' philosophy of existentialism was seen as a way to react against depersonalisation caused by modern world's dehumanizing of the individual. In one passage he describes how "words had disappeared and with them the meaning of things, the methods of using them, the feeble landmarks which men have traced on their surface" (Sartre, 1965; p. 181). He goes on to describe how the veil is torn away, how he has *seen* (p. 181); existence had unveiled itself. His mind went on to try and put words to this, to describe and categorise and relate the trees around him:

Each of them escaped from the relationship in which I tried to close it, isolated itself, overflowed. I was aware of the arbitrary nature of these relationships, which I insisted on maintaining in order to delay the collapse of the human world of measures, of quantities, of bearings; they no longer had any grip on things.

(Sartre, 1965; p. 184)

Sartre (1965) seems to be saying the same things as Tolstoy, that the mind's capacity to quantify and categorise is what causes the difficulty in surrendering to the experience of nature and the nurturance that provides. Likewise, where Taylor (1989) suggests that romantic expressivism is a source of self, this can be thwarted by a moral or ethical dilemma, where the mind insists on categorising or judging, as good or bad, events that occur. That is, affect as a mediator and expression of self, becomes overruled by cognitive processes which can lead to depersonalisation. Sartre (1965) and colleagues proposed existentialism as an antidote to depersonalisation caused by modernity. Experiencing the world and the concomitant affects was a way of experiencing self.

Other works portraying individual experiences of depersonalisation include Albert Camus *The Stranger*, Doris Lessing *The Singing Grass* and *The Memoirs of a Survivor*, Aldous Huxley *The Doors of Perception*, Nietzsche *Thus Spoke*

Zarathustra, whilst films such as *The Matrix*, *Apocalypse Now*, and *The Shipping News* show how the individual interacts with a depersonalising rationalising social force to produce automatons, such as those depicted by Lowry in *Going to Work*. The arts and literature have shown the links between rationalising forces and depersonalisation and furthermore provide ways of imagining differently. Indeed, Levin (1991) suggests that Descartes himself suffered from something similar to depersonalisation as he looked out of his window from self-isolation and "all he could see were self-moving machines instead of people" (Levin, 1991; p. 56).

In this section we have seen that the language of depersonalisation can be related to that of suffering and perhaps provide more descriptors, as appropriate. The language of detachment has been linked to processes of the mind, to the categorical imperative, with its focus on attention and encoding and ignoring of affect and emotion. This could be seen as a process of dehumanisation which predisposes individuals to seeking instrumental sources of self, particularly in health professional education, which thereby could predispose them to depersonalisation. The circular nature of depersonalisation and the language used in health professional training and practice are features which mean that health professionals could languish in finding the words to say in response to suffering of patients. Sinclair (1997) noted these predispositions and perhaps this is why he included the following quote at the beginning of his book:

> One might say that the learning of the medical role consists of a separation, almost an alienation, of the student from the lay medical world; a passing through the mirror so that one looks out on the world from behind it, and sees things in mirror writing.
>
> (Everett Hughes, 1984; p. 399 cited in Sinclair, 1997; p. 1)

Sinclair's (1997) work focused on providing an account of "passing through the mirror," yet although he was alerted to the probability of mental illness caused by medical training, he never related this to depersonalisation specifically, even though it appears as though he was aware of this from the above quote.

6.4.1.3 Burnout

Clinician burnout was described in Section 1.8.2 as the physical and emotional exhaustion from working within a challenging system that is inescapable and intolerable, to the point of detachment and depersonalisation (Dean et al., 2020). There are links here with both PTSD – inescapable and intolerable – as well as depersonalisation. Implicated in causing burnout are moral questions, ideas about the self, training, relationships with colleagues, patients and families and workplace conditions. However, suffering and moral issues tend not to be recognised as formative of the self as described earlier in this chapter. Instead, the self is left to flounder in existential anguish, not knowing what to say, or questioning one's own identity, all of which can cause structural dissociation. This must be due in part to the silence in medical training on issues of suffering and self as well as a focus on instrumentalist sources of self.

Surely, if awareness and understanding of suffering and the suffering self were included in medical training, we might know more about how to answers the question of "How do we live in a world of immense suffering?" (Viessière, 2011; p. 39) so that instead of becoming burnt out and de-personalised through exposure to too much suffering, where suffering is interpreted "within biomedicalized metaphors of 'diabetes', 'blood pressure', and the 'rotting' of her kidneys" (Viessière, 2011; p. 50), there was an understanding of how both patients and health professionals are exposed to relentless suffering through the machinery of colonialist empire building and thereby became complicit with consumerist desires and ghosts of that machine (Viessière, 2011).

However, therein lies a difficulty because it is through our complicit acts, our desires to become in an instrumentalist sense, that we also refuse a sociological and psychological understanding of what that may mean. Sinclair (1997) believes that medical students are not characterised by "existential angst" in relation to the training they undergo and resulting transformation, or even less affected by any uncertainties they face because they want to reduce any internal conflicts; "there is also within the profession the pervasive cultural aversion to investigation of social and psychological matters" (Sinclair, 1997; p. 303).

Avoiding disagreeable internal emotional states from the arising of cognitive dissonance, due to perhaps social (peer pressure) or political (hierarchical organisation) aspects of their practice, means that they may not have cognitive awareness or choose to compartmentalise these issues. There is a general professional lack of introspection; doctors for whom "the personal is a 'no-go area'– in some cases terra incognita" (Sinclair, 1997; p. 307). Any reflection can be carried out with a sense of a tick-box exercise or a fear for future repercussions if they were honest (Cook, 2018). According to Sinclair (1997), the lack of interest by the students in themselves reflected a lack of interest in them by seniors and their training. Any awareness of anxiety and unpleasant internal experiences was most likely to be attributable to the individual's most immediate concrete experience rather than understanding the broader social-political context of their lives generally and the training specifically (Sinclair, 1997). The difficulty, therefore, in recognising and attending to suffering in both themselves and others is partly due to a lack of motivation and words inculcated by training, which can lead to depersonalisation and the sense of being a ghost.

Viessière (2011) explores the notions of ghosts in his analysis of the postcolonial empire, believing that we become complicit through a transnational economy of desire, violence and suffering:

> I contemplate the dynamics of mutual exploitation in which our bodies meet and our desires intersect – my desire, and her desire; desire for sex, love, life, meaning, adventure, emancipation, mobility, money, happiness – and consider the ghosts of race, class, nation, history, and geography that seem to animate our bodies in such radically different ways; the Ghosts of the Empire, as I come to call them, inherited from the past and the accident of birth.
>
> (Viessière, 2011; p. 15)

Viessière (2011) proposes that these intangible yet fashionable symbolic categories of race, class and nation are the hard truths of economies, borders that are negotiated in currencies of desire, suffering and mobilities. He suggests that we are all complicit in these symbolic categories through accidents of birth and by virtue of our bodies. Categories and bodies make for strategic silences and self-censorship that prevent deep reflexivity:

> It was one thing to engage in predictable degrees of mandatory reflexivity, and to acknowledge one's position of power in the structures battle against; it was also inconceivable, once one had acknowledged *desire* as one of the main forces that animate the machine one sought to dismantle, to acknowledge the existence of one's desire, and to inquire into its historical constitution ... but it was something entirely different and infinitely more difficult and improbable to interrogate the *consequences* of one's desire by acknowledging and deconstructing the *acts of violence* that had been committed through this desire.
>
> (Viessière, 2011; p. 142–3; emphasis original)

To ask medical students to engage in this deep form of reflexivity that questions their positioning or situatedness in the political economy in the service of understanding suffering is an enormous challenge for most and one that is met with resistance (Bleakely, 2017; Kumagai & Lypson, 2009; Sinclair, 1997). The temptation to focus on biomedical science to alleviate suffering through medication or surgery, for example, is understandable when many of these interventions work to do so.

The challenge for medical students and faculty is that there is also a reversal implicit in this inquiry into suffering:

> I had come to realise, a central aspect of *what had to be done* to revert these asymmetrical relations was not simply to improve the living conditions of the downtrodden (the *consumed*; the *mutilated*), but to tackle the mechanisms that produced the desire of the dominant (*the consumers*). Looking deeply inside one's desires and one's actions, then, could hold a partial key to a way forward.

This key, however, was out of my reach. The social and political projects in which I was too deeply embedded, like what I imagined of Paul Theroux, did not allow me to look deeply inside what the ghosts and fetishes had done to me, and what I was doing to the world as a result.

(Viessière, 2011; p. 143; emphasis original)

The key of turning to oneself as the object of inquiry – a double loop of reflexivity – rather than always focusing on what was wrong with the other is a key of liberation for people who suffer. However, as he notes, this is not easy and may be out of reach without the tools to think and imagine differently.

It is important to consider how Viessière (2011) performed a critical ethnography of his time researching suffering because turning back on oneself – using this as a key to understand suffering – is part of the moral anguish of fusion of self and role as discussed previously and which he demonstrated. The ontological and epistemological assumptions of critical ethnography include the following:

1   All cultural groups produce an intersubjective reality which is both "inherited" and continually constructed and reconstructed as it is lived or practiced. This shared cultural reality is external ... a distinct, lived historical tradition "objectified" through structuring practices (laws, public policies, cultural conventions) ... marked by a collective memory of particular ecological, geo-political, embodied, spaces/places;
2   A well-trained, reflexive investigator can know that historical, socially constructed reality in a partial, provisional sense through an intensive, experiential encounter with people who live by these cultural constructions of reality;
3   A reflexive investigator, who has experienced this unfamiliar cultural space and has dialogued with its practitioners, can portray this cultural space and its people in a provisionally accurate manner (Foley, 2002; p. 472–473).

However, as soon as Viessière (2011) started to write about his own em-beddedness and situatedness he came upon a block which he could not go past. That is, unless he was prepared to explore his own suffering, he could not proceed. This is what de Certeau (1984) was referring to when he stated that it was no good to proceed or write as if suffering were somewhere else; we are all implicated and enjoined by suffering.

Portraying the lived experience of people who suffer will therefore always be historical and call on ghosts of times past within one's self as well as within the people one is exploring with. Within these assumptions, reflexivity is described as

[T]he capacity of language and of thought – of any system of significa-tion – to turn or bend back upon itself, thus becoming an object to itself. Directing one's gaze at one's own experience makes it possible to regard oneself as "other". Through a constant mirroring of the self, one eventually becomes reflexive about the situated, socially constructed nature of the self, and by extension, the other. In this formulation, the self is a multiple, constructed self that it is always becoming and never quite fixed, and the ethnographic productions of such a self and the "cultural other" are always historically and culturally contingent....

Turning in on oneself in a critical manner tends to produce an awareness that there are no absolute distinctions between what is "real" and what is "fiction", between the "self" and the "other". Methodologically, this means that we are forced to explore the self-other relationships of fieldwork critically if we are to produce more discriminating, defensible interpretations.

(Foley, 2002; p. 473)

The belief that there are no absolute distinctions between what is real and fiction, between self and other, can be disturbing for some people. The qualities described above also carry hints of depersonalisation and this may be an abyss some people are not willing to enter.

There seems to be hints of depersonalisation in Viessière's writing, in his close encounter with suffering. By exploring his own complicity with re-producing empire, performing a reversal on usual discourses of alleviating suffering, Viessière (2011) comes to an existential aporia:

There is nothing left, at least nothing that I can *know* if I strip the ghosts and fetishes from my body, other bodies, and the world in which we have inflected meaning: I can "choose" to reject the ghosts and fetishes of Late-Capitalism, but then, there will be nothing left, no more meaning: there is no access to meaning beyond ghosts and fetishes.

(Viessière, 2011; p. 124; emphasis original)

This seems to be a description of the void, entered into by a close examination of one's self and the capitalist world in which we are all embedded, from a rationalist instrumentalist perspective. The fear of finding nothing at the bottom of these excursions is perhaps what underlies acts of resistance about reflexivity on the part of students and healthcare professionals and therefore what keeps them on the hamster wheel of the trans-national economy of desire, suffering and violence. Hence they are more predisposed to burnout and not able to respond to suffering. Fear of opening a Pandora's box through the key of examining one's own desires and linking these to suffering seems an entirely new notion about the political and pedagogical implications of reflexivity, albeit one that echoes Freire's (2000) pedagogy of the oppressed.

In this section of the symbiotic relationship between capitalism, race and trauma, we have explored the words used to describe the experiences of

PTSD, depersonalisation and burnout, as well as how these relate to suffering and medical training. The language of detachment during training seems to lend itself to depersonalisation and the encounter with the void and ghosts of racist empire. However, it is difficult to see how to counteract this move when there may be fear of and resistance to reflexivity and a return to one's self in students (thereby not finding one's self), faculty and clinicians alike. Paradoxically, existentialism may provide a light in the darkness, as offering an experience and affect that takes us beyond capitalists' cultural void by and through our desires if we are able to examine and discern amongst these for ghosts of the transnational economy of the empire. What we can know beyond these ghosts may mean returning to Indigenous health to see what we can learn.

6.5 Institutional racism

Earlier, in Section 6.3, we stated that Indigenous health in Australia is marred by substantially lower life expectancy and longer periods of ill-health comprising multiple chronic diseases such as diabetes, cardiovascular disease and chronic kidney disease compared with white Australians. Indigenous people have been subjected to horrific white Australians' government policies of extraction and removal and suffer terribly from this in terms of intergenerational trauma, PTSD and mental ill-health. Indigenous people are more likely to die in police custody and more likely to be arrested in the first place. Indigenous communities are marginalised and impoverished. Their situation is not unlike those described in Mendenhall's (2019) work on syndemic suffering where diabetes is seen as both a cause and effect of poverty, immigration, violence, depression and anxiety and abuse. The clustering of these conditions means that clinicians have to think critically about public health interventions and not oversell the individual behavioural interventions of diet and exercise, often to ill effect.

Considering individual behavioural interventions of diet and exercise in isolation from Black Anthropocene fault lines of consumerist culture means that suffering is interpreted via biomedical narratives of diabetes and blood pressure, which become further acts of violence. The violence comes from the language and tone of detachment and depersonalisation. The disease is extracted and abstracted from the context of peoples' lives. Given that health professionals are not trained nor encouraged in introspection, ideas around self, choice and agency tend to be fairly lightly understood and usually only in terms of compliance of an instrumentalist source of self.

However, such categories of self can be a source of institutional racism when assumptions are made about individuals' (abstracted from their social context) ability to adhere to behavioural interventions. Institutional racism is defined as differential access to the goods, services and opportunities by race, often evident as inaction in the face of need (Jones, 2000). Institutionalised racism creates an association between socioeconomic status and race, with race being a social construct that precisely captures the impact of racism, rather than a biological construct that reflects innate differences (Jones, 2000). Personally mediated racism refers to prejudice and discrimination, based on differential assumptions about the ability, motives and intentions of others based on race and differential action towards others according to race (Jones, 2000), for example, compliance with behavioural interventions. Internalised racism is internalisation by stigmatised races of white norms and rejection of their own cultural norms (Jones, 2000). Ideas of self therefore become complicated and undermining, as Singleton (2015) has shown in cultural melancholy.

Critical race theory in public health works to identify racial biases in the field to reduce health inequities (Ford & Airhihenbuwa, 2018). Four focus areas include contemporary race relations, knowledge production, conceptualisation and measurement of variables, and action. Each of these could be said to be lacking in UK medical schools. In some places the Black Lives Matter movement has created a window of opportunity for open critique of current inequalities in healthcare practices (Morse & Loscalzo, 2020): "Naming racism was one of the most important charges of the committee, and this challenge was sometimes met with defensiveness and silence" (p. 5). Clinical training has the potential to create a mindset that directly conflicts with the visions espoused by social movements. Such mindsets include those of urgency, a focus on short term goals and on fixing and curing, an expert identity with a distaste for being challenged, and risk aversion (Morse & Loscalzo, 2020).

Whereas a social movement based on transformation of mindsets requires long term vision, building power for enacting change over time rather than implementing rapid solutions, humility, a willingness to take chances despite uncertainty, and a learning mindset are what counts in the minds of people who are trying to enact change (Morse & Loscalzo, 2020). All these initiatives require building relationships founded on trust. For trust to develop there must be an acknowledgement of past trauma and how forms of knowledge production can perpetuate that trauma through denying sources of self and knowing that are not in mainstream medical education practices yet.

What this may mean is acknowledging and making suffering foundational to the curriculum as suggested in Chapter One. Knowledge production will be required to be more inclusive of critical race theory and streetwalker theory in the form of pilgrimages (Lugones, 2003). Understanding the role of affect in knowledge production is also important (Mahendran, 2020). All these suggestions to truly address inequities and injustices require a shift in thinking, of different ways of walking with suffering, through epistemological voids and veils and the echo of deep chasms. Trauma informed training that includes critical race theory is a must if inequities are not to be perpetuated by health professionals' inaction in the face of need. Understanding how categories may perpetuate inequities is the subject of the next section.

6.6 Epistemology of the suffering framework: experiential turn

PTSD as an example of the power of categorisation is examined in this section in order to demonstrate how constructs interact with relations of authority. This is not to deny the lived experience of people with PTSD as Young (1995) is at pains to point out; rather, it is to show how categories work to perpetuate inequities and the status quo. PTSD is a classification of distinct criteria whose defining feature is the etiological event (Young, 1995). The etiological event transforms non-specific symptoms into tokens of PTSD. In his anthropological research into treatment of Vietnam veterans, Young (1995) draws attention to the distinction between emotion and cognition – the faculty of knowing, perceiving and conceiving. Conventionally, emotion is positioned as opposite to cognition, a result of thinking rather than the cause. However, there are three interconnected components – a sensate element (affect), a behavioural element (action scripts, narratives) and a distinct cognitive element. Emotion foregrounds elements in the perceptual field producing cognitive work and meaning making. Emotions are organised around conception of self – both a psychological construct and a moral construct – with three features including the subject of experiences, locus of responsibility for and initiator of actions (Young, 1995).

The moral construct has relevance in situations where relations of authority dominate (Fiske, 1993; Haslam, 2012) (Table 1, Chapter One). A moral community and a moral economy develop and are used to instigate and perpetuate policies of extraction within a colonialist empire building. Moral superiority justifies the treatment and dehumanisation of people who are considered less than, and operates through categories of self, of who is considered a person, drawing on emotions of shame, guilt and anger (Young, 1995). These emotions, particularly a shared sense of shame, are at the centre of a moral community and economy. Shame and anger are connected by ideas and feelings about autonomy. Autonomy relies on the construct of choice and responsibility; when a person is deemed to lack capacity for autonomy, this is an injury to the self, and a loss of autonomy is seen as shameful (see Figure 6.2). These constructs could be seen to be operating in the film *Rabbit Proof Fence* when Molly was taken by the white men, to be shamed by categorisation, and then took autonomy by leaving and walking off into the bush.

These categories of self and associated notions of autonomy, responsibility and choice operate within healthcare, with the underlying emotions of shame, anger and guilt playing a role in the moral anguish described in the earlier part of the chapter. Similarly, the enactment of policies of removal relied on colonialist notions of moral superiority with the avoidance of shame by autonomous perpetrators and displacement onto indigenous people, with the result of much suffering.

Staying at the level of cognitive evaluation of self – a complex, symbolic, experiential, relational self embedded in a context – means that one's

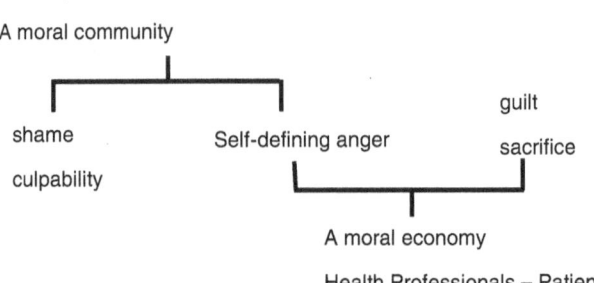

Figure 6.2 The deployment of the moral emotions at the centre (*Source: Adapted from* Young, 1995).

affective state is not made explicit (Kollareth et al., 2019). Experiences of shame involve a rational global negative self-evaluation as well as "an emotionally epistemic response that begins with (a) the sudden realisation (of which the subject may be unaware) that one is being seen (by the self or at least one other) as an aberrant member of one's epistemic community" and this may be accepted or rejected by both the subject and community (Mun, 2019; p. 27). Rational shame takes the form of instrumental rationality, epistemic rationality and evaluative rationality, related to decision-making, questions of truth and evidence, and justification in accordance with our personal values, respectively (Mun, 2019).

Experiences of shame are an emotion of self-assessment, logically entailed by a set of (normative) beliefs that are both the causes and the reasons for the holding of identificatory belief (Mun, 2019). This is an epistemic rationality about the truth of one's self. The experience of alterity, that shame always requires taking an outside perspective on one's self, means that shame is linked to depersonalisation. Drawing on the analogy of a mirror, Mun states:

> When standing in front of a fun house mirror, one sees a distorted image of oneself reflected back onto oneself. The distortion is an attribute of the mirror rather than the person who is reflected in the mirror. So, any subject's belief regarding the distorted image, other than the belief that the image is an image of the subject, would be about the mirror and not the subject.
>
> (Mun, 2019; p. 37)

However, in authoritarian relational contexts, the mirror of authority is likely to be internalised and disqualify the subject as a social rational agent. This affects our deep sense of self and identity by questioning our own sense of epistemic authority about ourselves and about the norms we share with our community. The valence of shame – whether it is seen as good or bad or somewhere in between – depends therefore on the context, on learning and critical dialogues to unpack what has happened (Candiotto, 2019).

Nietzsche presents shame as an affliction arising from humankind's attempts to renounce its instinctive and animal being (Herbert, 2019). This is particularly the case with Christianity, which suffers an excess of shame. Again, this can be seen in the film *The Rabbit Proof Fence*. Nietzsche opposed Schopenhauer, who believed that the empirical domain was nothing more than a phenomenal manifestation of an underlying reality, which he characterised as blind, insatiable will. This will was destined to remain in a state of unfulfilled desire, ceaseless striving and endless torment (Herbert, 2019). Affirming the will of desire brings both suffering and shame whilst making one complicit with the perpetuation of suffering:

> Christianity is the doctrine of the deep guilt of the human race by reason of its very existence, and of the heart's intense longing for salvation therefrom. That salvation, however, can be attained only by the heaviest sacrifices and by the denial of one's own self, hence by complete reform of man's nature.
>
> (Schopenhauer, 1966; p. 625; cited in Herbert, 2019; p. 122)

The tone of this piece of writing seems amply reflected in the white government policies enacted on Indigenous people and shown in the film *The Rabbit Proof* Fence. Herbert (2019) demonstrates how shame is inherently tied in with suffering and how we come to know ourselves in a community. The challenge is to withstand our own self-scrutiny without the need of comforting illusions. Shame is an important aspect of epistemology, but we need not be ashamed of ourselves when trying to recognise and appreciate life-affirming affects which have tended to be written out of medical discourses.

The challenge of self-scrutiny is enormous in an epistemology that seeks to know itself through reflexivity. Cartesian rationality withdraws into itself, to make itself the ground of all truth and being through a splitting of self, a refutation of embodiment and materiality, creating the affective and epistemological abyss between self and others (Levin, 1991). At the same time as enacting depersonalisation, there is also a grandiose sense of self-importance and uniqueness, defensive responses to perceived threats to integrity of a methodically reduced object-self which creates a deficient capacity for empathic responsiveness and social interaction (Levin, 1991). These ideas seem to trouble the notion of a double loop reflexivity (Foley, 2002) particularly in relation to Fareld's (2012) points about the recognition of the self as being more an experience of losing a part of the self in order to attain a self-relation, the self which does not find itself. Perhaps it is the instrumentalist self that does not find itself.

The trouble with self-scrutiny is perhaps mitigated by an embodied sense of self. A rationality grounded in a dialectic of socialisation and individuated self advocated by Merleau Ponty where the roots of justice are always already inherent in the body's order and need for relationships, reciprocity and mutual recognition, in the mirror of the flesh. Therefore we feel injustice in our body and being, as an affect: "it is the *logos* that is articulated in the transpositions and reversibilities of perception, and that constitutes, thereby, our initiation into the justice of reciprocity" (Levin, 1991; p. 72; emphasis original). It is therefore the body that resists forms of subjection and violence, as well as experiencing desire and will, that provides a level of reality against the nothingness of the instrumentalist self. Where domination prevails over principles of mutual recognition and participatory justice, there is a requirement to understand further how categories of self perpetuate these kinds of domination through transcendence. This necessitates a validation of pre-conceptual pre-categorical understanding of the reciprocity necessary for justice. The only way to do that seems to be to include experience and a pedagogy of encounter.

The epistemological dilemma of medical training is that it tends to produce people who seem slightly removed from the rest of the population (Sinclair, 1997), in the belief that they need to be, to do what they have to do; yet they then need to advise those people on how to live their lives whilst in all probability suffering from the effects of their training and practice without having the means to describe this. This dilemma can produce moments of intensity in practice. Moments of intensity in practice can mean the heightened awareness of sensations and affects which can profoundly alter the meaning and understanding of the encounter (Mahendran, 2020). These moments of intensity are called ruptures in standard practice where established ways of thinking or practice are disturbed;

> The knowing that emerges from these unexpected encounters with real practice, powerful and enduring, is grounded in the *thisness* of the experience, whereas established bodies of knowledge, for example curriculum or clinical guidelines, represent forms of knowing that are abstracted from actual experiences of practice.
>
> (Mahendran, 2020; p. 9; emphasis original)

The traditional transcendence economy of health professional curricula sidesteps moral anguish and suffering; so that any rupture is necessarily internalised by the health professional.

Part of that internalisation is seen as a becoming undone in the uncertainty of the moment, where the self is risked in an attempt to grasp a strange experience: "The 'risk' relates to being forced to respond, act and think in ways that fracture the security of established knowledge and methods" (Mahendran, 2020; p. 10). The encounter is where the individual comes to know something through language, images or senses – a prehension – that is inescapable and unanticipated. The slowing down and suspension in that prehension of the encounter occurs in the speechlessness of experience, before language, logic and reflection kick in (Mahendran, 2020). Attention is paid to affective states, where the subject encounters practice in ways that are pre-cognitive and non-rational. The affective dimension of experience enables the subject to come to know the event (Mahendran, 2020). It could be that this is what is required for health professionals to understand suffering.

Mahendran (2020) defines affect as "unconsciously experienced forces that arise from and within our continuous encounters of the world, exceeding the emergence of feelings and emotions" (p. 24). Affects drive us to respond, think, feel, act and emote; they are the feeling of what happens (Damasio, 1999). Affect is somewhat ethereal but it can be thought of as a mood, an ennui. Health professionals are talking about affects when they tune in to patients, sensing where to pitch information before the patient has necessarily even spoken (Lowe et al., 2014). As such, affective forces are intensities, non-conscious (or pre-verbal) and prior to emotion – a surge of energy or a rush (Mahendran, 2020). These tiny eruptions or microshocks anticipate and prepare us for the unknown that is yet to come: "Our bodies act like *resonating chambers* for the emerging affects that flow from an encounter – and which constitute the context of the encounter – bringing about a change or difference to our lives" (Mahendran, 2020; p. 29; emphasis original). This in-bracing is preparation for a response, a bracing for the unknown, where bodies enfold the context of an encounter (Mahendran, 2020). Understanding at this embodied level must play a prime role when encountering suffering as it exemplifies the speechlessness of suffering; of what cannot be said.

When encountering suffering, a different way of being with people and ourselves is necessary. Mahendran (2020) suggests that during ruptures to practice, we use a "knowing on the inside as it emerges from within events of practice" (p. 36). This is a knowing which is immanent to events; that is existing, intrinsic, inherent, or operating and a philosophical notion explored by Kant, Hussel and Deleuze (Mahendran, 2020). Knowing on the inside requires a detranscendentalisation of knowledge:

> Let us posit, as Vattimo does (1994:100), a difference between epistemology, as "the construction of a body of rigorous knowledge and a solution of problems in the light of paradigms that lay down the rules for verifications of propositions" (which seem to correspond to Nietzsche's picture of the conceptual universe of a given culture) and hermeneutics, as "the activity that takes place during the encounter with different paradigmatic horizons, which do not allow themselves to be assessed on the basis of some kind of conformity (to rules, or in the final analysis, to the thing) but exist as 'poetic' proposals of other worlds, of the establishment of new rules."
>
> (Vattimo, 1997:79, cited in Eco, 2014; p. 580)

These new rules that need to be established are about how we know and the self that knows. That rather than conform to rules of an instrumentalist self we must understand how that self suffers as part of the self. The existence of suffering necessitates hermeneutic understanding. Eco (2014) suggests that there is a hardcore of being (p. 581) – not an essentialised kernel – but rather lines of resistances that render some of our approaches fruitless. That is, in suffering, the lines of resistance to an approach based on an instrumentalist source of self and rational logical form of enquiry may manifest as the desire not to be objectified in a task focused approach.

A pre-categorical pre-cognitive approach is therefore necessary to understanding suffering, to what is already given:

> Stating that there are lines of resistance simply means that, even if it appears as an effect of language, the World always presents us with something that is *already given* and not *posited* by us. What is *already given* are precisely the lines of resistance.
>
> (Eco, 2014; p. 584)

What is already given in healthcare is the likelihood of suffering which resists the techno-rationalist approach health professionals are trained in. A precategorical pre-cognitive approach moves backwards and forwards between what is already given, and what becomes constructed by us, a moving between the figure-ground of a techno-rationalist curriculum and the lived experience of the patient, where the forest is not lost for the trees. Suffering requires us to take on experience in the totality of the situation (Orange, 2011). She cites Kohut who states that "we are dealing with a psychological universe, with an introspectively and empathically grasped universe, and the abstractions are code words for that experienced psychological universe" (Kohut et al., 1996 cited in Orange, 2011; p. 197). Therefore we need both a technorationalist and hermeneutic understanding of practice.

Thinking about how to represent this thinking between the figure-ground in medical education, Mahendran (2020) draws on a metaphor of a waterfall to explain affect: standing within a waterfall represents the immanent nature of experience, flows of affect and emotion; whereas standing outside on the river bank as an observer is a more detached experience. There is another interpretation of this metaphor: that in addition to the observer on the river bank, the waterfall of affect, emotion or experience; there is also the rock behind the waterfall, core consciousness, the feeling of what happens, pre-categorical and pre-cognitive, that experiences all these different levels of participation and awareness. We move between all of these different levels and states, caught perhaps between a rock and a hard place, sometimes a detached depersonalised observer, sometimes flooded with affect. The movement between figure-ground perception is vital to acknowledge that suffering occurs in this context.

These ideas of knowing on the inside, lines of resistance, in-bracing, affect, shame, and guilt help prepare us for encounters with suffering and contain the process. Knowing that experiences may be characterised as a void, or abyss, or chasm or as echoes of former selves helps us to accompany people who are suffering as we have a context in which to place ourselves, the encounter and the process. Knowing that suffering takes place within a context of Black Anthropocene helps us not to shy away from immense suffering and may prevent us from enacting this in the future. These ways of knowing help form a container for not trying the fix the unfixable, but for accompaniment along the path of suffering.

6.7 Pilgrimages around conceptual aspects of suffering framework

Behar (1996) suggests that we put ourselves in the way of a culture which bodies forth and enmeshes us, especially when "we feel complicitous with structures of power, or helpless to release another from suffering, or at a loss as to whether to act or observe" (p. 6). "To write vulnerably is to open a Pandora's box" (p. 11) where forms of knowing are no longer easily separable in a dialectic between connection and otherness, between selves, in the service of justice: this is a hard path to take. To provide some structure to taking this path, I draw on MacFarlane (2013; 2018), Lugones (2003) and the mythopoetic curriculum (Leonard & Willis, 2010).

MacFarlane (2013) offers some suggestions on walking as a way of knowing, building on non-Western cultures who see footfall as knowledge with Canadian terms for "knowledge" and "footprint" being used interchangeably. MacFarlane (2013) cites Wittengenstein who saw footlines of enquiry, with ideas that have been brought into being by means of motion along a path. Then of course there are the Indigenous Australian's vision of the songlines: oral history that connects places and creation narratives with ritual – the labyrinth of invisible pathways which meander all over Australia and that provide a source of escape from colonialist policies.

Learning is to follow a track (MacFarlane, 2013). He states the Spanish palindrome on the subject of pilgrimage "*La ruta nos aportó otro paso natural* – The path provides the natural step" (p. 277), a chiasmic form which acknowledges the transformative consequences of the foot pilgrimage of the mind turning back on itself returning the traveller to their origin, so that the pilgrim is at the same time unchanged as well as profoundly redirected. By walking the path, the pilgrim accessed the "keyless chamber of the brain" (p. 341) through instinct and body, knowing in ways the conscious mind cannot. Learning in this way was through atmospheres or metereologies of the mind. A model of thought, of self, not as something rooted in place and growing steadily over time. But as a shifting set of properties complemented and depleted by our passage through the world.

This embodied knowing is a function of displacement and mobility, in contrast to dwelling and belonging; where the world acts upon our senses, to draw us out beyond our thinking. Both perplexing and perforating, the world acts on us by pressing upon and into our bodies (MacFarlane, 2013). This is where the body is the first boundary with the world, even though our walking thinking may extend out into the world along these paths of learning. These are different ideas about ourselves and the world, in stark contrast to rational forms of belonging and dwelling, of roles and selves that congeal in moral anguish of fusion by precipitous circumstances of the civic nature. The displacement and mobility are forms of efficacious meanderings that offer alternatives to categories that congeal (Lather, 1991). This may be what Hollis (1996) is meaning when he believes that Antigone offers a category of self that secures a precarious space between the social factors and the inner world, as a response to suffering.

Efficacious meanderings in a precarious space along wandering lines (de Certeau, 1984) means experiencing a crossing over, a chiasma, in order to access the keyless chambers of the mind (MacFarlane, 2013). In this Black Anthropocene era, a key has been suggested as that of looking at our desires that enjoin us to be complicit with a consumerist society (Viessière, 2011). Keyless chambers of the brain, or perhaps a Pandora's box, have been feared for the ghosts they will loosen based on colonialist categorisation of humans by gender, race and poverty. The fear of facing the void of suffering, the salt lake of the landscape, where there seems to be nothing else, from a rationalist sense, denies the embodied affects and knowing from the inside. Moral constructs of the colonialist era helped to create this void and deny the plurality of selves and knowing.

The void of what white settlers in Australia call a "hideous blank," "the same dreadful dreary, dismal desert" (MacFarlane, 2016), is to Indigenous people a lived experience, of seeing much more, naming, mythologizing; in short, creating and inhabiting an epistemology of their own. Putting words to what we see as the void or abyss of suffering is a way of walking with suffering. "Walking becomes a means to a certain kind of knowledge – one of the constituents of which is an awareness of ignorance" (MacFarlane, 2016; p. 240). Walking with mindfulness with a focus on the details anchors perceptions in a context of vastness which is sometimes what the landscape of suffering can feel like. Using touch or haptic sense to know the world enables us to live all the way through suffering.

Walking in this way means also streetwalking, crossing over, to go through the confines of the normal (Lugones, 2003). This means hanging out in subjectivity as a strategic tactic: "The streetwalker theorist keeps both logics in interpretation but valorises the logic of resistance as she inhabits differentiated geographies carrying with others contestatory meanings to praxical completion" (Lugones, 2003; p. 218). *La Callejera*, the streetwalker, senses both the reality and the fiction of meanings and spaces which become concrete as they are crisscrossed by a multiplicity of meanings.

Streetwalker theorizing is an embodied practice of sustained intersubjective attention: oppressions are "not merely an ideological mechanisms, but the categorial training of human beings into homogenous fragments grounded in categorial mind frame" (Lugones, 2003; p. 223). Disentangling the hold of coupling of oppressions means perceiving and resisting oppressions as intermeshed, by cultivating a multiplicity and depth of perception and connection, sustained even in the midst of the concrete. *La Callejera* knows how to survive by uncovering, considering, learning and passing on knowledge of multiple tools of tactical strategists through deep spatio-temporal insights into the social (Lugones, 2003).

Lugones (2003) constructs the self subject as "I-we" – as both semi-solitary "I" and embedded in the social "we." However, she resists the seductive notions of collective sense making:

> There is no common language, no common expectations, no reason to assume trustworthiness, no comfortable womb-warm sense of safety and of having come home. What prompts one is a risk-full sense of opportunities, of possibilities, to be rendered artfully concrete, imminently social, insidiously and positively pragmatic.
>
> (Lugones, 2003; p. 229)

She warns against demanding equality, respect and justice without the realisation that these demands, within a particular dominant construal of sense, are mechanisms congruent with fragmentation and domination.

Lugones (2003) maintains that streetwalker theorists persevere with conscious critical resistance with uncertainty:

> Concepts, ways of doing things, institutions, values that conceptually, materially, and politically determine, decree, regulate, and justify oppression submerge, surround, inundate, constitute, circumscribe the streetwalker theorist. They form a deep, invisible, framework, encasing every move and gesture, every justification. The streetwalker theorist must break out of these "confines of the normal". These confines are the background and texture of the lonely, genial, unaccompanied, self-important, "self-made" subjectivity that constitutes modern agency. ... The streetwalker asks over and over again: Within which conceptual, axiological, institutional, material set of limitations is the meaning of the possible being construed?
>
> (Lugones, 2003; p. 231)

This may seem a very difficult path to tread in the confines of a structured environment of medicine and healthcare in order for health professionals to rescue a sense of themselves from the institutionalisation that occurs. Knowing how we know in a spatio-temporal sense means understanding how concrete concepts through to narratives, metaphors, symbols and abstraction form our paths of learning within the context of the Black Anthropocene. Once we are aware of the how measurement, categorisation, patterns, models and schemata are devised to support the status quo, we can move around in an embodied sense attending to the unknown in service of suffering.

The self formation in this case is in working in the crossover, the chiasma, in service of suffering and justice yet not wanting to add to injustice by being complicit with consumerism and the Black Anthropocene. Working with suffering means working with affect and emotion, and that includes the imaginal – of symbols and images from the imagination. There is just no way around this. To be able to work with suffering, as a human and a health professional, one has to be available to different ways of experiencing and surviving. Sometimes the only way through a crisis and extreme suffering is to hold onto an image, produced perhaps by the unconscious that will enable us to survive. Sustaining the ethic of the social contract implicit in professionalism requires more than a technical or rational understanding of the rules and values inherent in such a contract. Commitment to this ethic arises fundamentally from a deep sense of self, from attention to less conscious and visible forces brewing within (Dirkx, 2010; p. 66).

The romantic expressivism of the self combined with streetwalker tactics and strategies make for a dynamic and creative role of the unconscious or core self walking with extended consciousness. Focusing on embodiment, emplacement and enactment of knowledge, of knowing bodies, is challenging but necessary in response to the homelessness that pure reason teaches:

> When teachers step out from behind the façade of consistency, certainty, and coherence that has taken on almost sacred importance in modern pedagogies, even for a moment, they may initiate productive forms of confusion that can bring into empathetic inquiry the myth at the core of modern reason.
>
> (Davison, 2010; p. 53)

These are the sorts of strategies and practices that must be taken, whilst remaining critically aware, alongside traditional healthcare professional training if we are to begin the unbegun places of living; to know how to be with suffering.

In fact, in the shadow of hope, Bishop (2010) writes that multiple ways of knowing, valuing and imagining are necessary to go beyond traditional stereotypical teaching. The type of imagination required is more profound that just a faculty of individual creativity because it is rooted in suffering and therefore must be critical: "Studies of genocide and trauma gesture in the direction of imagination" and "Reconciliation, as a social process aims to break the cycle of revenge and heal the effects of traumatic events that produce guilt, anxiety, resentment and injustice" (Bishop Leonard 2010; p. 32). A reconciliation imagination takes on the formidable difficulties of acknowledgement and forgiveness "It was not my strength that needed nursing ... it was my imagination that wanted soothing" (Gourevitch, 1998; p. 7). A mythopoetic curriculum re-mythologises Western systems of knowledge and finds ways that do not replicate nor serve the system of oppression to be overcome (Bishop, 2010). By situating itself in the underbelly or shadow of the dominant culture, mythopoetics turns to depths of images, to insearch, for deeper meaning in the face of suffering:

> In the emancipatory praxis informed by postcolonial and critical theory, the shadow side, or suffering and oppression, form an insistent matrix of daily life against which and from the struggle occurs. There is a dialectic between, on the one hand grief-outrage and a kind of mourning-melancholy, and, on the other, a struggle for hope.
>
> (Bishop, 2010; p. 37)

This means including disturbing emotions, memories, responsibilities and a lack of closure. But without doing this, we lose the possibility of finding a portal through gross injustice, suffering and oppression.

The imaginal work does not shy away from images of fear, loss and grief as we are forced to descend through these: "the modern curse is the loss of a doorway into the imaginal realm, plus forgetting that such a doorway and such a realm even exist" (Bishop, 2010; p. 40). The imaginal stimulates latent but inherent qualities of the mind to find a way through, to find out what else is possible. This may mean drinking in some darkness so that not only can we begin to see, but we also become visible to others and ourselves (Bishop, 2010). There are many different types of imaginal knowing (Bishop, 2010; Ochieng, 2018) but whatever forms are drawn upon, they must address twin concerns of social justice and reflexive self-transformation.

The mythopoetic curriculum is therefore, at the same time, both de-mythologizing and demystifying, as well as deliteralizing. Demythologizing or interpretive approaches work on meaning, an ontological process of understanding and interpreting the world as it is experienced. Demystifying or critical approaches work on understanding how knowledge as theory is generated and used to serve particular human interests to reduce illusion (Holland & Garman, 2010). Both are required for a complete range of vision and adequate depth perception.

> Mythic knowledge derives from the unconscious self in wordless communication with its own apprehension of the elemental human life force; it is a sensing of sacred truth about the human experience.
>
> (Holland & Garman, 2010; p. 17)

The power of transforming reality into awareness of reality, the becoming aware of things as they are – of health professional trainings and practice as they are – is considered the minimum basis for imagination. But this requires an act of mind, in which is borne the principle of form or order. This is in turn prompted by an inner violence of consciousness emerging, as all the while the mind resists and arrests the awareness of reality. Individual and social responsibility for suffering is therefore about containing overwhelm by the violence of consciousness emerging and the provision or realisation of a context to reach a greater understanding.

6.8 Pedagogy of suffering

Suffering is what can not be said, the unspeakable, experiencing yourself on the other side of life as it should be, and distress that threatens the intactness of the self (Frank, 2001). Suffering is an understorey to the main business of healthcare because it is rarely spoken about either to or with patients or between health professionals. The dimensions of suffering include that between self and other and another between languishing and acting. In the experience of suffering there may be a fear of being misunderstood and a concomitant withdrawal from the world resulting in isolation. Being left with unbearable feelings and not having the words to articulate these instigates self-doubt and judgment. The loss of language requires us to use the imaginal to communicate. The eliminated may come back in disguise in the form of PTSD, Depersonalisation and burnout.

This work stitches together understandings from the field of medical humanities, sociology and medical education arguing that an interdisciplinary approach is necessary to understand suffering that is both individually experienced and socially constructed. In this way, the work is unique because it goes beyond responses that traditionally are located in one discipline or another: in education, pedagogy of the oppressed (Freire, 2000) is the seminal work on suffering yet there is little about the lived embodied phenomenological experience; there is work on a pedagogy of compassion (Gilbert & Mascaro, 2017; Worline & Dutton, 2017) but at the same time there is also a compassion gap in both higher education and healthcare (Waddington, 2016):

> But what are we doing about the compassion gap in universities that educate the people who go on to be the professionals who work in the NHS? The nurses, doctors, social workers and psychologists? If they don't experience a compassionate learning environment in universities it's no surprise that there is a compassion gap in practice!
>
> (Waddington, 2016; p. 1)

Medicine and social justice are the two main sources of addressing suffering yet the impact of these sources is mitigated by the profound upswell of suffering due to global pandemics, climate change, economic mismanagement, wars, terrorism, the displacement of millions of people and natural disasters. How can medical humanities help to understand and live with immense suffering?

Medical humanities has a natural affinity with compassion, as a way of understanding the human condition in its many forms through art, film, drama and literature. Compassion as "a sensitivity to suffering in self and others with a commitment to try and alleviate and prevent it" (Gilbert, 2017; p. 11) means attending to distress and having courage to do so. However, there is a difficulty because much of the success of medicine has been through a focus on biomedical components at the expense of the patient experience (Gilles, 2018). Yet the biomedical components also arose as a response to suffering. Medication and surgery are interventions that address suffering by relieving pain, inflammation and other disease processes. The biomedical focus relies on categorisation and conceptualisation to function. And some of these conceptualisations and categorisations are inherent to the perception of inequalities in health. Moreover, a focus on these types of conceptualisations has obscured the consumerism, individualism and scientific reductionism that has impoverished thinking of students as well as faculty within universities (Gilles, 2018).

Unless these drivers are acknowledged, then, it is difficult to see how we can truly be compassionate with patients when all the time health professional training and practice perpetuates the status quo. Compassion as an approach has competencies, social mentalities and motivations, as well as an overall meta level of reflection, that is self-referential and could find a home in medical humanities, yet it is not often included in medical humanities' compendiums. Compassion can determine how to reflect on and learn to take action with a deeper focus into the nature of reality (Gilbert, 2017). Deep listening and attending to another person is also another hallmark of compassion (Epstein, 2017). The self-referential nature of the reflexive turn means that both self and other are included in the approach and action (White, 2017). However, compassion must go further conceptually to understand suffering and how this is perpetuated racially and stereotypically in communities through adherence to specific types and sources of self.

However, medical humanities could help in crossing the lacunae of suffering by thinking differently about how we think about suffering. This is a craft – an exploration of depth and breadth of the body as sensorium and an attunement; an art – because it is an adventure on the very outer edges and limits of imagination across different cultures and races; and a praxis because it enjoins mind-body-social context (Ochieng, 2018). A pedagogy of suffering could therefore crafted on some basic principles:

1   To address epistemic injustice, different forms of knowing must be made explicit with the abject specifically named.

2   Critical race theories about and understanding of Black Anthropocene capitalism and post-colonial impact on suffering must form the foundation of health professional curricula.
3   Semantic expressions, classification and categorisation of knowledge must be explicit to show how concepts, schemata, patterns and models served the colonialist project.
4   The causal problematic must be enlarged to include dispositions, syndemic suffering and relational theory; to demonstrate how responses to suffering are mediated by contextual social forms of relation.
5   The epistemic break between life, death and suffering must be made explicit.
6   The medical matrix must be shown as to how it contributes to suffering in a way that implicates clinicians with patients in a shared suffering.
7   The suffering self must be envisioned as the self in order to include the experience within how we know what we know.
8   The best kind of curriculum as preparation for times of psychological and ethical duress is one that affords participants the ability to stay with as much as their experience as possible.
9   Suffering as gendered must be included in any analysis to know how people respond to and suffer differently.

Therefore some aims for a pedagogy of suffering curriculum could be the following:

1   To acknowledge how concepts of suffering are perpetuated by power differentials and honour that in order to demonstrate response-ability.
2   To recognise ruptures and reversals in knowledge, narratives and the social life.
3   To recognise the impact of moral anguish of fusion of self and role, and consequent exposure of self.
4   To identify one's own wandering lines within institutional structures/matrix.
5   To not be afraid of one's own solitude as an antidote to hungry ghost-isms.

Further information is in Appendix 1 on how to conceptualise a curriculum based on these principles and aims.

   Drawing on critical race theory to make explicit the use of assumptions, concepts, measurements, patterns and models in knowledge production is a way to directly address suffering in the training of health professionals. By being able to call into question the way we use knowledge and concepts, often to other's detriment, we may be able to envision a new way of practice. This will not be simple or straightforward.

6.9 Racial disparities in COVID-19 morbidity and mortality

The striking feature of the COVID-19 pandemic is how, in the UK and US, the disease prevalence and severity has highlighted already existing inequities in health particularly for the Black, Asian and Minority Ethnic (BAME) communities in London and beyond (Apea et al., 2020; Aldridge et al., 2020; Khunti et al., 2020; Thebault et al., 2020; Resnick et al., 2020). There have been various suggestions about why this may be so from biological risk factors such as a heightened inflammatory response or pre-existing health conditions to environmental and institutional racism as well as poverty and deprivation (Apea et al., 2020). It is difficult to think about this form of suffering without reinforcing race as a discriminatory category, yet when the categories used to classify patients in the NHS are scrutinised, they can be seen to be so broad and indeterminant that there seems to be little discernment as to what is actually happening. Categories are contested as reinforcing discrimination or of speaking to something that does not actually exist (Mallon, 2006; Shea, 2019). The risk of essentialising the experience of minority groups in the service of highlighting inequities and suffering has been debated (Platt & Nandi, 2020). The limitations of the existing categories are that they themselves send messages about key social divisions, racial thinking and hierarchies and have little relation to how people view their own identities. Any categories in use have to be scrutinised as to the function they perform and to assist in defining further categories that are more meaningful for the question being asked (Platt & Nandi, 2020). This scrutinisation requires us to be aware of our own cognitive and affective processes in the choices we make in a meta-analytic process.

In teaching research on critical race identity, the meta cognitive and meta affective strategies were identified from student reflections as follows:

- honest self-awareness and articulation of flawed self-assessments
- ability to see and name what one didn't previously know
- metacognitive awareness, or self-knowledge
- self-awareness of feelings with/about the generalisations and assumptions made
- self-awareness of feelings
- setting aside self-judgment so it won't derail the learning process
- ability to contextualise information and see it from a larger perspective
- ability to tolerate discomfort in order to learn so I don't run from the discomfort, but rather embrace it and try to acknowledge and understand what triggers certain emotions/thoughts (Chick et al., 2009).

These strategies were challenging and required insight into one's own behaviour. However, it is difficult to see how anything other than these sorts of metacognitive strategies can be used when working with people who suffer.

In learning to think differently about how we think about suffering, we know that although there are relationships and tensions between self and other; there are different sources of self and hence different perceptions of self and other – a moral dyad of intentional agent and a suffering moral patient (Gray et al., 2012) – between health professional and patient. A health professional may be operating more from an instrumentalist sense of self due to their role and may suffer from a moral anguish due to a fusion of self and role, when a person can't separate out the both but feel a need to act on a more humane level. A patient may feel a lack of trust, a need to not be objectified, and have a sense of being part of a fiction when that does occur. Responses to suffering affect a person's identity and sense of self. All of these factors form a cognitive and affective template for future experiences. How we think and feel about that template is a metacognitive strategy that has moral and professional identity implications.

Most health professionals have little training, experience in or awareness of metacognition in relation to themselves or their practice. This becomes challenging when considering issues to do with race and institutional racism. Students struggle with being able to reconcile taught biological information (on risk factors for disease), with social determinants of health: racism and discrimination, for example. The struggle is around accepting that both can be true at the same time, that both biological and social factors are implicated in the disease process, biological categories are created to analyse phenomena but are themselves products of meaning of the social context. "Broad population categories can be discerned genetically when enough polymorphisms are analysed … so these categories are not devoid of biological meaning" (Jorde & Wooding, 2004; p. S31). But these classifications are thought to be due more to ancestry and geography, and ancestry is not equivalent to race. The difficulty comes when instead of being able to stand back and see how the biological and social contribute to the disease process in a syndemic, students and health professionals feel forced to choose one over the other in the process of becoming a health professional.

Students, for example, fear not adhering to National Institute for Health and Care Excellence (NICE) guidelines for consequences from professional bodies and detrimental outcomes for patients. These issues are of course extremely important. However, these issues also form a stumbling block to see the forms of institutional racism that are being perpetuated and to perform a metacognitive analysis of the situation. Naturally, they will want to adhere to guidelines as part of their professional practice. Yet part of their professional practice is also about tailoring information to specific patients and their circumstances as well as being discerning in their thinking. Using racial categories as a heuristic for treatment decision making may not be appropriate and may perpetuate discrimination: "an individual's population affiliation would often be a faulty indicator of the presence or absence of an allele related to diagnosis or drug response" (Jorde & Wooding, 2004; p. S32). Nongenetic factors play a role in susceptibility to disease and response to medication as well. Health professionals' focus on the biological aspects of disease means that the social performative aspect of medicine then disappears from view.

To relate these considerations to the recent disparities in death rates from COVID-19 by ethnic groups, the question must be asked, "how does race as a concept work at a metacognitive level to explain these differences?" The concept of race works at both the object level and the meta level of understanding psychological cognitions and affects (Shea, 2019). At the object level of categorisation, while there is perhaps a biological meaning, there is no distinct category of race except for the socially constructed ones (Mallon, 2006); "Connecting these two issues – the metaphysics of race and the permissibility or desirability of 'race' talk – requires some argument" (p. 527). Social constructionist accounts of race argue that there is no such thing as race but admit that "race" talk exists:

> One might coherently hold, for example, that racial labels and concepts do not refer but that we should continue to use them anyway because the practical benefits are so great. Or alternatively, one might think that racial labels and concepts do refer but we ought not use them because we risk being misunderstood as legitimating oppression.

> If, for example, we decide that the use of 'race' talk is deeply oppressive, no argument to the effect that such talk refers to a biological population or a social construction would be of sufficient weight to merit the continuation of this practice. In contrast, if we decided that the use of 'race' talk is morally required, or carries enormous epistemic benefits, skeptical arguments that racial terms do not strictly speaking, refer to anything would be appropriately ignored in deciding how we use these terms.
>
> (Mallon, 2006; p. 549–50)

The trouble then arises because on the one hand, activitists argue that there is no such thing as essentialised racial categories in order to halt oppressive practices. On the other hand, categories of race are used to defend oppressed people who have been historically categorised and oppressed in this way. This is being played out at the moment in relation to COVID-19 deaths and disparities.

While the semantic and metaphysical aspects of race talk are evident, they don't address the real pragmatic effects of racism:

> there is profound disagreement over the practical and moral import of 'race' talk. Resolving this disagreement requires a complex

assessment of many factors, including, the epistemic value of 'race' talk in various domains, the benefits and costs of racial identification and of the social enforcement of such identification, the value of racialized identities and communities fostered by 'race' talk, the role of 'race' talk in promoting or undermining racism, the benefits or costs of 'race' talk in a process of rectification for past injustice, the cognitive or aesthetic value of 'race' talk, and the degree of entrenchment of 'race' talk in everyday discourse. The point is that it is on the basis of these and similar considerations that the issue of what to do with 'race' talk will be decided.

(Mallon, 2006; p. 550)

Medicine has been practised based on differentiation through race (Seth, 2018). Differentiation is a primary dynamic cognitive process that produces social effects and which was used for specific purposes during colonialism. Socially derived categories have been used to describe disparities in infection rates, disease outcomes, treatment and deaths from COVID-19 in the UK but these do not hold in other countries where contact tracing has been used aggressively based on previous experiences with pandemics (Moore, 2020).

Inequities in death from COVID-19 between different ethnic groups and the suffering involved in that is perhaps more a reflection of a syndemic of suffering that reflects the history of colonialism (Mendenhall, 2019). On the one hand, there is little genetic evidence for differences in ethnicity and as to why there should be differences in death rates. On the other hand, many people are saying that the differences are due to racism and discrimination, which is hard to conceptualise and may only reinforce oppressive categories. Health professionals get caught up in the middle of this with policies, guidelines and professional mandates. Getting caught up in this maelstrom is stressful when working with patients who are dying from what could be seen as preventable because of the helplessness to make any difference. There is no place to be in the middle of this, to make a difference. Knowing about the allostatic load due to racism links the biological and structural concepts together but does little to change the context (Allen et al., 2019). If we feel a sense of justice in our bodies, then we must feel the injustice, too. Categorisation of any sort has the potential to be dehumanising and depersonalising; people could feel like they are in a downward trauma spiral with the current state of affairs. There must be a way through this by the systematic scrutiny of policies and practices to ensure that they are not discriminatory. Thus whilst patients suffer directly from the effects of violence, discrimination, immigration and racism, health professionals caught between a professional identity on the one hand and reacting to patients as humans can also suffer with them.

There is a trauma to being caught up in conflicting ideologies where choices have to be made and there are not the resources, will, energy or time to work through the necessary processes. This can contribute to burnout on the part of health professionals and further suffering on the part of patients. Thus, it is difficult to know what to say.

Box 6.1   Reflection

Given the difficulties and protracted nature of inequities in health which seem to have only been highlighted by the categorical imperative of colour, the question remains of how to address these inequities in a meaningful way that doesn't reinforce difference. Referring to our common nature as human beings runs the risk of whitewashing historical and cultural racism and thereby performing another disservice to people that have suffered. Yet the field of health is awash with inequities and Indigenous people know this. People speak of the "revolving white car syndrome" – I have heard this said in both Africa and Australia – where those in power visit communities briefly in their white landcruisers and then disappear off into the horizon again in a cloud of dust. Human rights agendas bestow the most benefit to those in charge and the institutions they represent, which are generally colonialist empire building monoliths.

Talking to a woman one day, she spoke of how she had been taken as a child to a hospital to mend her broken leg. She did not return to her family for four years. When she did return, it was too late as everything had changed in that time and she no longer had a place there. "You can't go back," she had stated.

To have spoken at that time about public health advice to increase walking and physical activity would have been to commit a violence against her obvious suffering. These moments can only be endured with each other, to come undone if necessary. To be prepared for the onslaught of emotions and affects in an ethical response for past traumas which continue to affect people in the present.

To be able to be with people as they are is a powerful act which can be restorative if trust and relationship are established. At the same time, there are enough saviours left in the world from missionary times that can continue to re-enact sacrifice and redemption if awareness is not kept. Keeping both eyes open as to the ways in which the archetypal saviour and hero myth is enacted perhaps through the sacrificial trope of the self is important in order not to re-enact colonialist fantasies. Being aware of likely projections and introjects is key whenever there is a charged situation. Getting closer to the intersection of the axes of self-other and languishing-acting means entering a zone of disorientation and destabilisation.

Questions for reflection

1   What acts as an anchor for you in the zones of potential disorientation and destabilisation?

---

2   What are your thoughts and beliefs about inequities in health and how do they affect your practice?
3   How do you work with categories and concepts – do you stand by them or do you have a more fluid relationship with them?
4   What have you sacrificed to be able to do your job?
5   How do you manage the emotional residue from that sacrifice?

Further Resources
Rebecca Solnit. 2017. *A Field Guide to Getting Lost*. Canongate Books: London.
Pray the Devil Back to Hell. 2008. A film by Abigail E. Disney and Gini Reticker
Latcho Drom. 1993. Film directed by Tony Gatlif.
MacFarlane. 2013. *The Old Ways: A Journey on Foot*. Penguin: London.

References

Abugel J. 2010. *Stranger to My Self. Inside Depersonalization: The Hidden Epidemic*. Johns Road Publishing: Virginia.

Aldridge R.W., Lewer D, Katikireddi S.V. et al. 2020. Black, Asian and Minority Ethnic groups in England are at increased risk of death from COVID-19: Indirect standardisation of NHS mortality data [version 1; peer review: Awaiting peer review] *Wellcome Open Research*; *88*:5. https://doi.org/10.12688/wellcomeopenres.15922.1.

Allen A.M., Wang Y., Chae D.H., Price M.M., Powell W., Steed T.C., Black A.R., Dhabhar F.S., Marquez-Magaña L., Woods-Giscombe C.L. 2019. Racial discrimination, the superwoman schema, and allostatic load: Exploring an integrative stress-coping model among African American women. *Annals of the New York Academy of Sciences*; *1457*:104–127.

Allen M., Donkin, A. 2015. The Impact of adverse experiences in the home on the health of children and young people, and inequalities in prevalence and effects. 48. Retrieved from http://cdn.basw.co.uk/upload/basw_13257-1.pdf

Anzaldúa G. 1999. *Borderlands La Frontera*; The New Mestiza. Aunt Lute Books: San Francisco.

Apea V.J., Wan Y.I., Dhairyawan R., Puthucheary Z.A., Pearse R.M., Orkin C.M., Prowle J.R. 2020. Ethnicity and outcomes in patients hospitalised with COVID-19 infection in East London: An observational cohort study. medRxiv 2020.06.10.20127621.

Australian Institute of Health and Welfare. 2019. *Australia's Welfare 2019 in Brief. Cat. No. AUS 227*. AIHW: Canberra.

Barad K. 2007. *Meeting the Universe Halfway: Quantum Physics and the Entanglement of Matter and Meaning*. Duke University Press Books: New York.

Behar R. 1996. *The Vulnerable Observer: Anthropology that Breaks Your Heart*. Beacon Press: Boston.

Bishop P. 2010. The shadow of hope: Reconciliation and imaginal pedagogies. Chapter 3 in Leonard T., Willis P. (eds). *Pedagogies of the Imagination: Mythopoetic Curriculum in Educational Practice.* Springer: Chicago.

Bleakely A. 2017. The perils and rewards of critical consciousness raising in Medical Education. Academic Medicine; 37(7):289–291.

Brideson T. 2004. Moving beyond a 'Seasonal Work Syndrome' in mental health: Service responsibilities for Aboriginal and Torres Strait Islander populations. *Australian e-Journal for the Advancement of Mental Health; 3*(3). www.auseinet.com.journal/vol3iss3/bridesoneditorial.pdf.

Brideson T., Kanowski L. 2004. The struggle for systematic 'adulthood' for Aboriginal Mental Health in the mainstream: The Djirruwang Aboriginal and Torres Strait Islander Mental Health Program. *Australian e-Journal for the Advancement of Mental Health; 3*(3). www.auseinet.com/jounral/vol3iss3/bridesonkanowski.pdf.

Brohi K., Vulliamy P., Marsden M., Carden R., Griffiths M., Bew D., Carver M. 2019. A Public Health Approach to Knife Violence Reduction: Immunize, Protect & Rescue. London Major Trauma System, February 2019. V.10. k.brohi@qmul.ac.uk.

Butler J.P. 2005. *Giving an Account of Oneself.* Fordham University Press: USA.

Butler J. 1993. *Bodies that Matter.* Routledge: New York.

Butler P., Campbell D., Siddique H. 2019. Not just schools: Five public service areas struggling with cuts. Guardian Newspaper. https://www.theguardian.com/society/2019/mar/08/not-just-schools-five-public-service-areas-struggling-with-cuts.

Candiotto L. 2019. The virtues of epistemic shame in critical dialogue. Chapter Four in Mun C. (ed). *Interdisciplinary Perspectives on Shame: Methods, Theories, Norms, Cultures and Politics.* Lexington Books: London.

Chick N., Karis T., Kernahan C. 2009. Learning from their own learning: How metacognitive and meta-affective reflections enhance learning in race-related courses. *International Journal for the Scholarship of Teaching and Learning.* http://www.georgiasouthern.edu/ijsotl 3(1) ISSN 1931-4744 @ Georgia Southern University.

Clarke P.A. 2007. Indigenous spirit and ghost folklore of "settled" Australia. *Folklore; 118*(2):141–161.

Courtois C.A., Ford J.D. 2009. *Treating Complex Traumatic Stress Disorders: An Evidence-based Guide.* The Guildford Press: New York.

CSDH 2008. *Closing the Gap in a Generation: Health Equity Through Action on the Social Determinants of Health. Final Report of the Commission on Social Determinants of Health.* Health Organisation: Geneva.

Commonwealth of Australia. 1997. Bringing them home. Report of the National Inquiry into the Separation of Aboriginal and Torres Strait Islander Children from Their Families.

Cook J. 2018. GMC unveils advice on safe reflection in wake of Bawa-Garba case. GP Online. https://www.gponline.com/gmc-unveils-advice-safe-reflection-wake-bawa-garba-case/article/1492585.

Coomber R., Moyle L. 2017. The changing shape of street-level heroin and crack supply in England: commuting, holidaying and cuckooing drug dealers across 'county lines'. *British Journal of Criminology.* doi: 10.1037/a45d7867.

Corbett R. 2016. *You Must Change Your Life: The Story of Rainer Maria Rilke and Auguste Rodin*. W.W. Norton & Company Ltd: London.

Cunningham N., Savage M. 2017. An intensifying and elite city: New geographies of social class and inequality in contemporary London. *City*; 21(1):25–46. doi: 10.1080/13604813.2016.1263490.

Damasio A. 2010. *Self Comes to Mind. Constructing the Conscious Brain*. Vintage Books: London.

Damasio A. 1999. *The Feeling of What Happens: Body, Emotion and the Making of Consciousness*. Vintage: London.

Davison A. 2010. Myth in the practice of reason: The production of education and productive confusion. Chapter Four in *Pedagogies of the Imagination: Mythopoetic Curriculum in Educational Practice*. Leonard T., Willis P. (eds). Springer: Chicago.

Dean W., Talbot S.G., Caplan A. 2020. Clarifying the language of clinician distress. *JAMA*; 323(10):923–924.

De Certeau M. 1984. *The Practice of Everyday Life*. University of California Press: California.

Devisch I., Vanheule S., Deveugele M. Nola I., Civaner M., Pype P. 2017. Victims of disaster: Can ethical debriefings be of help to care for their suffering? *Medical Health Care and Philosophy*; 20:257–267.

Dirkx J.M. 2010. Care of the self: Mythopoetic dimensions of professional preparation and development. Chapter Five in *Pedagogies of the Imagination: Mythopoetic Curriculum in Educational Practice*. Leonard T., Willis P. (eds). Springer: Chicago.

Eades S.J. 2000. Reconciliation, social equity and Indigenous Health. *Medical Journal of Australia*; 172:468–469.

Eco U. 2014. *From the Tree to the Labyrinth: Historical Studies on the Sign and Interpretation*. Harvard University Press: New York.

Elliott-Farrelly T. 2004. Australian aboriginal suicide: The need for an Aboriginal suicidology? *Australian e-Journal for the Advancement of Mental Health*; 3(3). www.auseinet.com/journal/vol3iss3/elliottfarrelly.pdf Downloaded 9th June, 2005 4.

Ellis R. 2000. Inequalities in health - The twelfth national health promotion conference. *Aboriginal and Islander Health Worker Journal*; 24(6):25–31.

Emmerson G. 2007. *Ego State Therapy*. Crown House Publishing: Carmarthen.

Epstein R. 2017. *Attending: Medicine, Mindfulness, and Humanity*. Scribner: New York.

Fareld V. 2012. The *re-* in recognition: Hegelian returns. *Distinktion: Scandinavian Journal of Social Theory*; 13(1):125–138.

Felitti V.J. 2019. Origins of the ACE study. *American Journal of Preventive Medicine*. doi:10.1016/j.amepre.2019.02.011.

Felitti V.J., Anda R.F., Nordenberg D., Williamson D.F., Spitz A.M., Edwards V., ... Marks J.S. 1998. Relationship of childhood abuse and household dysfunction to many of the leading causes of death in adults: The Adverse Childhood Experiences (ACE) Study. *American Journal of Preventive Medicine*, 14(4): 245–258.

Fisher J. 2017. *Healing the Fragmented Selves of Trauma Survivors: Overcoming Internal Self-alienation*. Routledge: London.

Fiske A.P. 1993. *Structures of Social Life: The Four Elementary Forms of Human Relations*. The Free Press: New York.

Foley D.E. 2002. Critical ethnography: The reflexive turn. *Qualitative Studies in Education*; 15(5):469–490.

Ford C.L., Airhihenbuwa C.O. 2018. Commentary: Just what is critical race theory and what's it doing in a progressive field like public health? *Ethnicity & Disease*; 28(Suppl 1):223–230. doi:10.18865/ed.28.S1.223.

Forgash C., Copeley M. (Eds). 2008. *Healing the Heart of Trauma and Dissociation with EMDR and Ego State Therapy*. Springer Publishing Company: New York.

Frank A.W. 2001. Can we research suffering? *Qualitative Health Research*; 11(3): 353–362.

Freire P. 2000. *Pedagogy of the Oppressed*. 30th Anniversary Edition. The Continuum International Publishing Group Ltd.: New York

Gilbert P. 2017. Compassion: Definition and controversies. In *Compassion: Concepts, Research and Applications. Gilbert P. (ed)*. pp. 3–15. Routledge: London.

Gilbert P., Mascaro J. 2017. Compassion Fears, Blocks and Resistances: An Evolutionary Investigation. In *The Oxford Handbook of Compassion Science. Seppala E., Simon-Thomas E., Brown SL., Worline SL., Cameron CD., Doty JR. (eds.)*, pp. 399–418. Oxford University Press: New York.

Gilles J. 2018. Compassion, medical humanities and medical education. *Education for Primary Care*; 29(2):68–70.

Gourevitch P. 1998. *We Wish to Inform You that Tomorrow We Will be Killed with Our Families: Stories from Rwanda*. Farrar, Strauss & Giroux: New York.

Gray K., Young L., Waytz A. 2012. Mind perception is the essence of morality. *Psychological Inquiry*; 23(2):101–124.

Haslam N. (Ed). 2012. *Relational Models Theory: A Contemporary Overview*. Routledge: London.

Hill D. 2008. *The Forgotten Children: Fairbridge Farm School and Its Betrayal of Britain's Child Migrants to Australia*. Random House Australia: Sydney.

Herbert D.R. 2019. Nietzsche, shame and the seal of liberation. Chapter Six in *Interdisciplinary Perspectives on Shame: Methods, Theories, Norms, Cultures and Politics*. Mun C. (ed). Lexington Books: London.

Herman J.L. 2001. *Trauma and Recovery: From Domestic Abuse to Political Terror*. Pandora: London.

Hinch B.T. 2014, Aug 1. Adult implications of childhood maltreatment. *Psychiatric Times*; 31(8):10.

Holmes E.A, Brown R.J, Mansell W, et al. 2005. Are there two qualitatively distinct forms of dissociation? A review and some clinical implications. *Clinical Psychology Review*; 25(1):1–23. doi:10.1016/j.cpr.2004.08.006.

Holland P.E., Garman N.B. 2010. Watching with two eyes: The place of the mythopoetic in curriculum inquiry. Chapter Two in *Pedagogies of the Imagination: Mythopoetic Curriculum in Educational Practice. Leonard T., Willis P. (eds)*. Springer.

Hollis M. 1996. Of masks and men. Chapter 10 in *The Category of Person: Anthropology, Philosophy, History. Carrithers M., Collins S., Lukes S. (eds).*, 216–233. Cambridge University Press: Cambridge.

Hooks B. 1994. *Teaching to Transgress: Education as the Practice of Freedom.* Routledge: New York.

Hughes K., Bellis M.A., Hardcastle K.A., Sethi D., Butchart A., Mikton C., ... Dunne M.P. 2017. The effect of multiple adverse childhood experiences on health: A systematic review and meta-analysis. *The Lancet Public Health;* 2(8):e356–e366. doi:10.1016/S2468-2667(17)30118-4.

Hunter E. 2004. Commonality, difference and confusion: Changing constructions of Indigenous mental health. *Australian e-Journal for the Advancement of Mental Health;* 3(3). www.auseinet.com/jounral/vol3iss3/huntereditorial.pdf.

Hunter E. 1993. *Aboriginal Health and History – Power and Prejudice in Remote Australia.* Cambridge University Press: Cambridge.

Jackson L.R., Ward J.E. 1999. Aboriginal health: Why is reconciliation necessary? *Medical Journal of Australia;* 170(3 May):437–440.

Jones C.P. 2000. Levels of racism: A theoretic framework and a gardener's tale. *American Journal of Public Health;* 90(8):1212–1215.

Jorde L.B., Wooding S.P. 2004. Genetic variation, classification and 'race'. *Nature Genetics Supplement;* 36(11):S28–S33.

Khunti K., Singh A.K., Pareek M., Hanif W. 2020. Is ethnicity linked to incidence or outcomes of covid-19? Preliminary signals must be explored urgently. *BMJ;* 369:m1548. doi: 10.1136/bmj.m1548.

Kohut H., Tolpin P., Tolpin M. 1996. *Heinz Kohut: The Chicago Institute Lectures.* Analytic Press: Hillsdale, NJ.

Kohut H. 1984. *How Does Analysis Cure?* University of Chicago Press: Chicago.

Kollareth D., Kikutani M., Russell J.A. 2019. Shame is a folk term unsuitable as a technical term in science. Chapter One in *Interdisciplinary Perspectives on Shame: Methods, Theories, Norms, Cultures and Politics.* Mun C. (ed). Lexington Books: London.

Kristeva J. 1982. *Powers of Horror – An Essay on Abjection.* Columbia University Press: New York.

Kumagai A.K., Lypson M.L. 2009. Beyond cultural competence: Critical consciousness, social justice and multicultural education. *Academic Medicine; 84:* 782–787.

Latcho D. 1993. Film directed by Tony Gatlif.

Lather P. 1991. *Getting Smart – Feminist Research and Pedagogy with/in the Postmodern.* Routledge, Chapman and Hall: New York.

Laughey W.F., Brown M.E.L., Finn G.M. 2020. 'I'm sorry to hear that' – Empathy and empathic dissonance: The perspectives of PA students. *Medical Science Educator.* doi:10.1007/s40670-020-00979-0.

Laville S. 2017. *Man Sent as Child From UK to Australia Tells Abuse Inquiry: Name the Villains.* https://www.theguardian.com/uk-news/2017/feb/27/child-abuse-survivor-inquiry-name-villains-children-australia.

Leonard T., Willis P. (Eds). 2010. *Pedagogies of the Imagination: Mythopoetic Curriculum in Educational Practice.* Springer: Chicago.

Levin D.M. 1991. *Visions of Narcissism: Intersubjectivity and the Reversals of Reflection.* Chapter 3 in Merleau Ponty V., Dillon M.C. (ed). State University of New York Press: Albany.

Levine P. 2010. *In an Unspoken Voice: How the Body Releases Trauma and Restores Goodness.* North Atlantic Books: California.

Levine P. 1997. *Waking the Tiger: Healing Trauma*. North Atlantic Books: California.

Loach J. 2011. Oranges and Sunshine. Film.

Loff B., Anderson I. 2000. Aboriginal reconciliation still a long way to go. *The Lancet; 355*(9220):2070.

Lopez C., Nakul E., Preuss N., Elziere M., Mast F.W. 2018. Distorted own-body representations in patients with dizziness and during caloric vestibular stimulation. *Journal of Neurology; 265*(Suppl 1):S86–S94.

Lugones M. 2003. *Pilgrimages / Peregrinajes: Theorizing Coalition Against Multiple Oppressions*. Rowman & Littlefield Publishers Inc: Maryland.

Lowe W.A., Adams J., Ballinger C., Armstrong R., Lueddeke J., Protheroe J., McAffery K., Nutbeam D., Russell C. 2014. Patients' and health professionals' views, preferences and experiences of lower levels of literacy and musculoskeletal patient education: A qualitative analysis. Arthritis Research UK Report.

MacFarlane R. 2016. *Landmarks*. Penguin: London.

MacFarlane R. 2013. *The Old Ways: A Journey on Foot*. Penguin: London.

Mahendran A. 2020. *Moments of Rupture: The Importance of Affect in Medical Education and Surgical Training*. Routledge: London.

Mallon R. 2006. 'Race': Normative, not metaphysical or semantic. *Ethics; 116*: 525–551.

Marmot M., Allen J., Boyce T., Goldblatt P., Morrison J. 2020. *Health Equity in England: The Marmot Review 10 Years on*. Institute of Health Equity: London.

Marmot M, Steptoe A. 2008. Whitehall II and ELSA: Integrating Epidemiological and Psychobiological Approaches to the Assessment of Biological Indicators. In: National Research Council (US) Committee on Advances in Collecting and Utilizing Biological Indicators and Genetic Information in Social Science Surveys; Weinstein M, Vaupel JW, Wachter KW, editors. Biosocial Surveys. Washington (DC): National Academies Press (US). https://www.ncbi.nlm.nih.gov/books/NBK62431/.

Martin D. 2014. Doris Pilkington Garimara, Aboriginal Novelist, Dies at 76. The New York Times. https://www.nytimes.com/2014/04/21/arts/doris-pilkington-garimara-novelist-is-dead-at-76.html.

Martin G. 2004. Editorial. On social justice. *Australian e-Journal for the Advancement of Mental Health*; 3(3). www.auseinet.com/journal/vol3iss3/martin.pdf.

Maté G. 2018. *In the Realm of Hungry Ghosts: Close Encounters with Addiction*. North Atlantic Books: California.

Mendenhall E. 2019. *Rethinking Diabetes: Entanglement with Trauma, Poverty and HIV*. Cornell University Press: London.

Metz C., Calmet J.,Thevenot, A. 2019. Women subjected to domestic violence: The impossibility of separation. *Psychoanalytic Psychology*; 36(1):36–43.

Moore J. 2020. What African nations are teaching the west about fighting the coronavirus. *The New Yorker*. https://www.newyorker.com/news/news-desk/what-african-nations-are-teaching-the-west-about-fighting-the-coronavirus

Morse M., Loscalzo J. 2020. Creating Real Change at Academic Medical Centers — How Social Movements Can Be Timely Catalysts. NEJM; June. https://www.nejm.org/doi/full/10.1056/NEJMp2002502.

Moreton-Robinson, A. 2003. I still call Australia home: Indigenous belongings and place in a white postcolonizing society. In *Uprootings/Regroundings: Questions of Home and Migration*. Ahmed S., Castaneda C., Fortier A., Sheller M. (eds)., pp. 131–149. Berg: Oxford.

Mun C. 2019. Unification through rationalities and intentionalities of shame. Chapter Two in *Interdisciplinary Perspectives on Shame: Methods, Theories, Norms, Cultures and Politics*. Mun C. (ed). Lexington Books: London.

Nancy JL. [1997] 2002. *Hegel: The Restlessness of the Negative*. Trans. J. Smith and S. Miller. University of Minnesota Press: Minneapolis, MN.

Norton J., Whittaker G., Kennedy D.S., Jenkins J.M., Bew D. 2018. Shooting up? Analysis of 182 gunshot injuries presenting to a London major trauma centre over a seven-year period. *Annals of the Royal College of Surgeons of England*; 100:464–474 doi:10.1308/rcsann.2018.0037.

Ney A. 2019. *Metaphysics: An Introduction*. Routledge: London.

Noyce P. 2002. Rabbit Proof Fence.

Ochieng O. 2018. *The Intellectual Imagination: Knowledge and Aesthetics in North Atlantic and African Philosophy*. University of Nortre Dame: Indiana.

Orange D.M. 2011. *The Suffering Stranger: Hermeneutics for Everyday Clinical Practice*. Routledge: East Sussex.

Petchkovsky L., San Roque C., Napaljarri Jurra R., Butler S. 2004. Indigenous maps of subjectivity and attacks on linking: Forced separation and its psychiatric sequelae in Australia's Stolen Generation. *Australian e-Journal for the Advancement of Mental Health*; 3(3).

Public Health England. 2018. Research and Analysis Chapter 2: Trends in Mortality. https://www.gov.uk/government/publications/health-profile-for-england-2018/chapter-2-trends-in-mortality

Pendreigh B. 2003. Leaping the fence of Australia's past. IOFilm. http://www.iofilm.com/filmmaking/scriptwriting/2003-12-16-724-leaping-the-fence-of-australias-past

Platt L., Nandi A. 2020. Ethnic diversity in the UK: New opportunities and changing constraints, *Journal of Ethnic and Migration Studies*; 46(5):839–856. doi: 10.1080/1369183X.2018.1539229.

Porges S.W. 2011. *The Polyvagal theory: Neurophysiological foundations of emotions, attachment, communication, and self-regulation*. WW Norton & Company Inc: New York.

Price M., Legrand A.C., Brier Z.M.F., Gratton J., Skalka C. 2019. The short-term dynamics of posttraumatic stress disorder symptoms during the acute posttrauma period. Depress Anxiety; 1–8.

Purtle J., Corbin T.J., Rich L.J., Rich J.A. 2015. Hospitals as a locus for violence intervention. Chapter 3 in Donelly P.D., Ward C.L (eds). *Oxford Textbook of Violence Prevention: Epidemiology, Evidence and Policy*. Oxford University Press: Oxford.

Rebecca S. 2017. *A Field Guide to Getting Lost*. Canongate Books: London.

Resnick A., Galea S., Sivashanker K. 2020. Covid-19: The painful price of ignoring health inequities. BMJ Opinion. https://blogs.bmj.com/bmj/2020/03/18/covid-19-the-painfulprice-of-ignoring-health-inequities.

Riggs D.W. 2006. Queer(y)ing rights: Psychology, liberal individualism and colonization. *Australian Psychologist*; 41(2):95–103.

Riggs D.W. 2004. Challenging the monoculturalism of psychology: Towards a more socially accountable pedagogy and practice. *Australian Psychologist*; 39(2):118 – 126.

Roberts, S. 2019. The London killings of 2018: The story behind the numbers and some proposed solutions. *Crime Prevention and Community Safety*; 21:94–115. doi:10.1057/s41300-019-00064-8.

Ross G. 2007. Beyond the trauma vortex into the healing vortex: A guide for diplomats and NGOs.

Ross G. 2003. *Beyond the Trauma Vortex: The Media's Role in Healing Fear, Terror and Violence.* North Atlantic Books: California.

Rothschild B. 2000. *The Body Remembers: The Psychophysiology of Trauma and Trauma Treatment.* WW Norton & Company: New York.

Rozek L.S., Dolinoy D.C., Sartor M.A., Omenn G.S. 2014. Epigenetics: Relevance and implications for public health. *Annual Review of Public Health*; 35:105–122.

Saggers S., Gray D. 1991. *Aboriginal Health and Society. The Traditional and Contemporary Aboriginal Struggle for Better Health.* Allen and Unwin: Sydney.

Sartre J. 1965. *Nausea.* Penguin classics: London.

Scaer R. 2014. *The Body Bears the Burden: Trauma, Dissociation and Disease.* Third Edition. Routledge: New York.

Schopenhauer A. 1966. *The World as Will and Representation.*Translated from the German by E.F.J. Payne, Vol. 2, Dover Publications Inc: New York.

Scottish Government. 2019. Repeat Violent Victimisation: A Rapid Evidence Review. Crime & Justice. Social Research.

Scottish Violence Reduction Unit. 2020. http://www.svru.co.uk/aces/.

Seth S. 2018. *Difference and Disease: Medicine, Race, and the Eighteenth-Century British Empire.* Cambridge University Press: Cambridge.

Sharpe C. 2016. *In the Wake: On Blackness and Being.* Duke University Press: Durham.

Shea N. 2019. Concept-metacognition. *Mind and Language*; 1–18.

Simeon D., Abugel J. 2006. *Feeling Unreal: Depersonalization Disorder and the Loss of the Self.* Oxford University Press: New York.

Sinclair S. 1997. *Making Doctors: An Institutional Apprenticeship.* Bloomsbury Publishing: London.

Singleton J. 2015. *Cultural Melancholy: Readings of Race, Impossible Mourning, and African American Ritual.* University of Illinois Press: Illinois.

Sloterdijk P. 2013. *You Must Change Your Life.* Polity Press: Cambridge.

Substance Abuse and Mental Health Services Administration. (2014). SAMHSA's concept of trauma and guidance for a trauma-informed approach. HHS Publication No. (SMA) 14-4884. *U.S. Department of Health and Human Services*, (July), 1–27. Retrieved from https://store.samhsa.gov/system/files/sma14-4884.pdf.

Slutkin G., Ransford C., Zvetina D. 2018. How the health sector can reduce violence by treating it as a contagion. *AMA Journal of Ethics*; 20(1):47–55.

Stolorow R. 2010. Collective Trauma and Existential Anxiety. Huffpost. https://www.huffpost.com/entry/collective-trauma-and-exi_b_680945?guccounter=1&guce_referrer=aHR0cHM6Ly93d3cuZ29vZ2xlLmNvbS8&guce_referrer_sig=AQAAAEq5ObT1HCr5fKbRp-cqGzMQmIH7m3QaYQOyd2l3bvbOeZlEsgF086HmNoyl5tOd4Vh5vFWG5UPFZnopWplWxfkvNZ9hF1eu58WDDqGp8BY-BwEFwm4JbN4NSzIBfhLs1sOT6BEFKAcw735B09tgjR-82eh-_yg7Glz182DkEsUXs.

Stolorow R.D. 1999. The phenomenology of trauma and the absolutisms of everyday life: A personal journey. *Psychoanalytic Psychology*; 16:464–468.

Stolorow R.D., Atwood G.E. 1992. *Contexts of Being: The Intersubjective Foundations of Psychological Life.* Routledge: New York.

Vicary D., Westerman T. 2004. 'That's just the way he is: Some implications of Aboriginal mental health beliefs. *Australian e-Journal for the Advancement of Mental Health*; 3(3). www.auseinet.com/journal/vol3iss3/vicarywesterman.pdf Downloaded 9th June, 2007.

Taylor C. 1989. *Sources of the Self: The Making of the Modern Identity*. Harvard University Press: Cambridge.

Taylor G. 2000. Recent developments in alexithymia theory and research. *Canadian Journal of Psychiatry*; 45:134 – 142.

Thebault R., Tran A.B., Williams V. 2020. The coronavirus is infecting and killing black Americans at an alarmingly high rate. Washington Post Apr 7. https://www.washingtonpost.com/nation/2020/04/07/coronavirus-is-infecting-killing-black-americans-an-alarminglyhigh-rate-post-analysis-shows.

Trauma Audit and Research Network. 2020. Performance Comparison: Trauma Care. Trauma Care in England and Wales Care. https://www.tarn.ac.uk/Content.aspx?ca=15#:~:text=The%20Trauma%20Audit%20and%20Research%20Network&text=Every%20year%20across%20England%20and,non%2Dfatal%20injuries%20each%20year.

United Nations Development Programme (UNDP). 2019. Human Development Report 2019: Beyond income, beyond averages, beyond today: Inequalities in human development in the 21st century.

United Nations Development Programme (UNDP). 1997. Human Development Report 1997: Human Development to Eradicate Poverty. http://www.hdr.undp.org/en/content/human-development-report-1997.

United Nations Hugh Commissioner for Refugees (UNHCR). 2017. Global trends forced displacement in 2016.

Van der Hart O., Nijenhuis E.R.S., Steele K. 2006. *The Haunted Self: Structural Dissociation and the Treatment of Chronic Traumatization*. WW Norton & Company Ltd: London.

Van der Kolke B.A., McFarlane A.C., Weisaeth L (Eds). 2007. *Traumatic Stress: The Effects of Overwhelming Experience on Mind, Body, and Society*. The Guildford Press: London.

Vattimo G. 1997. *Beyond Interpretation: The meaning of hermeneutics for Philosophy*. Translated by David Webb. Stanford University Press: Stanford.

Viessière S. 2011. *The Ghosts of Empire: Violence, Suffering and Mobility in the Transatlantic Cultural Economy of Desire*. Transaction Publishers: London.

Yamada L., Chong S. 2017. Epigenetic studies in Developmental Origins of Health and Disease: Pitfalls and key considerations for study design and interpretation. *Journal of Developmental Origins of Health and Disease*; 8(1):30–43.

Young A. 1995. *The Harmony of Illusions: Inventing Post-Traumatic Stress Disorder*. Princeton University Press: Princeton.

Yusoff K. 2018. *A million Black Anthropocenes or none*. University of Minnesota Press: Minneapolis.

Waddington K. 2016. The compassion gap in UK universities. *International Practice Development Journal*; 6(1). https://www.fons.org/Resources/Documents/Journal/Vol6No1/IPDJ_0601_10.pdf.

Waddington K. 2017. Creating conditions for compassion. In *The Pedagogy of Compassion at the Heart of Higher Education*. Gibbs P. (ed)., pp. 49–70. London: Springer.

Weheliye A. 2002. Freenin' posthuman voices in contemporary black popular music. *Social Text*; 20(2):20–47.

Westerman T.G. 2004. Engagement of Indigenous clients in mental health services: What role do cultural differences play? *Australian e-Journal for the Advancement of Mental Health*; 3(3). www.auseinet.com/journal/vol3iss3/westermaneditorial.pdf.

White R. 2017. Compassion in Philosophy and Education. In *The Pedagogy of Compassion at the Heart of Higher Education*. Gibbs P. (ed)., pp. 19–33. London: Springer.

World Health Organisation Report. 2002. *Reducing Risks, Promoting Health Life*. Geneva: World Health Organisation.

World Health Organisation. 2017. Violence Info. HOMICIDE WHO Global Health Estimates (2015 update). https://apps.who.int/violence-info/homicide/.

Winnicott D.W. 1954. Mind and its relation to the psyche-soma. *The British Journal of Medical Psychology*; 27:201–209.

Worline M.C., Dutton J.E. 2017. *Awakening Compassion at Work*. Oakland, CA: Berrett-Koehler Publishers, Inc.

Worringer W. 1997. *Abstraction and Empathy: A Contribution to the Psychology of Style*. Ivan R. Dee Inc: Chicago.

7 Diving down deep

7.1 Introduction

Suffering is both an individual experience and a social construct. Therefore the individual embodied emotional experience is indicative of as well as formed and influenced by social events and relationships in a particular context. All types of knowing are necessary in order to encounter and understand suffering. Whilst suffering appears universal across contexts, clustering in syndemics, there are differences in how suffering is perceived and responded to by family and healthcare services and by different cultures, for example (Cain et al., 2018). The individual experience is located along a continuum of isolation and solitude on the one hand, and possibly interacting with healthcare services on the other hand. A sense of self and other is inherent in the experience of suffering, either by absence – a hole in what could be said – or as a yearning for salvation and redemption, a silent speechlessness of appeal that perhaps can be felt at the level of a resonant body. At the same time, there is an agonising push away from contact, borne of uncertainty in being able to trust the other. The push-pull dynamic inherent in suffering, both within the self and the social, is a conflict difficult to bear and endure on both sides and can feel like moral anguish.

For health professionals, bearing witness to this agonising suffering, this kind of conflicting impulse, is a challenge for which they are generally unprepared. Whilst they may be prepared for the tasks they have to do, there is little in any health professional curriculum that prepares them for the depth of this encounter, and they may feel as if they, their instrumentalist self, has come undone. The rupture can be felt at the level of affect, as a knowing on the inside and an in-bracing (Mahendran, 2020) of their body as container for resonance, as a feeling of what happens at a deep level of experience of their self. This work has sought to go down deep into this experience of self and other, to swim in the depths, in order to find a way of expressing and moving forward from here, that may help health professionals to understand what is necessary to know, be and do on these occasions; to help allay fears of swimming in unchartered waters. This intention works against the tide of transcendent medicine which tries to apply universalised abstracted guidelines to the particular and may end up pulling ourselves out of ourselves. In order to dive down deep, I have drawn on medical humanities, sociology and medical education to show ways of thinking differently, how stitching together is important, in understanding sociological patterns of injustice and suffering, to suggest a pedagogy of suffering.

Medical humanities' role is to provide a map for both the pilgrimage of wandering lines and the diving into the depths of the matter:

> *La facultad* is the capacity to see in the surface phenomena the meaning of deeper realities, to see the deep structure below the surface. It is an instant "sensing"; a quick perception arrived at without conscious reasoning. It is an acute awareness mediated by part of the psyche that does not speak, that communicates in images and symbols which are the faces of feelings, that is, behind which feelings reside/hide. The one processing this sensitivity is excruciatingly alive to the world.
>
> (Anzaldúa, 1999; p. 60; emphasis original)

La facultad is a way of surviving "that people caught between the worlds, unknowingly cultivate" (Anzaldúa, 1999; p. 61). Surviving health requires strategies to endure the understorey of suffering, to better able to be with patients, to bring to the surface the conflicts and anguish of speechlessness, in order to live again. But this is not an easy journey.

Travelling in the underworld of suffering requires strength of a different kind to that generated by the instrumentalist source of self:

> Miro que estoy encabronada, miro la Resistencia – resistance to knowing, to letting go, to that deep ocean where I once dived into death. I am afraid of drowning. Resistance to sex, intimate touching, opening myself to alien other where I am out of control, not on patrol. The outcome on the other side unknown, the reins falling and the horses plunging blindly over the crumbling path rimming the edge of the cliff, plunging into its thousand foot drop.
>
> (Anzaldúa, 1999; p. 70)

The art of travelling the underworld of suffering is part of medicine, the pre-cognitive pre-categorical faculty we all have before we learn to conceptualise and abstract. We have just forgotten or lost the ability to dive down deep into matters, to see beyond the false binaries to the unity that is always there in our knowing.

The contributions of medical humanities, sociology and medical education are all required to understand the construction of suffering. Medical humanities is core to thinking differently about suffering, for being prepared to enter through the portal of suffering in the first place and then to provide images and symbols as ways through the entering of some darkness, to provide the imaginal at the very edge of our experience. Sociology enables the understanding of social justice, inequalities in health and the geologic patterns of the Black Anthropocene, stratified deep in the earth by a consumerism that won't go away, perpetuated by extraction and displacement of populations the world over. These stratifications create confusion around self and other at the level of binaries that structure the instrumentalist self through practices of exclusion and a democracy that seems to require the excess deaths of black asian and minority ethnic groups of people to maintain itself (Sharpe, 2016). Medical education can provide the lens on how we learn· and teach about the imaginal in service of suffering of both patients and health professionals. Including affect and multimodal forms of learning must now be a priority. In order to stitch these together, we have had to explore and become as clear as possible on a great number of concepts and schemata.

Throughout the stitching together, I have kept a thread on epistemology, on how we know what we know, using this as a tool to both dive down deep into conceptual analysis as well as stitching together across fault lines. Suffering provided a conceptual unity to enable this and seems to be a starting point for thinking about psychological aspects such as attitude and emotion, as well as affect (DeGrazia, 2014); these include embodied experiential notions of social justice as a crossing over as well as being socially constructed through culture, politics and governmentality. I have kept the descriptions of suffering in line with those of Frank (2001), Cassell (2004) and Devisch et al. (2017) in order to keep the experience of suffering close and not as something that occurs elsewhere. Abstract considerations of suffering suggest the following:

> In what we might call the objective sense of the term, suffering is roughly equivalent to misfortune. More precisely, the verb to suffer is treated as transitive: one suffers a misfortune. Now, one can suffer a misfortune without being aware of it, say if one's house is destroyed while one is away on vacation; and such a possibility highlights the distinction between this objective sense of suffering and the subjective sense that will be our topic. In the subjective sense, to suffer is an intransitive verb: one suffers, period, rather than suffering something. Such suffering is subjective in the sense of mind dependent: suffering is a type of mental state or occurrence. Moreover, suffering is consciously experienced, which is why it automatically lowers one's quality of life while it occurs. If suffering could occur without one's feeling it, it would not have this tight conceptual tie to experiential welfare.
>
> (DeGrazia, 2014; p. 135)

The tight conceptual tie of suffering to experiential welfare is important and is the link between biomedicine and inequalities in health. And there is also the sense whereby the experience of suffering is much more complicated because it can be displaced unconsciously, abstracted and extracted from the embedded and embodied person. The awareness of this requires understanding about concepts of self, consciousness, awareness itself, knowledge that are linked more through a network of beliefs than a dichotomous or labyrinth model of knowledge arrangement. In this chapter, I will review the progress made in each part of the book, reflect on surviving health, have a final review of epistemology and self before turning to a few final points to be made in the stitching together of the understorey of suffering.

7.2 Review of chapters

In Chapter One, I explored epistemology through the arrangement and classification of knowledge. How suffering is classified – according to its properties of self-other and languishing-acting begins to tell us about the kind of self that suffers. The self that suffers is speechless, profoundly affected and called to question existence and their experience of the world (Frank, 2001; Cassell, 2004; Devisch et al., 2017). It is a *person* who suffers:

> Suffering always involves self-conflict because persons are not "of a piece." The source of suffering is usually seen as outside the sufferer—the cause of the pain or the pain itself, or the circumstance or fate. The clue lies in the fact that meaning enters into suffering.
>
> (Cassell, 2014; p. 15)

The person or self must by default engage in a poetics of making do, to wrest back from institutional strategies, the ability to name the unnameable (de Certeau, 1984). The unnameable, or the void, has been consistently apparent during this writing, in the name of impossible speech. This naming requires an awareness of reversals in epistemology, particularly in healthcare around who benefits from the speeches on poverty and inequities in health.

Epistemic injustice necessitates the inclusion of critical race theory in any work on poverty and inequities. To take care over any universalisms of suffering so that those who suffer are not exposed to further manipulation and abuse by institutions, grounded in neo-liberal economic policies (Butt, 2002). Living on the edge of our experiences due to the deeply ingrained cultural and social norms inculcated by consumerism encourages abjection of those who do not fit the norms. Thinking about this is destabilising and disorienting. Coming closer to the intersection of the self-other and languishing-agency axes means navigating increasingly unstable and disorienting regions, but this is necessary in order to link social sciences, ethics, humanities, and biomedicine when considering suffering. Ideas about choice, responsibility and control become increasingly unstable the closer we get to the experience of suffering. These disturbances are the ground of inquiry (Devereaux, 1967). When thinking about ideas on choice, responsibility and control and the disturbances these thoughts bring, we create a ground that requires both an immersion in the local and a stepping back to view the wider perspective. Stepping back provides a unity, a consilience, to the relations of types of knowing (Wilson, 1998). To know that biomedicine is founded on difference, differential categories (Seth, 2018), enables us to see beyond this to prevent further injustice by making suffering an organisational principle in our thinking.

The theoretical struggles of writing from this principle means a constant movement between opening up to what lies outside as well as a focus on what is reproducing itself within. This dynamic form of theory making requires a methodological plurality to include both the suffering stranger (Orange, 2011) alongside the syndemics of suffering (Mendenhall, 2019). Since syndemics involve the clustering of conditions at both an individual and social community level, there is a need for both experiential and social levels of analyses. Health professionals are caught between attending to individual patients and conforming to institutional, professional and governmental requirements. The principles of the latter are seemingly abstract, often have a virtual existence, and yet they determine behaviour and response to suffering as much as anything else. This abstract virtual level of existence ensures theory making is a struggle in a profession that is attached to concrete facts.

Authoritarian relations of the type governing healthcare institutions predominate. Particular ideologies and perceived benefits place the sufferer in specific locations requiring redemption and salvation (Gastaldo, 1997), the typical sorts of Western Christian biblical response to suffering (Engelhardt, 2014). These sorts of relations keep people tied into their own subjectivity in relations of dependence and are formative of their identity. Identity in suffering is formed around a hole, an unconscionable loss that is displaced unconsciously onto the ego and which resists awareness (Singleton, 2015). Metaphoric mediators abound, perhaps in an unconscious attempt to cross the uncrossable. The uncrossable hole is around the colonial centre with the interlocutors of the others having disappeared in the speechlessness of suffering. Metaphors help us to know and are one of the places where medical humanities excels. Metaphors can reach across differences and help provide unity, connection and remembering.

Chapter Two reviewed patterns of inequity in health and poverty with trends in the widening of inequity only set to continue. Medicalisation of symptoms of poverty is a worrying trend as is the lurching of the NHS from one crisis to another. Trends of rising co-morbidities – the syndemics of suffering – have been exacerbated by COVID-19 with the rehabilitation needs of very sick patients causing concern. Any budgetary constraints have been blown out of the water by COVID-19 as hospitals, GP surgeries and communities have scrambled to meet the acute demand whilst also knowing the delay in treating patients, who would otherwise attend for pre-existing conditions, will have consequences in the form of increased severity and prevalence of morbidity and mortality. NHS staff morale has waxed and waned appreciating public support but wary of false promises by the government and a lack of practical action in following up cases of COVID-19 and preparation for the second wave.

The long haul of the suffering from COVID-19 is becoming more apparent as a marathon rather than a sprint. Widening inequities in health have been exacerbated by COVID-19 with people from black asian and minority ethnic communities affected much more in the UK and US. Healthcare workers, especially those from black asian and ethnic minorities, have been affected most of all. This is a clear statement that suffering is inseparable between health workers and patients. In addition, there is a real concern about the mental health effects of working in systems with patients who have COVID-19. Health professionals speak of being haunted by what they have seen, worrying about people's ongoing recovery and rehabilitation and desperate over the inability of loved ones to be with patients in what are perhaps their last moments.

The level of responsibility carried by health professionals, their self-assumed culpability for events beyond their control, a system of training that encourages depersonalisation and the limited language available to talk about their suffering all contribute to the likelihood of suffering emotional and physical anguish during moments of fusion of self and role. Yet apparently this is difficult to address given the seemingly recalcitrant ways that resist thinking and working differently, about how workforces are organised and how this organisation impacts on mental health. Workforce issues impact patient care through the mediators of self, roles, ethical decisions and behaviour. At the same time as being a source of self, work can also be a source of undoing of that same self. Burnout, moral injury, depersonalisation co-exist within the very same self structures that enable agency and care. Therefore a more nuanced understanding of these terms is necessary if we are to avoid shallow thinking. In order to progress how we think about suffering, there mustn't be a premature foreclosure, working as a sleight of hand, operating as a fiction and indicating an inability to be with suffering.

Unfortunately for those who like to believe in trivial moralities, humane chumminess and wellness programmes (Sloterdijk, 2013), suffering is not an aberration of self; it is formative of self. This demands that we incorporate our own contingent embodiment by attending to our body. Being on the front line of care without having the means to attend to suffering in one's self and others makes for an alienating environment. Health professionals don't always know if they are allowed to or how to encounter suffering in the fullest sense for themselves or patients. Chapter Three puts words to the categories and definitions of suffering so that health professionals have a richer vocabulary to draw from. Mapping out the biographical break, understanding the coagulated lived experience and appreciating the unrecognizability of this experience, gives health professionals more tools to work with.

Given that human existence is the concrete, personal, individual starting point for experience – Merleau Ponty stated:

> I am the absolute source, my existence does not stem from my antecedents, from my physical and social environment; instead it moves out towards them and sustains them, for I alone bring into being for myself (and therefore into being in the only sense that the word can

have for me) the tradition which I elect to carry on, or the horizon whose distance from me would be abolished – since that distance is not one of its properties – if I were not there to scan it with my gaze. Scientific points of view, according to which my existence is a moment of the world's, are always both naïve and at the same time dishonest, because they take for granted, without explicitly mentioning it, the other point of view, namely that of consciousness, through which from the outset a world forms itself around me and begins to exist for me. To return things to themselves is to return to that world which precedes knowledge, of which knowledge always *speaks*, and in relation to which every scientific schematization is an abstract and derivative sign-language, as is geography in relation to the countryside in which we have learnt beforehand what a forest, a prairie or a river is.

(Merleau Ponty, 1962; p. ix)(emphasis original)

Within this starting point is the conundrum given by the individual social interaction – there is both a constraint by being and making choices that are limited within current conditions of choosing, as well as the compulsion to live as if we are in control. Depending on your perspective, matters to do with medicine may seem like a constraint and medical humanities may seem like a freedom, or vice versa. Sociology has struggled to progress a theory of suffering from an intrigue of its own making (Wilkinson, 2005), perhaps by staying at the level of categories and patterns.

In contrast, attending to the localised characteristics and properties of suffering within a context of racialised colonialised self, Singleton (2015) provides us with a way of moving forward. By drawing on understandings of cultural melancholy and the holy trinity of disavowed loss, unconscious displacement of that unconscionable loss of self onto the ego and avowed and hidden affect, Singleton (2015) shows how black being is always racialised with the colonial white self. Re-enactment of the hole at the colonial centre of self through social crisis, ritual and process of subject formation produces a stable, coherent self at one level, at the same time as being insecure, contradictory, and disoriented because we have come closer to the intersecting axes of the self-other and languishing-acting continuums and closer to the centre of intersecting disciplines.

Only by understanding the experience of suffering in this way can we come closer to understanding the dynamic occurring between health professionals and patients. By attending to the marginalised abject experience, we may come closer to understanding the reversals and introjects of racialised suffering. Where the white ego demands to see itself through difference, it is also struggling to bar loss of self from recognition. This understanding could account for the sense of the sufferer appealing for help while at the same time withdrawing from relationship in order to refuse recognition of loss. It seems as though little progress will be made until we can understand this forceful dynamic.

Understanding suffering is hard, incomplete and disruptive (Orange, 2011). Relying on others in the unreliability is a challenge. These characteristics are the very nature of suffering which is primed by distress, reciprocity, reversal, tension, conflict and an embodied felt sense of social (in)justice. And these experiences of suffering are situated in a world and healthcare that focuses on cognition as a way of managing. Stitching these all together in a framework of understanding means attending to the process of stitching across fault lines and matrices, fragmentation, overwhelm and traumatism of responsibility as well as keeping in mind questions and the art of thinking about thinking. Such a framework can provide a container through the use of metaphors for survival and art as a manifestation of the self. As we approach the centre of the self-other and languishing-acting axes – a region characterised by instability and disorientation – the medical humanities can provide an anchor.

Inherent in current work in medical humanities is the role of medical education to integrate different ways of thinking. Chapter Four explored how working across disciplines requires a different mindset and specific skills to traverse minefields and uncertainty. Understanding how the medical mind has been trained and how it works is crucial to any proposed integration. That is, knowing that medical minds have been trained through evidence based practice means being able to accept and integrate that understanding into medical humanities practice. Perhaps the confusion is not so much a matter of exclusion of medical humanities, although that is a consideration, but more a matter of the rejection of medical minds' reality of evidence based practice by medical humanities. If evidence based practice is seen as the last bastion standing between medicine and unremitting chaos, then any attempt to critique it will be seen as a threat.

Instead medical humanities may be wiser to focus on the pedagogical process of how we come to know what we know in relation to suffering by researching the relationship between analysis and synthesis. From theory to practice, there is much that medical humanities can do. The current epistemic crisis in medicine (Altschuler, 2018) is an opportunity to enrich knowledge production (Ford & Airhihenbuwa, 2018) and connection in a consilience view of unity (Wilson, 1998). A consilience perspective is metacognition of the translation of medical knowledge as an applied science. There is art to and art of knowledge translation. The art is an ethical engagement that is process as well as product. Primary in both process and product is the imagination.

The imagination is the capacity to represent an object, to perceive and interpret experience, to evoke what is not present, and to create a subjective world of personal consciousness through the elaboration of schema, intellect and judgment. In this understanding, art and science are inseparable. The places where they differ is in the judgment of perception from the legislative activity of the intellect (Eco, 2014). Conversely, the intertextual reality impinges on experience only along the edges of the fabric of our beliefs. The boundary conditions of experience are tested when it comes to suffering, when it appears that the sufferer feels they are on the wrong side of the fault line of life and so is rendered mute (Frank, 2001). The existence of the pre-categorical pre-cognitive state is perhaps closer to the boundary experience of someone suffering, when they feel beyond the dichotomies of art or science and just want to be acknowledged as they are.

Empathy has traditionally been the focus of medical humanities (Graham et al., 2016; Haidet et al., 2016). Yet there is still much to learn about the value of medical humanities in exploring empathy with students. Without providing granularity of what exactly empathy is and when it is appropriate, efforts in this regard can come across as patronising in the face of unremitting suffering due to poverty, racial disparities and inequities in health. Perhaps more dedication is necessary to understanding how a psychological level of explanation fits in with a neuroscientific level of analysis and how these are both affected (Decety 2014; Ekman & Krasner, 2016; Garland & Howard, 2014) and this may provide more traction for an epistemology that works across fault lines of suffering. Being a companion in suffering means understanding and drawing from a pedagogy of suffering that begins and ends with an understanding of consumerism, the neo-liberal human subject and the colonial project that sought to achieve economic and social advantage over others.

Using imagination in the meta-discourse about curriculum in medical education and medical humanities means understanding colonial projects and the archetypes invoked. Understanding vulnerability to displacement, destabilisation and deindustrialisation through political policies aimed at dismantling the welfare state is crucial in the UK (Walsh et al., 2016). Poverty as the underlying force of health inequities in areas of inequality is crucial (Mendenhall, 2019). These findings reinforce that immigration, violence, depression, abuse, anxieties and diabetes cluster together in syndemics of suffering. Being able to imagine how all these factors cluster together in suffering means being able to draw on a wide range of perspectives that support understanding of how these are formative of a person's self. These factors are constitutive and play a large role in how health is valued at an individual and social level. Imagination is necessary to see both the individual and social effects of suffering together whilst considering how to address these:

> How might it be possible to bear moral witness to the suffering endured through experience, and also to set this within a sociologically meaningful framework that equips people with the knowledge to take actions to transform the conditions of their existence?
>
> (Wilkinson & Kleinman, 2016; p. 86)

These considerations apply to both health professionals and patients. The imagination is necessary because science has removed the cognisant subject (awareness of social injustice) from the knowledge making process:

Analytical reflection starts from our experience of the world and goes back to the subject as to a condition of possibility distinct from that experience, revealing the all-embracing synthesis as that without which there would be no world

(Merleau Ponty, 1962; p. ix)

Imagining how to create a world beyond the Black Anthropocene in a synthesis requires us to go back to ourselves, back to our own subjectivity.

In Chapter Five, we started drilling down into what constitutes or what are sources for a self, with a particular emphasis on the suffering self. The crossing over of the individual experience of suffering as well as how the social construction of that suffering implicates both health professional and patient is a crucial notion to hold that honours the involvement of both in suffering. Ideas about the self show different levels of analysis and understanding from a felt sense, to a concept of self and finally to a category of self. Each level and the interplay between them constitute different levels of awareness and therefore require different disciplinary knowledges to understand them. In a category of self drawn from theistic sources, medieval religious women's experiences of suffering were explored because they included life, suffering and death, thereby avoiding an epistemic break. Identity and role were bound up in redemption and suffering. Experiencing the body was more important than controlling it (Bynum, 1987). Images were of profound deepenings encouraging women to become more human in their expanded suffering as a way of retrieving their sense of self. The digestion of moral dilemmas in an embodied manner meant food for the self. They feasted on anguish in a formation of their self in order to gain entry into experiences that deepened ordinary reality (Bynum, 1987).

In contrast, health professionals professed to an idealised self as being in control and able to exercise choice even though they themselves often struggled at work with the self-policing and self-regulation required to fit this norm. They seemed to not know how to be with suffering either their own or others. Health professionals were subject to manipulation through categorisation and the practice of exclusion as were patients. Health professionals developed an instrumental self from their role which requires disengaged rationality, disengaged from matters of social justice, for example. Many metaphors were used to describe the body; one in particular was that of the health professional required to be the balancing point on which healthcare hinged. The instrumentalist approach seems to require an "us" and "them" mentality. Punitive ways of dealing with distress, teaching through humiliation, ridicule of people perceived as not fitting the idealised norm were all ways of reinforcing categories, separation and disembodiment. Health professionals were instruments of a system that was not necessarily equipped for being with suffering and in fact may have contributed to suffering.

These circumstances require health professionals to work at the limits of the dominant constructions of self. Understanding that the ways health professionals are trained and how practice is constructed out of dominant perspectives of the self as an instrument means that health professionals are compelled to connect in this way with patients who are constructed and categorised as particular at risk groups of people (Wilkinson, 2006). In this sea of construction and discrimination, there is the necessity to know that there is something else other than the constructions, a pre-categorical pre-cognitive self that can survive through suffering and may perhaps be where imagination arises to process social constructions. There is the constructed self, as well as the experiential self – the feeling of what happens (Damasio, 1999) – as well as the consciousness underlying all this (Damasio, 2010). Links between embodiment, self and sociocultural context must be made in order to mitigate the sociocultural void around suffering. Consilience is therefore an act of restoration through linking experience, words and images whilst being on the edge of those experiences. What seems to go missing in suffering is the interlocutor of the instrumentalist self.

Restoring the interlocutor seems to require an admission of the suffering self as the self. That is, no longer living in denial of suffering, which means not living a fiction that the instrumentalist self is all there is. Acknowledging that in order to survive health, health professionals must shut down, dis-embody and fuse their role with their self and that this must have im-plications for knowing what to say and do to someone who is suffering. Chapter Six explored the fusion of self and role further through a romantic expressivism ethical source of self. Ethical dilemmas can produce cognitive dissonance which can then also produce identity dissonance.

Identity dissonance occurs when identity is built on a sense of agency as the sole source of self. Viewing identity in this limited way may reinforce the epistemic break at the level of embodied symbolic cognition. The epistemic break manifests as a moral anguish in knowing what to say or do – "Who am I to be in this room?" This sort of moral anguish resists rationalisation, requiring an in-depth or inseeing into the situation to un-derstand more. Inseeing demands that we look differently at ourselves, our world and the precarious intersubjective space we occupy. The romantic expressivism sources of self requires imagination and an acceptance that we are more than instrument or role.

Understanding differently means also thinking about the return to self or recognition of the self as potentially a loss of the instrumentalist self (Fareld, 2012). The self that does not find itself is the one that has particular relevance for suffering. Paradoxically, in not finding itself, there can be resonance and attunement; "in each case it is the doing of pre-personal forms of consciousness, whose communication raises no problem, since it is demanded by the very definition of consciousness, meaning or truth" (Merleau Ponty, 1962; p. xi). In seeming to lose one's instrumentalist self, there is also the possibility of connecting in a pre-personal level of consciousness. In times of crisis, our collective imagi-nations require soothing. Caught between two poles of transcendence and immanence, and others of social good and evil, the precarious space we occupy calls for serious acrobatics to maintain our roles and instrumentalist self in the face of suffering.

Medical humanities must take into account the colonialist project through understanding how concepts of colour, measurement, as well as categorisation into roles and humanity have extracted and displaced peoples the world over. Such notions are inherently tied up with salvation and redemption through transcendence and abstraction from suffering. Health professionals are implicated in promoting lifestyle ideals that transcend the context of suffering in which patients are embedded. There is the perception that health professionals may have oversold the clinical benefits of diets and exercise without understanding the impact of displacement and poverty on peoples' lives (Mendenhall, 2019).

Poverty, violence, and trauma are mediators of worst health outcomes and co-morbidities for people who suffer the most and who may be the largest attenders of healthcare. There are many reasons why health professionals should be aware of the links between social deprivation and health outcomes. The most important reason seems to be the awareness of trauma so that healthcare services do not re-traumatise patients who present at GP surgeries and A&E departments. We seem now to be in an age of trauma as Stolorow (2010) suggests. The shattering of absolutisms that allowed us to function has been experienced on a global scale. Meetings as siblings in the darkness requires an acknowledgment of a shared ethical principle of our connected humanity.

Depersonalisation can also be seen as a thread running through suffering and has long been expressed in the literature and arts. The blow of the void is an existential crisis impacting on the ability to use words. The interlocutor disappears. The language of detachment has been linked to processes of the mind, to the categorical imperative, with its focus on attention and encoding whilst losing touch with affect. Dehumanisation predisposes people to seek instrumentalist sources of self which in turn predisposes them to depersonalisation. Becoming explicitly aware of suffering in healthcare may seem an unpalatable suggestion but may help prevent the instrumentalist self from floundering in existential anguish. However, such an awareness also requires an exploration of how desire contributes to the colonialist project and its influence on suffering.

Institutional categorisation of what counts as knowledge pursues transcendence. Therefore affects are generally not included which makes processing ethical dilemmas grounded in shame, guilt and anger difficult. The importance of this cannot be overstated. Healthcare services and training are rooted in a Christian doctrine of unacknowledged unconscious guilt, the grief of which has been displaced, transmuted into the heart's desire and intense longing for salvation. The instrumentalist self carries this load, seeing its own culpability yet unconscious about the sources of this seeing, the ghosts of colonialist times past (Viessière, 2011). Salvation seems to be achievable only by the heaviest of sacrifices and by the denial of one's own expressivist self. Health professional training institutions run on this ethic therefore any moral anguish must be viewed from this awareness. This ethic is what underlies the epistemic abyss between self and others.

The epistemological dilemma of medical training is that it tends to produce people who seem slightly removed from the rest of the population with the belief that they need to be in order to do what they have to do (Sinclair, 1997). Having to advise people how to live healthier lives whilst in all probability suffering from the effects of their training and practise without having the means to describe this leads to a reversal. Patients' experiences to them seem concrete, real and deterministic to their health as well as being embedded in a context. What health professionals say comes across as abstract and decontextualised. Conversely, health professionals have been trained to see experiences and emotions as abstract. Moreover, by providing general guidelines not tailored to specific patients, a decontextualisation occurs. These moments can be experienced as ruptures in practice and could conceivably impact of patient adherence.

Walking with suffering, using touch or haptic sense to know the world, enables living through ruptures and suffering. Streetwalker strategies rely on the deconstruction of concepts and categories as well as acceptance of the nomadic nature of this task. Walking this path means not belonging to any polarised community of categorisation. As a health professional streetwalker, holding the experience of suffering requires a dual awareness of both the focused biomedical training and inherent professional requirements, in addition to a wider stepped back perspective that also allows inseeing into the imaginal particularity of the patient and the moment. This is a matter of holding the question of how biomedicine and medical humanities can both be true at the same time. It means knowing what to do from a task focused perspective as well as knowing that that occurs in a context and with the experiential person in front of you.

Launer (2020) reflects on the possibility of using two approaches in medicine – digging holes and weaving a tapestry: "Digging a hole requires intense effort and single-mindedness. Weaving a tapestry involves immense delicacy and careful collaboration. One activity is practical, the other is aesthetic" (p. 307). Weaving a tapestry involves three main components – negative capability; "I know many doctors who have acquired such a capability through personal and professional experience, but feel slightly ashamed of it, as if they are committing a sin by suspending their belief in the received truths of their education" Launer, 2020; p. 307); – courteous curiosity; "This is an ability to ask in detail about someone's subjective experience and to try and understand it through the patient's own words, without judging or categorising anything, or reframing it in a more official way" (ibid); –and unrelenting positivity "holding on to the belief that every narrative has its own momentum; if it is explored with respect and kindness, and allowed enough freedom, it will reveal a potential to surprise both doctor and patient alike" (ibid).

Streetwalker strategies retrieve from the institutional effects the means to be able to occupy precarity and efficacious meanderings, through having gone down deep into matters. This means being able to sense both the reality and fiction of meanings and spaces within the vastness and detail of suffering. One of the tactics to be with suffering is to be both/and – non-dual – and not identified with either polarity of biomedicine or medical humanities exclusively. This seems particularly important for addressing the experience of being on the wrong side of the fault line of life, the feared objectivisation, when individuals who suffer may feel they are beyond any type of classification based on gender, race, ethnicity or socioeconomic status. In those moments of extreme suffering, these sorts of classifications and differentiations seem to fall away, and there is the raw palpable humanity present.

Biomedicine and medical education belong to the instrumentalist sources of self and other. Sociology has a role in deconstructing those roles across fault lines of poverty, displacement and destabilisation the closer we come to the intersection of the self-other and languishing-acting axes as a source of no self. Medical humanities is necessary to go underneath and beyond those to return to a self that is pre-cognitive and pre-categorical, that can insee into and beyond the situations of healthcare. Figure 7.1 shows a mermaid, diving deep, somewhat astonished and amazed that anyone would want to try and fit into a linguistic only box, a box of conceptual and categorical limitations. The elephant seems to celebrate sentient being or consciousness that feels, perceives or experiences sensations subjectively. This experience or being as described by Merleau Ponty (1962) is outside the box of scientific reasoning. The raw palpable humanity experienced when suffering is resonated with and there are no words.

7.3 Surviving health

Images like this, retrieved from the deep time of imagination, beyond the instrumentalist self, can provide an anchor for survival in difficult times. These images seem to come from a different source altogether than the intellect yet they are sustaining in the midst of disorientation and destabilisation. The images, metaphors and symbols can complement reasoning processes that conceptualise and categorise. Perhaps all of these processes of the self are mediators between self and other, in addition to the dynamic structuring brought about by language and institutional practices.

Figure 7.2 shows how this may work as we zoom in on the intersection of the self-other and languishing-acting axes. The mediators of concrete experience, narrative, metaphor and symbol (concepts to schemata) are all ways of learning from self and other, ways of communicating, and constitute the shared reality or intersubjective space. Yet these parallel vertical axes, linked in the crossover like a model of DNA, are also created and constrained by the matrix in which they are embedded, which is fractured

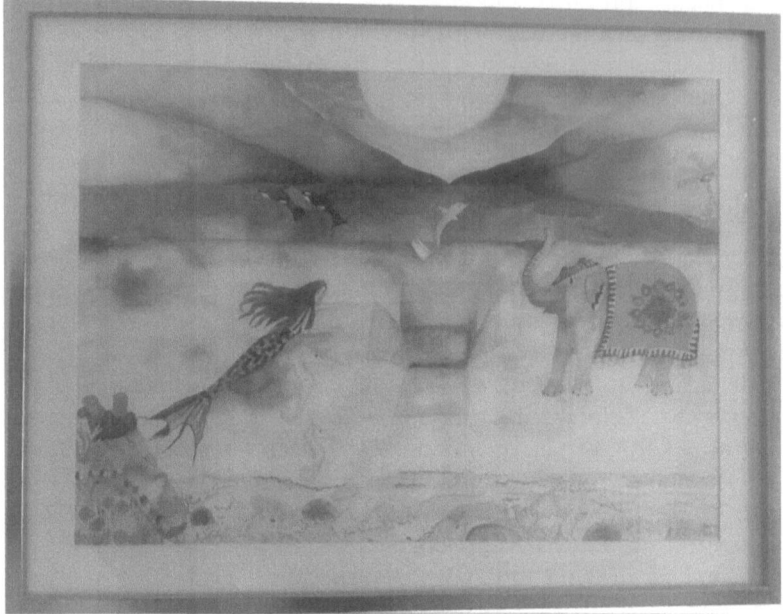

Figure 7.1 Diving deep and thinking outside a box.

along fault lines of the typically measured sociodemographics of poverty, gender, race, socioeconomic status and location as well as the less typically measured features such as violence, immigration, isolation, depression, diabetes, abuse and anxiety, i.e., the clusters of syndemic suffering (Mendenhall, 2019). The relations between (as shown in Table 1.1) bring together the individual and social through these mediators.

In times of destabilisation, disorientation, displacement and deindustrialisation where people are more vulnerable, they are more susceptible to worse health and therefore more susceptible to encountering the healthcare system. Healthcare care can be a place of compassion (Dempsey, 2018), and it can also be a place of the void where individuals' felt sense of reality, or their suffering, is not responded to. In fact, at times, there can be an impingement – unwilled and unchosen – to a subjectivity that is non-narrativizable, a responsibility which can be considered relational but about which there is vulnerability and trauma (Butler, 2005). A range of affective responses happen at the moment of impingement of self-other (Butler, 2005; Mahendran, 2020).

These affects often register at a level that is not always fully recoverable because there is little validation and acknowledgment of them as a source of knowing. Or, worse, responders may be aware of these affects of suffering and use them to manipulate and abuse the sufferer (Butt, 2002). Butler (2005) calls

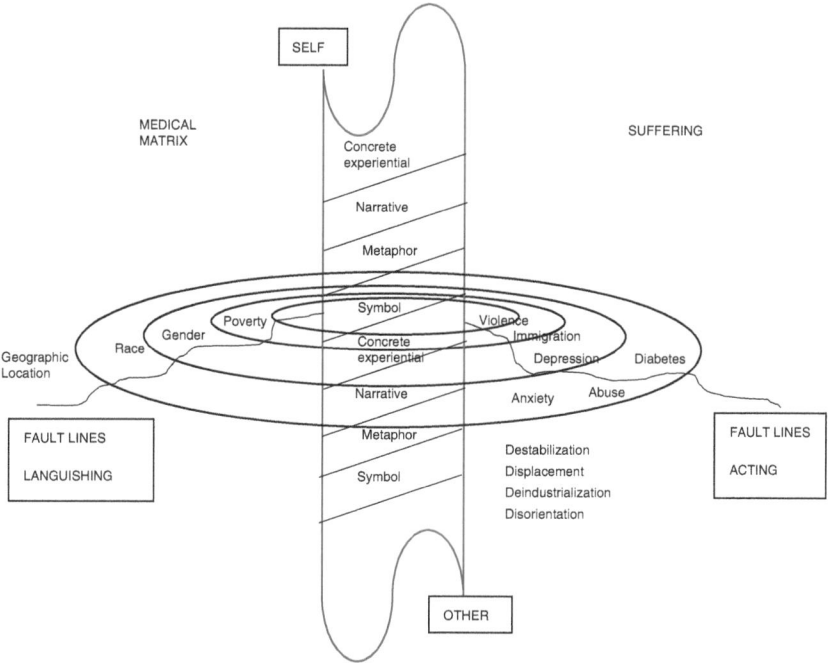

Figure 7.2 Detail of intersection of self-other and languishing-acting axes – lacunae.

for an ethical response to unwilled and unchosen impingement precisely because "we did not create it, and therefore it is what we must heed" (p. 101). While we may be the absolute source of our existence (Merleau Ponty, 1962), we are not responsible for what happens to us, but what does happen forms the horizon of choice, grounds our responsibility and creates the conditions under which we assume responsibility (Butler, 2005). "To be human seems to mean being in a predicament that one cannot solve" (Butler, 2005; p. 103). Therefore, these sorts of predicaments are what occur at the intersection of axes and why a multimodal perspective of knowing is so important. To refuse one form of knowing over another in this zone is to invalidate peoples' experience that may otherwise sustain them in difficult situations. This works both ways for biomedicine and medical humanities.

For example, patients or their family may have a sense of what is happening in relation to their healthcare or condition and may use images, words or metaphors to describe their understanding or suffering. They may hope to be met with resonance, attunement, understanding or validation of their affects. Instead, they may be met with reversals in the information or treatment regime provided. Worse, they may be met with health professionals who are more interested in their own agenda in a form of narcissistic preoccupation at maintaining narrative control. There is a sense of withdrawing healthcare at the same time of speaking the language of providing care as discussed in Chapter One. The void around the patients' and families' suffering which is difficult to cross becomes unspeakable. This occurs when there is no dialectic of socialisation and individuation because of the lack of echoing and mirroring (Levin, 1991) from health professionals. The patient then has little choice but to withdraw into self-containment and self-sufficiency.

A similar type of reversal occurs at an institutional level when services are offered to help people, then are withdrawn or are otherwise inaccessible to people who want help. Health promotion guidelines are not yet available for people who have a complicated relationship with their health behaviours and the conditions under which they live. There are simply not the guidelines, resources nor the activism necessary to address poverty or immigration effects on health, given the neo-liberal climate under which we all live. And, in fact, through the creation of hostile environments, the government has sought to manipulate and abuse those most in need. All of the above contribute to a sense of fiction with which people can be met in their suffering unfortunately.

A strategic withdrawal or disengagement in these times and circumstances is therefore a useful tactic to know about and do. In this case, morality is on the side of restraint, of not joining in and refraining from self-assertion (Butler, 2005). This is interesting because in terms of moral injury – claiming a "right" to not be so treated, as an entitlement – there is a narcissism in that, rather than accepting the "inevitability of injury; along with a moral predicament that emerges as a consequence of being injured" (Butler, 2005; p. 102) as part of being human; the narcissistic perspective believes they are entitled to not experience these predicaments or impingements:

> After all, if self-assertion becomes the assertion of the self at the expense of any consideration of the world, of consequence, and, indeed, of others, then it feeds a "moral narcissism" whose pleasure resides in its ability to transcend the concrete world that conditions its actions and is affected by them.
>
> (Butler, 2005; p. 105)

Thus in some ways, the withdrawal of the suffering self (Devisch et al., 2017) is a strategic strength because at some level there is a sensing of the potential for moral narcissism. Butler (2005) suggests "we become human in and through the destitution of our humanness" (p. 106). Through the fundamental inevitability of impingement, both health professionals and patients experience destitution at times, and this is part of life.

The idea of becoming more human through our destitution sounds similar to Bynum's (1987) description of medieval religious women who expanded their suffering to become more human. The focus is on the experiencing of suffering rather than controlling it by will. In fact, any "will" dominated discourse cannot hold, and this is perhaps what happens with health professionals overselling the idea of diet and exercise to patients in situations of precarity.

> [A]ny conception of the human that either defines the human by will or, alternately, robs the human of all will is a conception that cannot hold. Indeed, the "inhuman" emerges for Adorno as *both* a figure of pure will (eviscerated of vulnerability) and a figure of *no* will (reduced to destitution).
>
> (Butler, 2005; p. 107; emphasis original)

There is a dialectical inversion (or reversal) that takes place between moral purity and moral narcissism, between an ethics of conviction and a politics of persecution. The more morally pure a person presents themselves as, the more likely there is to be an inversion or reversal, the more narcissistic the person is likely to be and the more likely they are to use their assumed moral purity as a tool to persecute other people. This would seem typical in authoritarian types of relations where transcendence and abstraction are the norm of privileged locations.

There almost seems to be a type of descent necessary in order to counter moral purism (Figure 7.3). From the lofty abstracted transcended heights of the socially constructed instrumentalist self, there is an impingement – a human predicament that involves moral anguish. Moral injury or purity refuses this and asserts a right not to be impinged upon. Moral anguish on the other hand grapples with the very predicament as an ethical source of self – "Who am I to be in this room?" This is the zone of disorientation and destabilisation. Then further down the descent, through embodied experiential knowing, there is core consciousness or direct experience of self; inseeing.

This figure echoes Orange's words of "Who am I, so inconstant, that not withstanding, you count on me?" (Orange, 2011; pp. 50–51). The self-other axis is a zone of instability and unreliability, of potential moral narcissism and moral anguish. These are places where we can all come undone in encountering suffering. Yet we are compelled to encounter these reversals and reciprocities, and ideas about the self and sources of self, because they are all we have as we try to survive on the edge of our experience. In this place, we need to see with two eyes and both demystify and demythologise (Holland & Garman, 2010) as well as derealise ideas about self and other. This is because one of the major properties of suffering is that it calls into question what is normal, moral and right.

These are the questions we all sit with when we try to understand suffering as both an individual and a social construction. Moral anguish is not an aberration of suffering; it is formative of the self. The self is formed within a matrix of social suffering within the Black Anthropocene and consumerism. The Black Anthropocene is a place of extraction and

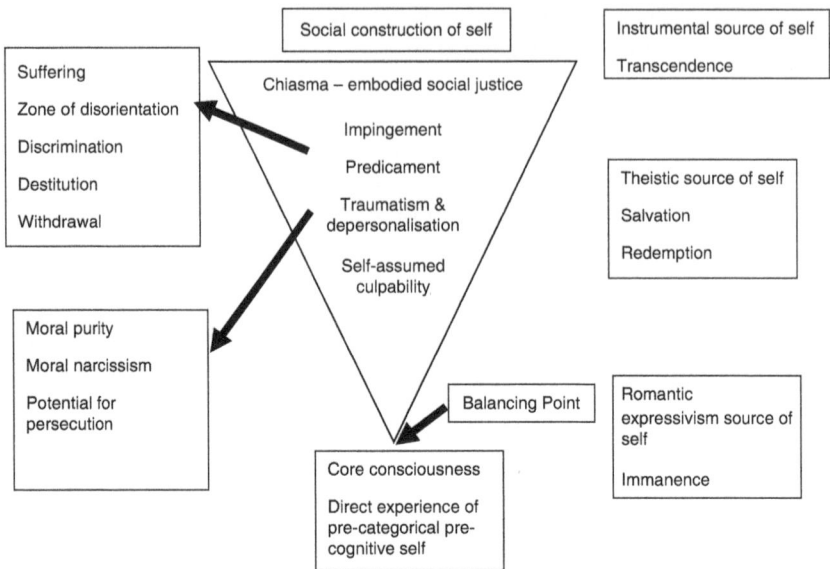

Figure 7.3 Processes of self at the zone of disorientation.

displacement. Understanding both the individual experience and the social construction of suffering through these different ideas presented in Figures 7.2 and 7.3 means that we are perhaps less inclined to believe the fiction of the neo-liberal individual as an ideal to aspire to. This in turn means that in order to practice as a health professional, a companion to suffering, we may feel more inclined to look at theory and practices that work outside the norm, such as critical race theory and streetwalker tactics.

Initially I presented some questions posed by health professionals: "How do we even begin to ask the right questions?" "What do you say when ...?" and "Who am I to be in this room?" To begin to think about these questions and how to answer them for one's self, I have provided tools on sources of self, ideas on reversals, reciprocity, resonance and attunement. I have also responded with ideas about the social matrix in which these notions arose and which must be considered as any context must in order to see the conditions under which we formulate responses.

To enter the social matrix of healthcare is to enter an archetypal situation where heroes, angels, witchy women, God's police, transcended and abstracted figureheads, desires, ghosts and the void are all in operation. To survive health, specific knowledge is required to identify practices of institutional and systemic oppression, as well as understanding moral anguish between self and role. It is necessary to have a strong sense of self through embodied experience to counter depersonalisation yet also retain a degree of disengaged rationalism. Awareness of suffering must be the foundation of training and practice; otherwise there is the danger of living a fiction. Awareness of both health professionals' and patients' suffering is crucial, to be aware of the crossing over and connection between each other's suffering. Most importantly, understanding how and where concepts and categories can be harmful through being able to recognise and deconstruct under- pinning assumptions is vital. These strategies help to counter depersonali- sation by keeping present to the current moment and relating to personhood personally.

Thinking about "How do we even begin to ask the right questions?" it should be apparent by now that the analysis in this book on suffering shows that there is more to understanding people and their conditions than surface appearances. Just as x-rays are used to understand what is happening at the level of bone structure, thinking about a pedagogy of suffering should help gain some traction on thinking about sources of self – what has gone missing? Where is the hole in the self? – as well as what sorts of moral anguish may be present. By being aware of the colonial past, the Black Anthropocene and discrimination through difference, there is a greater window of opportunity to connect with people through their suffering and not repeat impingements and intrusions, extractions and displacements of the past. Acknowledging and connecting with peoples' experiential reality – their concrete lived reality – will give them more opportunity to build relationship and trust. In that vein, being aware of reversals and fictions means that more choice is available to not react to them. Honouring people's right to make a tactical withdrawal is also necessary. These ideas should provide plenty of room to manoeuvre when thinking about questions.

Conversely, there may be no need or sense in asking questions. Questions may be a sign that soothing is required. In thinking about what to say in moments of extreme suffering, often words are not necessary. Instead a profound presence and silence is more powerful to show support and compassion in suffering. Sometimes in that profound silence and presence words may bubble up, more than consciously thinking about them, and these can be offered as a tentative gesture. Likewise, touch can be appro- priate to show presence, acknowledgement and acceptance (Orange, 2011). Being prepared for the hardness of this all and coming undone yet staying for an ethical response is enough and all that can be done at times.

And in situations of extreme suffering there is a requirement to attend to the self – Who am I to be in this room? – there are implicit questions here about worthiness, deserving, self-assumed culpability, shame, guilt and affect that can be processed later in a safe space. Knowing that there are opportunities to connect with patients at a different level, in addition to the instrumentalist self, which is more about their experiential lived concrete reality, may help in knowing who you are in the room. This connection at the level of subjectivity affirms their reality, keeps both health professional and patient in the here and now versus somewhat abstracted idealised future. These strategies all help to reduce the depersonalisation inherent in such situations. The processes are open ended questions to live with. In fact, Whyte (2014) suggests that one of the ways to live with a predicament is to think of a beautiful question that goes with it, for example, "how will I forgive myself?"

In giving an account of oneself by asking these sorts of questions, there are never straightforward easy answers. These sorts of questions are meant to be something struggled with. There is a cost to answering them in that in the act of knowing, something is always lost, as being outside the answer and field of possibilities (Butler, 2005). The more important point is to show the relationality between the rationality used and the way one lives one's life. Butler (2005) discusses Foucault's perspective "reflexivity, self-care, and self-mastery are all open-ended and unsatisfiable efforts to 'return' to a self from the situation of being foreign to oneself" (Butler, 2005; p. 129). There will always be an incompleteness about this return as Fareld (2012) suggested. Another question: "How much does it cost the subject to be able to tell the truth about itself?" is also worthy of consideration.

Therefore, asking these sorts of questions in relation to our thinking about suffering seems a good place to start. Furthermore, our capacity to reflect on these questions and our selves is limited by what we, and what the systems we are embedded in, allow us to say. The way we put the questions to ourselves is the art of metacognition. Butler (2005) ratifies the necessity of asking "Who are you?" "Who speaks to me?" "To whom do I speak when I speak to you?" (p. 135). These sorts of questions and demands "to give an account of oneself is a matter of fathoming at once the formation of the subject (self, ego, *moi*, first person perspective) and its relation to responsibility" (Butler, 2005; p. 135). Understanding one's own subjectivity and its relation to responsibility only make sense when we understand the conditions that make deliberation possible in the first place (Butler, 2005).

These are questions to *live* with rather than finding a specific answer or conclusion because answers are not always possible. Butler (2005) expects us not to find answers because the "I" is non-narrativizable especially under situations of moral duress:

> If I am not able to give an account of some of my actions, then I would rather die, because I cannot find myself as the author of these actions, and I cannot explain myself to those my actions may have hurt. ... where my repetitions enact again and again the site of my radical unself-knowingness. How am I to live under those circumstances?
>
> (Butler, 2005; p. 79)

The compulsion to re-enact the unknowingness is *La Coatlicue* (Anzaldúa, 1999). The hole in the answers of being able to give an account of ourselves is suffering. The non-narrativizability takes away agency and accountability whilst diminishing the grandiose notion of the transparent "I" presupposed as the ethical ideal. The anguish and opacity of the "I" is transferred to the other.

The anguish here seems at the heart of suffering, at the intersection of self-other and languishing-acting axes, the zone of disorientation and instability. The inability to given an account of the self leads to diminished agency. We may be non-narrativizable but we still exist, and in that there is hope. We still have a body, images, symbols, metaphors to carry us forward in our relations with others even though we cannot find words to narrate our story. Butler (2005) would perhaps suggest that in the intersection between health professional and patient, the crossing over is a humble "I am my relation to you" "given over to a 'you' without whom I cannot be and upon whom I depend to survive" (p. 81) much like Orange (2011) suggests that in our unreliability, our inconstancy, we are also the one who sufferers depend upon. From this perspective, there is no wonder that we do not know what to say in moments of extreme suffering. Yet we still carry on, still survive.

The sort of questions we can ask about what to say or do occur in this place of anguish and in some way cannot be answered. They are a direct statement of the inadequacy of the instrumentalist "I" to respond, where something else is necessary and must come in from the edge of our experiences. This is a risky business and perhaps why people resort to rhetoric and clichés. Living with a question, accepting that there may not be "an" answer is a moral ethical intention. And at the same time, in this limited fragmented "I," the existential angst of the subjective self, there is a yearning for self-regulation and soothing. But this does not mean that health professionals can be a substitute "breast" self-object (Winning, 2020) for patients either, for that would be a fiction. Rather there must be a facing up to suffering, accepting the lack of trust in health professionals (Devisch et al., 2017) in their unreliability as a sign of wisdom, an awareness of the hole at the centre of the instrumentalist self.

For many people, the idea of a soothing health professional, whilst laudable, and compassion is definitely preferential over neglect and abuse, must seem somewhat of a fantasy particularly if they have had a complex relationship with authority figures. It seems more honest to face up to what Sharpe (2016) believes about the system as reimagining and constituting itself through gratuitous violence at the level of structure that creates a nothingness, which constitutes the black as the constitutive outside. Surviving, continued vulnerability to inexplicable and overwhelming forces, overwhelms psychological theory that could see all relationships as being "nice" and reasonable, medicine as a source of relief from suffering and that there will always be solutions to problems. Perhaps it is more honest to believe that "while even as that terror visited on our bodies the realities of that terror are erased" (Sharpe, 2016; p. 15). Perhaps it is necessary to think about surviving suffering in solitude and what this might mean for a self that is beyond the instrumentalist sources.

This is perhaps the hole in the colonialist self; we tend not to know or speak of any other except perhaps for the pre-cognitive pre-categorical self. Butler (2005) struggles with the boundaries between self and other and conditions of possibility. Whilst on the one hand, she speaks of relying on the other in order to be, on the other hand, she speaks of any enunciation as a break in the narrative structure and control, as perhaps an opacity of that self that speaks but does not speak at the same time. Narrative control and manipulation is an attempt to stave off a threat of dissolution precipitated by acting. Perhaps a tactical withdrawal is an attempt to maintain narrative control on the part of the sufferer, be they a patient or a health professional. At some level, there is a truth here about dealing with suffering in solitude – somewhat akin to what Frank (2001) thinks about having to be with his suffering in order to maintain his integrity. This is perhaps the greatest insight of relevance to a healthcare that attempts to maintain narrative control through scientism. That is, while we may have theories about psychology and use compassion to respond to suffering, there is also the reality that doctors themselves tend to be with their own suffering through the mechanism of a psychological isolate within the medical matrix. To begin to imagine that some of that narrative control might be handed over to medical humanities or to the social determinants of health seems inconceivable. Therefore something else is necessary to survive health.

7.4 Epistemology

Each chapter of this book has sections on how we know what we know in order to show the inherent unity, or consilience, at the level of thinking about suffering. As shown in Figure 1.2 we require all of our faculties to think differently about suffering. We can no longer afford to think in silos without considering the relationships between social science, humanities and ethics, biomedicine and the environment. Each impacts the other; without relating them to each other, we create lacunae in what we know and do. This book has endeavoured to link the different disciplines in order to think more deeply about suffering. Part of the reason for thinking about suffering in silos may be to maintain narrative control in a form of moral narcissism. However, we must move beyond this, work through a zone of disorientation, in order to question and perhaps find answers to recalcitrant engrained issues that have resisted change.

While thinking about concepts, patterns, models and schemata may seem like an abstracted academic perspective to take, it is important to do so because this is the foundation of where our beliefs come from that influence practice so much. The culture of healthcare is such that students are required to believe in the biomedical model to the exclusion of other ways of thinking and knowing. They are expected to perform with certainty in their knowledge even though they will be operating in conditions of uncertainty.

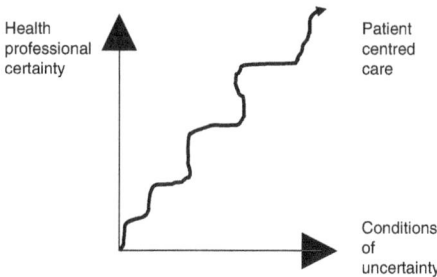

Health professional certainty

Patient centred care

Conditions of uncertainty

Figure 7.4 Relationship between operational necessity of certainty and uncertainty.

Figure 7.4 shows the relationships between these axes and patient care, where suffering may manifest.

The relationship between health professional certainty and conditions of uncertainty can affect the trajectory of patient-centred care through more or less suffering. Trying to maintain narrative control in conditions of uncertainty can exacerbate suffering from the sense of living a fiction; it is far more worthwhile to admit to not knowing and being with the patient in the conditions of uncertainty than to perpetuate untruths or false reassurance.

Gaining entry into a healthcare profession requires knowledge, understanding, skills and beliefs in the certainty of your practice. As Mary, one of the research participants referred to in Chapter Five, stated – you had to believe strongly in your models in order to succeed:

> To be successful in psychiatry there, I think having a conceptual framework and believing in it, being able to intellectualize and have that understanding of whatever the medical system has at the moment of the brain and psychiatry and so on. If you really have that theoretical framework and believe it, then you can do this thing of categorizing people and giving them labels and giving them medications and you know advising treatment. I guess my problem is I don't believe *laughs* and that's where I have the issue.

> Umm, yeah its about believing in what you do. I think the people who do really well, really believe it, they really apply it and in that way it works. People know where they stand, they have got a position, they have got a diagnosis, they have got a plan.
>
> (Mary)(Lowe, 2010)

Therefore because it is necessary to have concepts and work from them, we also must be aware of how these concepts work to advantage and disadvantage people. These strong beliefs, necessary for success, can make dealing with uncertainty challenging (George & Lowe, 2019). Moreover, the system of beliefs related to medical science can encourage self-objectification, where how we know what we know is believed to be perceived, interpreted, understood and mediated by a neutral detached objective observer. This perspective can dehumanise health professionals, leading to depersonalisation and it is also a hallmark of scientific practice. Health professionals are encouraged to take an objective stance in an intention to provide an ethical neutral service based on evidence-based medicine. Its not that health professionals are dragged along unwillingly in training to do this. Evidence-based medicine is embraced in order to provide the best treatment possible. However, this is not just an individual's choice or responsibility as there are systemic influences, too. In all these factors, there are always both social and individual influences. Therefore how the self is conceived is of primary importance for the formation of concepts, interpretations of patterns and development of models.

According to Nussbaum (1995), a person is objectified if one or more of the following properties apply to him or her:

1 Instrumentality – treating the person as a tool for another's purpose; the health professional is trained as a tool for healthcare and best possible treatment of patients, thereby developing an instrumentalist source of self;

2 Denial of autonomy and self-determination – healthcare professionals are embedded in institutional, organisational and governing bodies rules and regulations that deny their ability to operate except within narrow confined parameters;

3 Inertness – lacking in agency or activity – health professionals seem to have agency when it comes to patient care but lack agency when it comes to their working conditions or changing the conditions of possibility for inequities in health; activism is still rare;

4 Fungibility – treating the person as interchangeable with other objects – health professionals are interchangeable with each other in rosters, rotations and placements in the way they are treated by some NHS Trusts with the added burden of having to compete with each other to be treated this way;

5 Violability – treating the person as lacking in boundary, integrity and violable – as something that is permissible to break up, smash and break into – workloads of health professionals generally and working in a system of overwhelm lends itself to a kind of frenzy to getting work done; this is a cultural norm;

6 Ownership – if they can be bought, sold, owned – this happens on a number of different levels from undergraduate training – having to bid for placements and projects; placements in NHS Trusts, outsourcing to private firms, and submitting applications for research funding. The

marketisation of healthcare encourages the idea of ownership and health itself as a commodity to be bought and sold;

7   Denial of subjectivity – treating the person as though there is no need for concern of their experience and feelings – this does not enter undergraduate training where the focus is on passing exams and obtaining a high aggregate of personal exam score over the years, and in continuing professional development that focuses on technical skills (Nussbaum, 1995);

8   Reduction to a body – the treatment of a person as identified with the body or body parts – the biomedical model is based on the body as a machine;

9   Reduction to appearance – treatment in terms of how a person looks – the uniform of health professionals where communication is based on what position they occupy in the system;

10   Silencing – treating the person as if they were silent, lacking the capacity to speak; generally there is an atmosphere in healthcare where there is a strict unwritten rule book of who can say what to whom and when (Langton, 2009).

Health professionals by their training and practice therefore have plenty of opportunity for objectification, depersonalisation and dehumanisation. This is particularly salient because different channels for knowing and understanding experience have been silenced. Some of the consequences and correlates of that is that patients will continue to be objectivised whilst health professionals cannot recognise their own objectification and complicity in order to provide the best possible practice. A more nuanced approach is required to bring awareness to and tease out which aspects of training and practice are non negotiable for objectification such as carrying out techniques and those which have more room for negotiation.

The instrumentalist self, in order to be able to be with suffering, therefore must be enjoined with thinking through issues and it seems as though medical humanities and ethics could facilitate this. Sociology is useful for unpacking structures and practices that become habitual but may inadvertently reinforce categories and discrimination, with its alignment with the medical model. Where experience can be included in the curriculum and how the study of that influences how we know what we know is of crucial importance in being with suffering. Understanding how the traditional arrangement of knowledge encourages unconscious objectification and exclusion of consciousness of the second half of the binary – subjectification – means that we know what is missing from the instrumentalist self.

Medical humanities can provide the missing pieces of the bricolage. Since in suffering, the unimaginable happens, there is a shock to the mind that literally cannot imagine how or what can be. Talking through what has happened and using the imagination to assist in that can be soothing. It may be that the existential questions are more a request for soothing of the imagination. By tapping into deeper ways of knowing, images and words may arise that activate the imagination as a resource for both health professional and patient. Connections are made that were not available previously in a restorative movement. Or there may be no words, as in the speechlessness of suffering, yet still an image may arise that is a resource for survival that enables the person to carry on. Giving up narrative control as the health professional means that one can assume and activate the knowing of the patient. This all depends on the understanding presented in the first chapter and subsequently that people have pre-cognitive pre-categorical knowing that will help them through these difficult times. We all need this as we navigate these times of heightened anxiety and precarity during a pandemic.

COVID-19 has provided a unique urgency to sorting out our multimodal ways of knowing and the relationship between them. We can no longer work in silos or use activism to reactivate old polarities that regress to the lowest denominator. Different ways of thinking about suffering are necessary now more than ever. There is not one area of life that is not touched by suffering. We have to think through more deeply and more differently by working across fault lines and pursuing understandings provided by marginalised groups of people. This includes perceptions like McGarvey's (2017) insights on the poverty industry and Butt's (2002) that the people who benefit most from health inequalities and human rights rhetoric tend to be those in power.

I have deliberately included writings from traditionally marginalised people in order to reinforce this requirement to think differently about suffering. Including writers from peoples that have suffered so much, that exemplify the effects of the Black Anthropocene, as a way of moving forward in the hope that we can learn from those who have trodden this path for so long. Understanding cultural melancholy may help us to acknowledge our own hungry ghosts in order not to perpetuate colonialism when it comes to suffering, and how we are all complicit with consumerism. By doing so I have made explicit the embodied experience of suffering in its racialised form; the crossover in the embodied experience of social justice and how health professionals and patient are tied in together in this chiasma.

Stitching together different understandings of the suffering self and sources of the self means that we can see the relevance of different cultures' religiosity on suffering and what expectations may be present in relation to transcendence, salvation, redemption and restoration. Instead of the rescuer-victim-persecutor triangle (Baum, 1993), we may move to the witness-companion-interlocutor of suffering. This triangle is more likely to be able to bypass getting caught up in the archetypes within healthcare services and an ability to bear witness to moral anguish of the deepest kind. Going down deep means understanding ruptures, reversals, reciprocities, knowing on the inside and affects in an economy of suffering. Medical humanities cannot be used without an appreciation of this knowing-on-the-inside of social justice and must incorporate inequities in health in its thinking and knowing.

In this book, I have explored how to know and understand what form and shape suffering takes. I have aimed to pull together the threads of medical humanities, sociology and medical education through the unifying experience of suffering in order that we may know what is involved and explore our response to that. I have introduced different concepts and theories related to suffering by drawing on medical humanities and sociology to demonstrate how they can be used to attend to and encounter suffering. Going down into the detail of suffering as well as across syndemics of suffering has been a way of surviving; a resource addressing grieving and loss as a form of praise:

> This is because true praise (the beauty and art that arise from the capacity to grieve) needs to know the details of all the functions and forms of the myriad things of the world ... because you need to have enough details of the world's tactile reality to even minimally express grief in the first place, much less graduate to the natural human impulse to praise. In order to give life's inevitable losses a face whose voice speaks a beauty that can keep us all from this spiritual deep freeze, these details of life truly seen and loved must be there for us to begin to speak.
>
> (Prechtel, 2015; p. 156–157)

Box 7.1 Reflection

When the unimaginable happens, thinking can stop or it can become a frenzy in order to deal with projected outcomes and likely scenarios. Either way, these are natural normal responses. Staying with the experience of suffering is so necessary. We do not speak about suffering enough. We do not acknowledge suffering enough. When we run from the experience of suffering, there is more likelihood of blame, shame or attacking other people in order not to feel the embodied experience. By being able to stay with and explore the experience of suffering – what is the wordlessness like? What texture is there to the silence? What tone do the lacunae have? – we can get to know both the local and universal experience of suffering. This exploring is different from categorising or labelling.

Rilke talks of the clarifying force of sadness and of cultivating the capacity to be alone with our experiences in a fertile solitude. Like Jung, he believed that the relationship between what we processed on an inner level had an effect in the outer world. If we can have courage for the most difficult experiences in our lives and live to that principle of holding to the difficult, then we will learn we can trust the most

---

that which seems the most difficult. This means opening a door to vast silences and a journey, a pilgrimage, across vast unfamiliar landscapes, with the unsayable. Conversations from living on the edge and between, enlivened and engaged, even in the midst of suffering.

Once, seeing light dancing on the underside of a boat, reflected from the water, I thought that we are like that light, an awareness of the reflection that we are, always dancing on the underside of our being, generated by the existential sea of uncertainty. We dance between affect, core consciousness and the detached observer.

Anne Boyer writes: "Before I got sick, I'd been making plans for a place for public weeping, hoping to install in major cities a temple where anyone who needed it could get together to cry in good company and with the proper equipment. It would be a precisely imagined architecture of sadness: gargoyles made of night sweat, moldings made of longest minutes, support beams made of I-can't-go-on-I-must-go-on.

When planning the temple, I remembered the existence of people who hate those they call crybabies, and how they might respond with rage to a place full of distraught strangers—a place that exposed suffering as what is shared. It would have been something tremendous to offer those sufferers the exquisite comforts of stately marble troughs in which to collectivise their tears. But I never did this."
Questions for reflection

1   What shared suffering can you subscribe to? What do you reject?
2   What becomes narrowed and gossamer about suffering to you?
3   How do you use your imagination?
4   What perspective do you have on solitude and being alone with your experiences?
5   What lost words of suffering can you re-imagine?
6   What redemption songs from suffering do you hold from your ancestry?

Further Resources

Boyer A. 2019. What cancer takes away. New Yorker Magazine https://www.newyorker.com/magazine/2019/04/15/what-cancer-takes-away

Prechtel M. 2015. *The Smell of Rain on Dust: Grief and Praise*. North Atlantic Books: Berkeley, California.

Rilke R.M. 2016. *Letters to a Young Poet*. Penguin Little Black Classics: London.

References

Altschuler S. 2018. *The Medical Imagination: Literature and Health in the Early United States*. University of Pennsylvania Press: Philadelphia.

Anzaldúa G. 1999. *Borderlands La Frontera; The New Mestiza*. Aunt Lute Books: San Francisco.

Baum F.E. 1993. Healthy cities and change: Social movement or bureaucratic tool? *Health Promotion International*; 8(1):31–40.

Bynum C.W. 1987. *Holy Feast and Holy Fast: The Religious Significance of Food to Medieval Women*. University of California Press: Berkely.

Butler J. 2005. *Giving an Account of Oneself*. Fordham University Press: USA.

Butt L. 2002. The suffering stranger: Medical anthropology and international morality. *Medical Anthropology*; 21(1):1–24; discussion 25–33. doi: 10.1080/01459740210619.

Cain C.L., Surbone A., Elk R., Kagawa-Singer M. 2018. Culture and palliative care: Preferences, communication, meaning, and mutual decision making. *Journal of Pain & Symptom Management*; 55(5):1408–1419.

Cassell E.J. 2014. *Suffering and human dignity*. Chapter 1 in *Suffering and Bioethics*. Green RM., Palpant NJ. (eds). *Oxford Scholarship Online*: November 2014. doi: 10.1093/acprof:oso/9780199926176.001.0001.

Cassell E.J. 2004. *The Nature of Suffering and the Goals of Medicine*. Oxford University Press: Oxford.

Damasio A. 2010. *Self Comes to Mind. Constructing the Conscious Brain*. Vintage Books: London.

Damasio A. 1999. *The Feeling of What Happens: Body, Emotion and the Making of Consciousness*. Vintage: London.

de Certeau, M. 1984. *The Practice of Everyday Life*. University of California Press: California.

DeGrazia D. 2014. *What is suffering and what sorts of beings can suffer? Chapter 7 in Suffering and Bioethics*. Green R.M., Palpant N.J. (eds). *Oxford Scholarship Online*: November 2014. doi: 10.1093/acprof.oso/9780199926176.001.0001.

Decety J. 2014. *Social neuroscience meets philosophy: Suffering, empathy, and moral cognition. Chapter 5 in Suffering and Bioethics*. Green R.M., Palpant N.J. (eds). *Oxford Scholarship Online*: November 2014. doi: 10.1093/acprof:oso/9780199926176.001.0001.

Dempsey C. 2018. *The Antidote to Suffering: How Compassionate Connected Care Can Improve Safety, Quality and Experience*. McGraw-Hill: New York.

Devereaux G. 1967. *From Anxiety to Method in the Behavioural Sciences*. Mouton & Co: Paris.

Devisch I., Vanheule S., Deveugele M. Nola I., Civaner M., Pype P. 2017. Victims of disaster: Can ethical debriefings be of help to care for their suffering? *Medical Health Care and Philosophy*; 20:257–267.

Eco U. 2014. *From the Tree to the Labyrinth: Historical Studies on the Sign and Interpretation*. Harvard University Press: New York.

Ekman E., Krasner M. 2016 Empathy in medicine: Neuroscience, education and challenges, Medical Teacher. doi: 10.1080/0142159X.2016.1248925.

Engelhardt H.T. 2014. *The Orthodox Christian View of Suffering. Chapter 11 in Suffering and Bioethics. Green R.M., Palpant N.J. (eds). Oxford Scholarship Online*: November 2014. doi: 10.1093/acprof:oso/9780199926176.001.0001.

Fareld V. 2012. The *re-* in recognition: Hegelian returns. *Distinktion: Scandinavian Journal of Social Theory*; 13(1):125–138.

Ford C.L., Airhihenbuwa C.O. 2018. Commentary: Just what is critical race theory and what's it doing in a progressive field like public health? *Ethnicity & Disease*; 28(Suppl 1):223–230; doi:10.18865/ed.28.S1.223.

Frank A.W. 2001. Can we research suffering? *Qualitative Health Research*; 11(3):353–362.

Fredrikson B.L., Roberts T.A. 1997. Objectification theory: Toward understanding women's lived experiences and mental health risks. *Psychology of Women Quarterly*; 21: 173–206.

Gastaldo D. 1997. Is health education good for you? Re-thinking health education through the concept of bio-power. Chapter 6 in *Foucault – Health and Medicine*. Petersen, A., and Bunton, R. (eds). Routledge: New York.

Garland E.L., Howard M.O. 2014. A transdiagnostic perspective on cognitive, affective, and neurobiological processes underlying human suffering. *Research on Social Work Practice*; 24(1):142–151.

Graham J., Benson L., Swanson J., Potyk D., Daratha K., Roberts K. 2016. Medical humanities coursework is associated with greater measured empathy in medical students. *American Journal of Medicine*; 129(12):1334–1337.

George R.E., Lowe W.A. 2019. Well-being and uncertainty in health care practice. *Clinical Teacher*; 16:298–305.

Haidet P., Jarecke J., Adams N., Stuckey H., Green M., Shapiro D., Teal C.R., Wolpaw D.R. 2016 A guiding framework to maximise the power of the arts in medical education: A systematic review and metasynthesis. *Medical Education*; 50(3):320–331.

Holland P.E., Garman N.B. 2010. Watching with two eyes: The place of the mythopoetic in curriculum inquiry. Chapter Two in *Pedagogies of the Imagination* Leonard T., Willis P (eds). Springer Science + Business Media BV: Chicago.

Langton R. 2009. *Sexual Solipsism: Philosophical Essays on Pornography and Objectification*. Oxford University Press: Oxford.

Launer J. 2020. Digging holes and weaving tapestries: Two approaches to the clinical encounter. *Postgraduate Medical Journal*; 96:307–308.

Levin D.M. 1991. Visions of narcissism: Intersubjectivity and the reversals of reflection. Chapter 3 in *Merleau Ponty Vivant*. Dillon M.C. (ed). State University of New York Press: Albany.

Lowe W.A. 2014. Complexity or meaning in health professional education and practice? *Health Education Journal*; 73(1):3–8.

Lowe W.A. 2010. *Health and 'I': An analysis of Curricular Phenomena in Health Professional Education Through the Focus of Critical Pedagogy*. Unpublished Thesis. School of Education. Murdoch University: Western Australia.

McGarvey D. 2017. *Poverty Safari: Understanding the Anger of Britain's Underclass*. Picador: Edinburgh.

Mahendran A. 2020. *Moments of Rupture: The Importance of Affect in Medical Education and Surgical Training*. Routledge: London.

Mendenhall E. 2019. *Rethinking Diabetes: Entanglement with Trauma, Poverty and HIV*. Cornell University Press: London.

Merleau Ponty M. 1962. *Phenomenology of Perception*. Routledge Keegan Paul: London.

Nussbaum M.C. 1995. Objectification. *Philosophy & Public Affairs*; 24(4):249–291.

Orange D.M. 2011. *The Suffering Stranger: Hermeneutics for Everyday Clinical Practice*. Routledge: New York.

Posttraumatic Stress Disorder: Issues and Controversies, edited by Gerald Rosen, John Wiley & Sons, Incorporated. 2004. ProQuest Ebook Central. https://ebookcentral.proquest.com/lib/gmul-ebooks/detail.action?docID=210566.

Seth S. 2018. *Difference and Disease: Medicine, Race, and the Eighteenth-Century British Empire*. Cambridge University Press: Cambridge.

Sharpe C. 2016. *In the Wake: On Blackness and Being*. Duke University Press: Durham.

Singleton J. 2015. *Cultural Melancholy: Readings of Race, Impossible Mourning, and African American Ritual*. University of Illinois Press: Illinois.

Sloterdijk P. 2013. *You Must Change Your Life*. Polity Press: Cambridge.

Stolorow R. 2010. Collective Trauma and Existential Anxiety. Huffpost. https://www.huffpost.com/entry/collective-trauma-and-exi_b_680945?guccounter=1&guce_referrer=aHR0cHM6Ly93d3cuZ29vZ2xlLmNvbS8&guce_referrer_sig=AQAAAEq5ObT1HCr5fKbRp-cqGzMQmIH7m3QaYQOyd2l3bvbOeZlEsgF086HmNoyl5tOd4Vh5vFWG5UPFZnopWplWxfkvNZ9hF1eu58WDDqGp8BYBwEF-wm4JbN4NSzIBfhLs1sOT6BEFKAcw735B09tgjR-82eh-_yg7Glz182DkEsUXs.

Sinclair S. 1997. *Making Doctors: An Institutional Apprenticeship*. Bloomsbury Publishing: London.

Viessière S. 2011. *The Ghosts of Empire: Violence, Suffering and Mobility in the Transatlantic Cultural Economy of Desire*. Transaction Publishers: London.

Walsh D., McCartney G., Collins C., Taulbut M., Batty G.D. 2016. History, politics and vulnerability: Explaining excess mortality. Glasgow Centre for Population Health.

Whyte D. 2014. *Solace – The Art of Asking the Beautiful Question*. CD. Many Rivers Company: Vancouver, British Columbia.

Wilkinson I. 2006. Health, risk and 'social suffering'. *Health, Risk & Society*; 8(1):1–8.

Wilkinson I. 2005. *Suffering: A Sociological Introduction*. Polity Press: Cambridge.

Wilkinson I., Kleinman A. 2016. *A Passion for Society: How We Think about Human Suffering*. University of California Press: Berkeley.

Wilson E.O. 1998. *Consilience: The Unity of Knowledge*. Abacus: London.

Winning J. 2020. The use of an object: Exploring physician burnout through object relations theory. Medical Humanities Published Online First: 28 May 2020. doi: 10.1136/medhum-2019-011752.

Appendix

Curriculum for a pedagogy of suffering

Meta-curriculum

Ontology	Being human – what does it mean to be human?	Being suffering – what does it mean to suffer?
Epistemology	Questions around Truth (evidence) – how do I know what I know?	How do I understand life? What grand (Truth) narratives am I involved in?

Meta-curriculum statements: Questions Around Truth and Reality (evidence) – how do I know what I know?

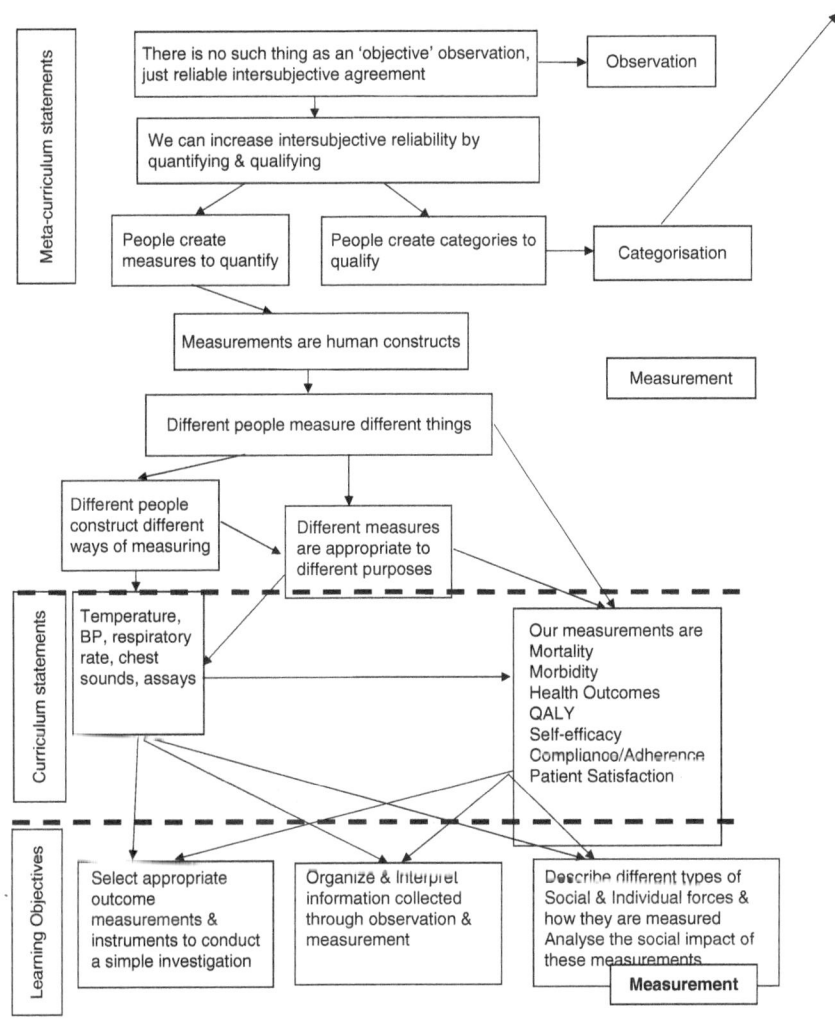

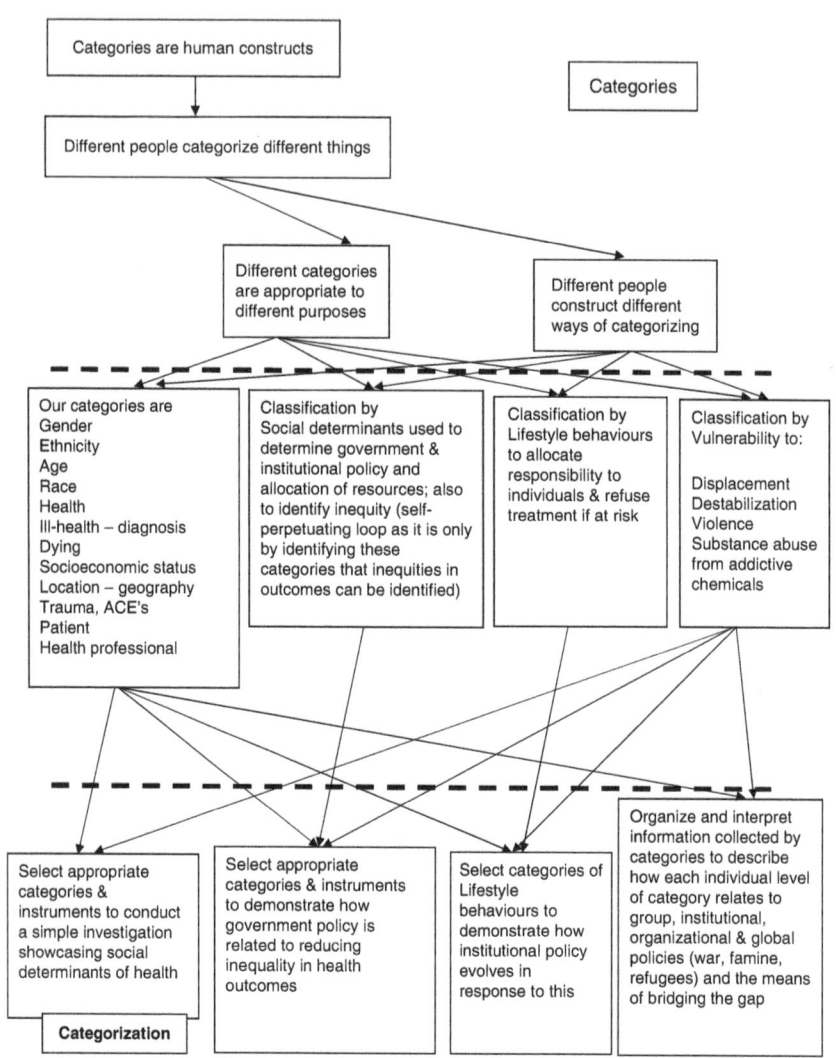

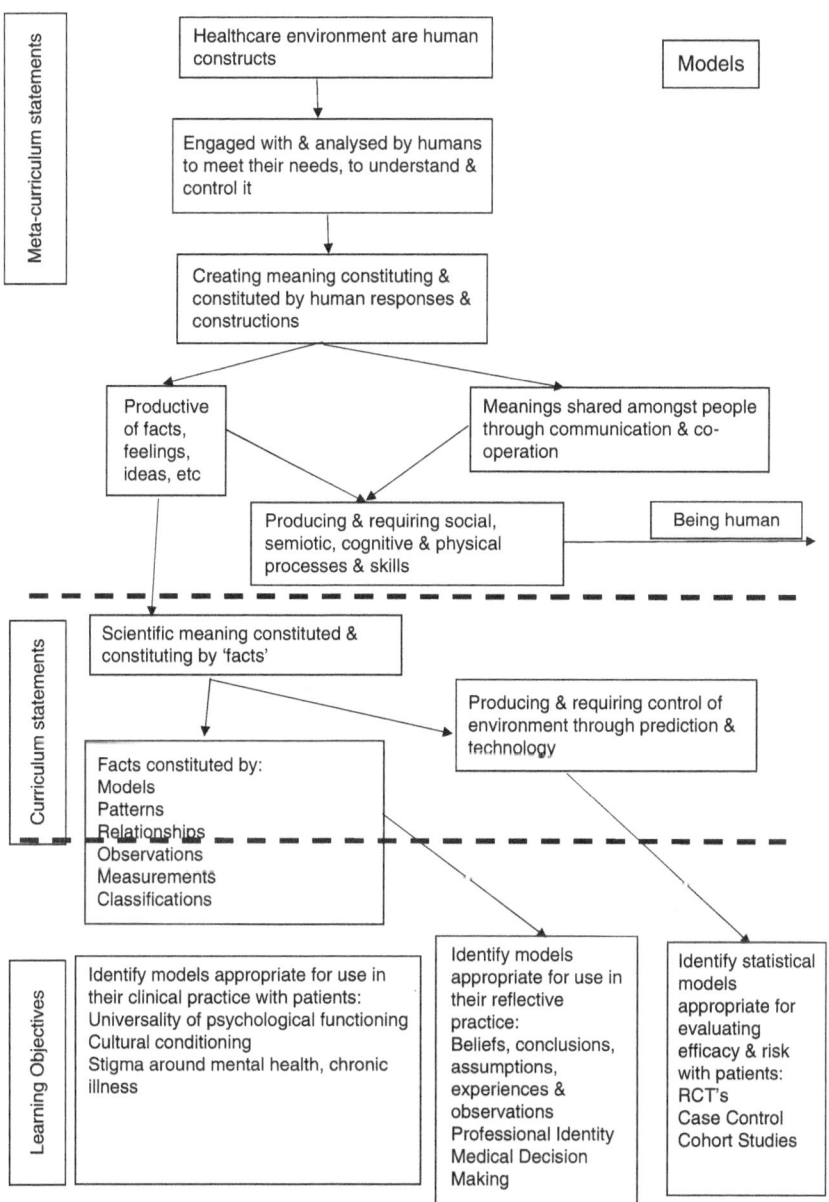

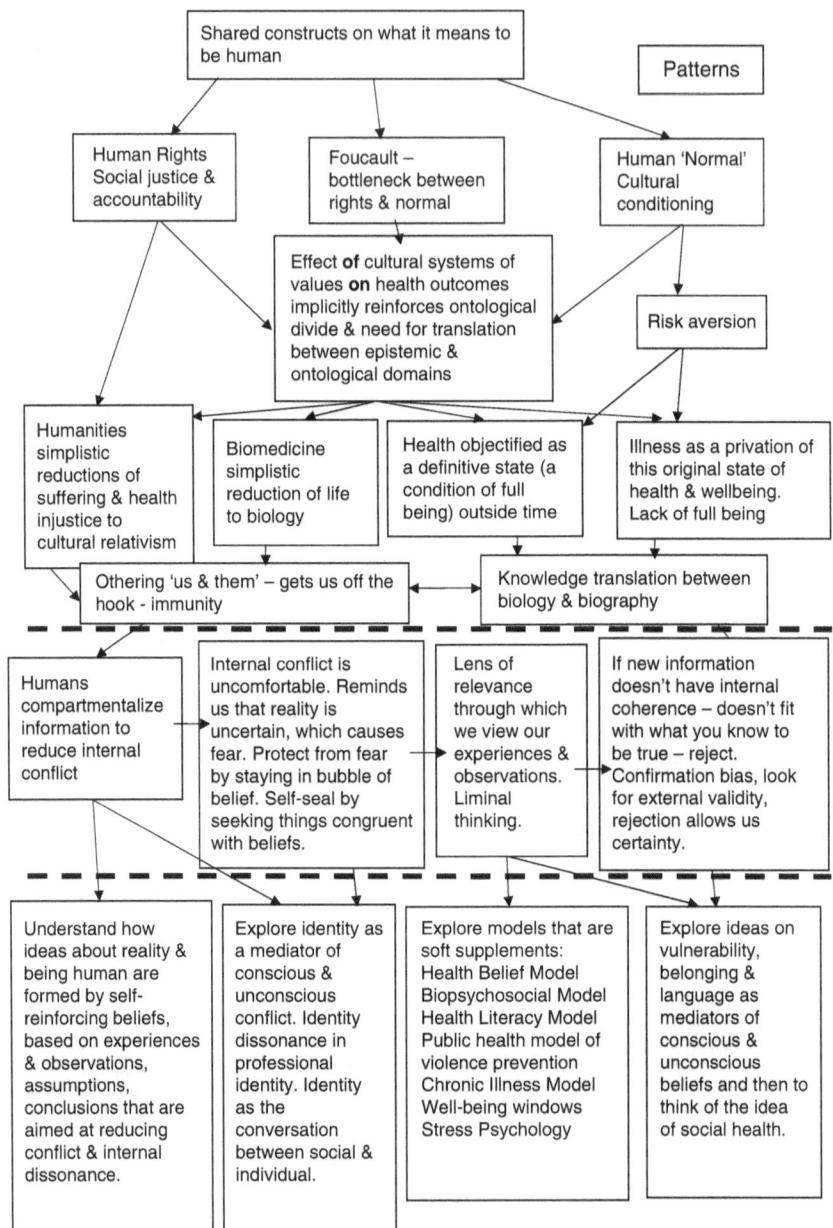

1 Necessary concepts, skills, attitudes (beliefs) to topics

Learning outcomes

Measurement

Select appropriate outcome measurements & instruments to conduct a simple investigation.

Organise & interpret information collected through observation & measurement.

Describe different types of social & individual forces & how they are measured.

Analyze the social impact of these measurements of difference in the context of the Black Anthropocene and consumerism.

Categorisation

Select appropriate categories & instruments to conduct a simple investigation showcasing social determinants of health.

Select appropriate categories & instruments to demonstrate how government policy is related to reducing inequality in health outcomes.

Select categories of lifestyle behaviours to demonstrate how institutional policy evolves in response to this.

Organise and interpret information collected by categories to describe how each individual level of category relates to group, institutional, organisational & global policies (war, famine, refugees) and any means of bridging the gap.

Models

Identify models appropriate for use in their clinical practice with patients:
   Syndemic suffering – VIDDA model
   Trauma Informed Care Model
   Cultural conditioning of colonial influence on measurements, categories and models of difference
   Stigma and racialisation around mental health, chronic illness

Identify models appropriate for use in their reflective practice:
   Beliefs, conclusions, assumptions, experiences & observations
   Professional Identity

Patterns

Students will understand how ideas about reality & being human are formed by self-reinforcing beliefs, based on experiences & observations, assumptions, conclusions that are aimed at reducing conflict & internal dissonance.

Students will explore identity as a mediator of conscious & unconscious conflict. Identity dissonance in professional identity. Identity as the conversation between social & individual.

Students will explore ideas on vulnerability, belonging & language as mediators of conscious & unconscious beliefs and then to think of the idea of social health.

2 Topics, generalisations, concepts, topics, skills and attitudes

Understanding of process of knowledge making through sensing, perception, interpretation, concept, schemata, model.

Arrangement of knowledge – tree, encyclopedia, labyrinth, networks.

Consilience – unity of knowledge – medical humanities, social sciences, biomedicine and environment all necessary.

Suffering – definitions, cultural melancholy, self-other and languishing-acting axes, sources of the self (instrumentalist, theistic, romantic expressivism), relations, religious responses, moral anguish.

Professional sources of suffering – patient anguish, death and dying, systemic oppression, systemic overwhelm, dehumanisation, depersonalisation.

Professional expressions of suffering – burnout, PTSD, depersonalisation, moral anguish.

Medical humanities – ways of thinking differently, inseeing, in-bracing, knowing on the inside, ruptures, ethical response.

Mythopoetic curriculum – demythologising, demystifying, seeing with two eyes – dual awareness, imaginal, siblings of the darkness.

Streetwalker tactics – pilgrimages, and diving down deep – *La Callajera*.

Dissonance – lack of internal coherence at two levels – classification used to determine inequity in health outcomes forms a self-perpetuating loop as it is only by identifying these categories that these categories are reinforced.

The simplistic reduction of suffering and health injustice to cultural relativism through categories is the antithesis of the biopsychosocial model, which is not deconstructive but a vision of how life and health should be.

Combined Subject and Author Index